HEALTH CARE FINANCE

and the Mechanics of Insurance and Reimbursement

MICHAEL K. HARRINGTON, MSHA, RHIA, CHP

Faculty
Department of Health Administration
St. Joseph's College of Maine
Standish, Maine

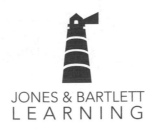

JONES & BARTLETT
LEARNING

World Headquarters
Jones & Bartlett Learning
5 Wall Street
Burlington, MA 01803
978-443-5000
info@jblearning.com
www.jblearning.com

Jones & Bartlett Learning books and products are available through most bookstores and online booksellers. To contact Jones & Bartlett Learning directly, call 800-832-0034, fax 978-443-8000, or visit our website, www.jblearning.com.

Substantial discounts on bulk quantities of Jones & Bartlett Learning publications are available to corporations, professional associations, and other qualified organizations. For details and specific discount information, contact the special sales department at Jones & Bartlett Learning via the above contact information or send an email to specialsales@jblearning.com.

The content, statements, views, and opinions herein are the sole expression of the respective authors and not that of Jones & Bartlett Learning, LLC. Reference herein to any specific commercial product, process, or service by trade name, trademark, manufacturer, or otherwise does not constitute or imply its endorsement or recommendation by Jones & Bartlett Learning, LLC and such reference shall not be used for advertising or product endorsement purposes. All trademarks displayed are the trademarks of the parties noted herein. *Health Care Finance and the Mechanics of Insurance and Reimbursement* is an independent publication and has not been authorized, sponsored, or otherwise approved by the owners of the trademarks or service marks referenced in this product.

There may be images in this book that feature models; these models do not necessarily endorse, represent, or participate in the activities represented in the images. Any screenshots in this product are for educational and instructive purposes only. Any individuals and scenarios featured in the case studies throughout this product may be real or fictitious, but are used for instructional purposes only.

This publication is designed to provide accurate and authoritative information in regard to the Subject Matter covered. It is sold with the understanding that the publisher is not engaged in rendering legal, accounting, or other professional service. If legal advice or other expert assistance is required, the service of a competent professional person should be sought.

Production Credits
VP, Executive Publisher: David Cella
Publisher: Michael Brown
Associate Editor: Lindsey Mawhiney
Associate Production Editor: Rebekah Linga
Rights and Media Manager: Joanna Lundeen
Media Development Assistant: Shannon Sheehan
Senior Marketing Manager: Sophie Fleck Teague
Manufacturing and Inventory Control Supervisor: Amy Bacus
Composition: Cenveo Publisher Services
Cover Design: Kristin E. Parker
Rights and Media Coordinator: Mary Flatley
Cover Image: © HelenStocker/iStock/Thinkstock
Printing and Binding: Edwards Brothers Malloy
Cover Printing: Edwards Brothers Malloy

08625-6

Library of Congress Cataloging-in-Publication Data
Harrington, Michael K., author.
  Health care finance and the mechanics of insurance and reimbursement / Michael K. Harrington.
     p. ; cm.
  Includes bibliographical references and index.
  ISBN 978-1-284-02612-2 (paper)
  I. Title.
  [DNLM: 1. Insurance, Health, Reimbursement--United States. 2. Financial Management--methods--United States. 3. Insurance Claim Reporting--United States. W 275 AA1]
  RA412.3
  368.38'200681--dc23
                                     2014038076
6048
Printed in the United States of America
19 18 17 16 15   10 9 8 7 6 5 4 3 2

Dedication

This book is dedicated to the people in my life who unfortunately have passed away, but along their way in life they provided me with insight, understanding, patience, love, and most important, the ability to know that what one receives in life must be shared with others, or the tremendous gift they gave me would be lost.

Vincent J. Harrington
Winifred Harrington
George E. Donahue
John E. Vaughan

Contents

Preface

In our current healthcare delivery model, the healthcare administrator needs to be more adept in managing not only the financial end of the facility such as appropriate debits, credits, ratios, and trial balances, but the reimbursement end that is a feeder to these reports and transactions as well. As a matter of fact, the financial end has become more involved with, and reliant on, the reimbursement process unlike in years past. To add to the confusion, the overall profitability of the healthcare organization rests entirely on their shoulders and is tied to reimbursement and the quality of care provided to the patient. It is imperative that the healthcare administrator know about all of these areas through the education process and from their first job post-graduation be aware of these complex reimbursement issues on day one of their employment and not wait until they can learn on the job.

In my years of teaching at the undergraduate and graduate levels covering healthcare finance and healthcare reimbursement, there are several healthcare finance books that I looked at for the courses I taught and they all focused on accounting and only touched on a few areas of reimbursement. However, with the rapidly changing environment where reimbursement is the driving force of healthcare facilities, we need to give faculty the tools necessary to educate their students and have them ready to make an impact in the field that they have chosen to pursue. The graduates from programs that come out having received a solid and comprehensive education in healthcare finance, along with healthcare reimbursement, will be far more marketable as professionals than those without any formal education in healthcare reimbursement. It is clearer now than ever before that a healthcare facility is not only responsible for quality care, but is fully responsible for the profit or loss on any given patient stay. This responsibility comes from the integration of the Revenue Cycle into the daily management function of the Healthcare Administrator and that of the Health Information Management professional. All departments are not only worried about their annual budget, but they are concerned about driving quality, reducing costs, and improving access for the patients. This is happening because the focus on reimbursement is now the driving force in healthcare facilities; processes are integrated across the continuum of care which makes everyone responsible for the financial success of the facility.

The current topics that a healthcare administrator has to deal with when it comes to reimbursement are the different types of payment arrangements such as block payments, capitation, and Managed Care. Synonymous with reimbursement these days are Diagnosis Related Groups (DRGs) and prospective payment systems for acute, inpatient rehab, skilled nursing facilities, home care, outpatient settings, and ambulatory surgical centers. As if the different payment types were not enough, the healthcare administrator has to deal with readmissions, and case mix index and the Recovery Audit Contractors (RAC) who look for overpayments made to a facility.

■ What the Text Does for the Student

Health Care Finance and the Mechanics of Insurance and Reimbursement introduces reimbursement to the healthcare administrator and provides them a comprehensive outlook on who are the payers in health care, the payment systems in health care, basic coding instruction, revenue cycle management, what fraud and abuse is and how it can have a negative impact on your facility, some key tools that can have a negative impact on your facility if they are not managed daily such as transfer cases and high cost outliers, and tomorrow's trends. Reimbursement has evolved from a process where hospitals and other healthcare providers were paid for what they did for the patient. This type of retrospective payment system, fee-for-service, is one of the main causes of healthcare costs spiraling out of control in the 70s and 80s. Now we have a prospective payment system for many of the types of care such as Inpatient Prospective Payment System (IPPS) and Hospital Outpatient Prospective Payment System (HOPPS). These payment systems allow the healthcare facility to be in full control of their profit or loss on any given patient. Unless the healthcare administrator has a solid foundation of finance and reimbursement, they will not have the necessary skillsets to effectively manage in today's environment.

Other healthcare finance books cover all basic functions of accounting such as business transactions, general ledger, financial statements, depreciation, payroll, expenses, inventories, and interpretation of financial statements. *Health Care Finance and the Mechanics of Insurance and Reimbursement* will not only cover the basic financial accounting process, but it will also cover things like interpretation of financial statements in the healthcare arena, which is crucial for the healthcare administrator as they will need to manage their facilities with these financial statements. Understanding the different ways an insurance company can pay a facility will help the healthcare administrator become more involved in the contract negotiation process and work towards a more favorable contract or better manage the population that is being served.

Along with this, the different types of insurance coverage will be addressed. This will include traditional insurance, managed care, HMOs, Medicaid, and Medicare. Understanding how these payers work is instrumental to the healthcare administrator so that they can better manage their contracts and reimbursement levels so that the facility can remain profitable. This text will help the healthcare manager to better understand Managed Care Organizations, Staff Models, Closed Networks, Exclusive Provider Organizations, and Preferred Provider Organizations just to name a few. Understanding Managed Care Organizations and all of their unique characteristics is critical to the healthcare manager so they can effectively plan budgets, negotiate contracts, and understand the projected utilization versus actual utilization needed to break-even servicing the MCO's patients or to show a profit from a particular payer.

Health Care Finance and the Mechanics of Insurance and Reimbursement not only addresses the basic finance and accounting tools for the healthcare administrator, but the full picture of reimbursement including Charge Description Master (CDM) and Revenue Cycle Management. The CDM is a tool that automatically manages up to 70 percent of the charges in a hospital. The CDM is managed by both the Finance Department and the Health Information Management Department. If this tool is not accurate, it is highly likely that the facility revenue will not be accurate. It can either be understated or overstated. If it is understated then costs need to be cut or programs that are not profitable need to be eliminated. But, without the CDM being accurate, some of the programs could be losing money or their revenue could be understated. With regards to overstating revenue, this usually generates a visit from your payers or the federal government (OIG or CMS) and can lead to charges of fraud, abuse, or both.

Revenue Cycle Management is not a new tool for the healthcare administrator, but a process that has evolved from a fragmented system of individual departments, each managing a single part of the revenue process of a system that has integrated all sections that handle the revenue process into one function called the Revenue Cycle. The revenue for a healthcare facility has evolved from an accounting and finance driven area with cost reports to a revenue cycle process in that insurance companies and other payers reimburse the facility based on the services provided to the patient. It is critical for the Finance Department and Health Information Management to communicate on a daily basis to see about charts that are not coded yet, audits from payers, and case mix index issues. If the healthcare administrator is not well versed in the Revenue Cycle, he or she stands to have a very short career in that healthcare facility.

Finally, the text addresses Electronic Medical Records (EMRs). This is generally a very expensive project to undertake, but it is also another way to get reimbursement from the government that can help to cover the expense of catching up to the electronic age. In *Health Care Finance and the Mechanics of Insurance and Reimbursement* the basics of healthcare finance will be covered along with EHR and Meaningful Use which will assist the healthcare administrator to not only be up to speed with current topics but able to act on and implement the changes necessary to meet the standards set forth in the recent health reform bill in the Obama Administration.

Now, it was clear to me that if we provide access to the information that includes Health Care Reimbursement to the Health Care Administration student, they will be better equipped to function in the healthcare environment today. This ever-changing environment has shifted from the process-oriented environment of cost reporting to a fully integrated Revenue Cycle Management-focused environment. I had to learn this process on my own, as did many of the current Vice Presidents of Health Care Finance and/or Vice Presidents of Revenue Cycle Management, because it is not offered in many of the Health Care Administration programs. However, there is one thing that none of us can forget. There is a patient in the middle of all of this and we need to keep our facilities providing the highest quality care for the patient, and at the same time understand the revenue streams and remain profitable and able to change with the times. This includes access, technology, reducing costs, and increasing the quality delivered to the patient. And, last but not least, the ability to survive in an era of Pay-for-Performance, Medical Home Models, and Value Based Purchasing where the Health Care Administration student needs to be well versed in all the future trends in health care. By bringing healthcare reimbursement to the forefront, this can have a huge impact in the education process of Health Care Administration programs because after 30 years of the same approach, I think it is time for a change.

Acknowledgments

I really do enjoy teaching and feel that everyone learns differently. I pride myself in taking the time to get to know all the students in the class and to make sure that I figure out how each one learns. This process is accomplished by timely and accurate communication in class through discussions, assignments, and e-mails. I find that my experience in the healthcare arena was started by someone who believed in me and mentored me through my early years. This person is my sister, Ruthann, and without her help I would not be where I am today. So, with that said, I do what I do in the healthcare field and the classroom because I want to give back what was given to me.

Others that were of great help along the way were Dr. Twila Weiszbrod from St. Joseph's College of Maine who is the Program Director for the Healthcare Administration Program. Twila was not only instrumental in supporting me with encouraging dialogue along the way, but she provided me with her insight to the needs for more focus on reimbursement in a healthcare administration program to support the current and future trends in the healthcare market. Her direction and insight were invaluable and I can't thank her enough. And there was a friend by the name of Josh Pechar. He was very helpful in guiding and introducing me to different models in health care such as predictive models and database management. Josh was always there when I needed a question answered or just to listen to me ramble on about what I was writing about.

Most importantly, I acknowledge my wife Kathy and our daughter Michaela. The time spent away from the family to complete this book was significant, and without their support and understanding none of this would be possible. So, I say thank you to Kathy and Michaela. And since the book is now complete, maybe we will stop eating out every night and start cooking again. Just a thought.

Foreword

The provision of healthcare services in the United States has grown increasingly complex over time. The reimbursement for services has become a critical element of care, alongside quality of care. To be effective, healthcare leaders must understand regular accounting and financial principles, as well as the specifics of reimbursement for services in an increasingly convoluted and complex system. It is not enough to be committed to the provision of quality healthcare services, because without being reimbursed for services, a healthcare system cannot survive.

There are many payers for healthcare services and rarely is the payer the one receiving the services. Few patients can or do pay for services privately. Each payer, whether they are a government payer like Medicare, Medicaid, or the Veteran's Administration, or a private payer like Blue Cross, Etna, and Cigna, has specific requirements that must be met in order for the healthcare provider to be paid. Attention to the details of the requirements makes the difference between whether or not a healthcare provider is reimbursed for services already provided. Failure to get it right will result in unpaid bills and financial instability for the organization.

This text combines financial principles that are unique to the healthcare setting, with the mechanics of reimbursement. The revenue cycle is explained in detail and correlated with regular management functions in a healthcare setting. Reimbursement is explained from capturing the charges at the initial point of care, through the claim submission and reconciliation process, to accounting procedures to keep track of revenue and expenses. Types of reimbursement and methods for calculating payments are explained in detail by payer type. Revenue cycle management has become a cornerstone of good healthcare leadership and this text provides everything a leader or aspiring leader will need to know to successfully lead a healthcare department or organization.

Dr. Twila Weiszbrod
Program Director
Healthcare Administration Programs
Saint Joseph's College

Foreword

I have been in the healthcare executive role for over 30 years focusing on executive management and finance, along with sales and technology leadership. When Kevin Harrington came to me and discussed the possibilities of writing a book for healthcare administration focusing on healthcare reimbursement I was very intrigued as to what approach he would take to educate the healthcare administration student. When he went over the outline of the book, the focus and forward thinking that was present in the material was clear. The outcome for this is that it would address past elements of health care to come up with an approach that will help the healthcare administrator in today's market enter the field with, what I feel to be, a greater understanding and will be better equipped with knowledge of the current finance and reimbursement systems to help them have a greater and immediate impact in the healthcare facility or field that they manage.

In the past, administrators could come out of college with their degree in management, or if they were fortunate enough, a degree in healthcare administration and go through a training program to bring them up to speed with the current operations of the hospital or other healthcare facility. Now, the new graduate and existing administrators with a bachelor's degree and those pursuing a master's degree, need to have a better understanding of the daily operations of a healthcare facility focusing on healthcare finance and reimbursement starting on day one. This book allows the student, at any level, to advance themselves into areas of importance such as the current activities in accounting, financial reporting, and most importantly Revenue Cycle Management almost immediately.

The information that is delivered in this book should prove to be a great resource for the student and will assist them in increasing their level of understanding in this ever changing healthcare environment that we currently work in and what it is to become in the future.

John L. Connolly
Chief Executive Officer
Anexinet

About the Author

Michael K. Harrington, MSHA, RHIA, CHP, has more than 30 years of experience in health care in areas such as Health Information Management, managing homecare companies on a local and regional level, and consulting in the post-acute sector. He is a leading authority on healthcare reimbursement and Revenue Cycle Management (RCM) and has extensive experience in implementing the RCM model in physician's offices and other healthcare organizations outside of the acute care setting.

After starting out in the healthcare field in a home care company as a coordinator, Harrington quickly advanced into managing home care companies that handled durable medical equipment, specialty home infusion, high-tech respiratory, and specialty biologicals and repositioned these companies by using reimbursement and quality clinical care as the cornerstones to his success. In addition to managing homecare companies, Harrington started to teach and was part of the adjunct faculty at Gwynedd Mercy College, Temple University, and St. Joseph's University in the Philadelphia area. His focus has always been in healthcare reimbursement when teaching, but has instructed in other areas such as Healthcare Policy, Healthcare Ethics, Healthcare Delivery, Computerized Medical Records, and Healthcare Law. Recently Harrington has become part of the full-time faculty at St. Joseph's College Online where he is assisting in the development of the online Health Information Management Program. In addition, Harrington has formed his own consulting firm called Professional Revenue Management Services, LLC, in 2013. He provides healthcare organizations with consulting services focused on healthcare reimbursement, specifically, Revenue Cycle Management services in the physician's office and other healthcare settings.

Harrington earned his bachelor's degree from LaSalle College and his master's degree from Independence University (formerly California College for Health Sciences). Harrington also earned his Registered Health Information Management (RHIA) credentials at Alabama State University. He is an active patient advocate and is a much sought after speaker in the areas of healthcare reimbursement, healthcare finance, and healthcare operations.

He can be reached at kevin@prmsllc.com.

Part I

Introduction to Healthcare Finance

Learning Outcomes

After reading this chapter, the student will be able to:

- Identify the different accounting authorities and their functions within the accounting process.
- Explain the process by which financial reports are generated and the accounting principles that govern this process.
- Describe the objectives for financial reporting and the impact this has on the management process of an organization.
- Identify the different types of financial transactions in a healthcare facility and the transactions in a healthcare facility that help to control the planning and forecasting of a healthcare organization.
- Describe the sources of financial data in a healthcare organization.
- Identify three uses of financial data and how they impact reimbursement in addition to planning and forecasting.
- Explain the various elements that make up the financial statements of the healthcare organization.
- Explain the different types of financial organizations, such as sole proprietorship, partnership, and corporation.
- Describe the characteristics of for-profit and not-for-profit organizations.

■ Introduction

Through the years, health care has evolved from paying cash to the physician at the time of the office visit or the visit to the home, and then the progression to insurance covering the visit. The changes that have occurred over the years have been from the patient having varying responsibilities with regards to payment for the services that ranged from paying the provider first and getting reimbursed from the insurance company in a major medical environment to paying a copayment or coinsurance amount to the provider and the insurance company paying the provider directly. This changing environment has placed many challenges on the healthcare provider and administrator. The timing on payment is different from most industries; for example, when you go to the store to buy lumber and supplies for a weekend project, you pay at the time of check-out in the form of cash or credit card. For health care, the patient receives services and leaves the facility, and the hospital or provider bills the insurance company several days later and waits for payment up to 45 days or longer. This process requires the healthcare administrator to be well versed in healthcare finance and general accounting principles.

This chapter will help to uncover some of the concepts and principles of the basics with regards to accounting by identifying and describing the accounting authorities that oversee financial transactions for federal and public organizations. Then the chapter will cover the objectives for financial reporting and the uses of financial information that will support the decision-making process in the running of an organization. This financial information that represents the data or transactions of an organization will help to compile various financial statements that will assist the for-profit or not-for-profit organization in their decision-making process. The sources of this data come from clinical services, patient accounts, the health information department, and administration. This financial data will help in the areas of reimbursement, control, and planning and forecasting for the healthcare organization.

■ Accounting Authorities

Federal Accounting Standards Advisory Board

The mission of the **Federal Accounting Standards Advisory Board (FASAB)** is that it "serves the public interest by improving federal **financial reporting** through issuing federal financial accounting standards and providing guidance after considering the needs of external and internal users of federal financial information" (FASAB 2014).

The FASAB is an independent organization that works towards setting the accounting standards for all businesses that operate in the private community (LaTour & Eichenwald Maki, 2013a, p. 766). The FASAB works to provide for public accountability through financial reports that include **financial statements** that are prepared in a format that is compatible with generally accepted accounting principles. The board for the FASAB plays a critical role in accomplishing the outcome of the government being accountable in the public's eye. The use of financial reports on the federal level will demonstrate the government's ability to show effective and efficient processes and social, political, and economic impact of various uses of federal resources.

The FASAB looks to improve the financial reporting of the federal government so as to meet its responsibilities to be accountable, and this is done through an independent process that is comprehensive and invites participation from all stakeholders. The FASAB strives to provide a timely and comprehensive study of issues, participation by various stakeholders involved in the standards-setting process, consideration of the costs involved with and the benefits of the financial information, common understanding of the information obtained via financial reporting, availability of informal and formal guidance for preparers and auditors, and holding itself accountable through transparency and comprehensive governance practices.

The FASAB sets the accounting standards for federal and other entities that will assist them in selecting the most applicable form of guidance to use in preparing and auditing accounting and financial reports and this is accomplished through two types of information sources labeled authoritative and other. The authoritative source is considered to be the *FASAB Handbook of Accounting Standards and Other Pronouncements*, or otherwise known as the *FASAB Handbook*. The other sources of information that the FASAB has developed include guides, reports, and other documents that are not considered to authoritative sources but can be appropriate if they are utilized in the proper environment.

Generally Accepted Accounting Principles

The term **Generally Accepted Accounting Principles (GAAP)** consists of accounting principles that are used in the preparation of financial reports and statements for businesses or entities. Generally Accepted Accounting Principles or GAAP "is often used to describe the body of rules and requirements that shape the preparation of the four primary financial statements" (Cleverley, 2012a, p. 182).

According to Wiley, GAAP establishes "the measurement of economic activity, time when such measurements are to be made and recorded, disclosures surrounding this activity, and preparation and presentation of summarized economic information in the form of financial statements" (Flood, 2014a, p. 2). GAAP comes into play when questions come about regarding how to best accomplish these items—and the end result is that GAAP will develop accounting and financial reporting standards. According to GAAP, there are two categories of accounting principles: recognition, which covers timing and measurement of items to enter the accounting cycle, and disclosure, which involves non-numeric issues such as reporting all data (Flood, 2014a, p. 2). If recognition and disclosure were not part of the financial statement process, the end result would be that statements would be misleading and would be missing information necessary for the person who is reading the statements to make or render a decision based on the information provided. Disclosure ultimately supports the recognition principles in that assumptions are explained that are part of the numeric information; these provide additional information to the person reading the financial reports.

Securities and Exchange Commission

The **Securities and Exchange Commission** (SEC) has a mission to "protect investors, maintain fair, orderly and efficient markets, and facilitate capital formation" (SEC 2014a). With the changing marketplace and the increasing amounts of new investors to the market who are looking towards the future on ways to pay for new homes and college tuition through these markets, it has become an even greater need to regulate the market to sustain continued economic growth.

Investing in the market can be exciting and rewarding, and at the same time it can be dangerous as well. Deposits in a bank may be guaranteed by the federal government, but stocks, bonds, and other types of securities can pose a risk for losing their value. The SEC strives to have a straightforward approach to the laws and regulations that govern the securities industry, in which they look to make sure that all investors, regardless of their size, have access to basic facts about a particular investment or multiple investments through the disclosure of meaningful, timely, and accurate information from the public companies to the public or individual investors. This way, the individual investors can determine on their own whether to buy, sell, or hold a particular investment or security.

The responsibility of the SEC is to interpret and enforce federal securities laws, issue new and amend existing rules, oversee the inspection of securities firms, oversee private regulatory organizations, and coordinate regulations with federal, state, and foreign authorities (SEC, 2014b).

The SEC oversees securities exchanges, securities brokers and dealers, investment advisors, and mutual funds to ensure disclosure of market-related information and protecting against fraud. The SEC accomplishes effective oversight through their ability to enforce the laws through civil enforcement actions against **corporations** and individuals that violate these laws. These violations include insider trading, fraud, and companies providing misleading information surrounding the securities they issue. The SEC works closely with a number of other institutions such as Congress, various federal agencies, stock exchanges, state securities regulators, and other private-sector organizations.

Internal Revenue Service

The **Internal Revenue Service** (IRS) "is a department of the United States Treasury and is considered to be one of the most efficient tax administrators and in 2012 alone the IRS processed over 237 million tax returns and collected more than $2.5 trillion dollars in revenue" (IRS, 2014a).

The mission of the IRS is to provide to the American taxpayers the highest quality services surrounding their personal taxes and business taxes and helping them understand their tax responsibilities and in the process of doing this, enforce the law fairly and with the highest integrity. Overall, the IRS helps the taxpayer understand the laws that Congress passes and makes sure that they are compliant and for those who are not compliant, the IRS will make sure that they comply and are responsible for their fair share.

The IRS "is organized under the Unites States Treasury under the Internal Revenue Code, section 7801, and the secretary has the full power to administer and enforce the laws associated with the IRS and also has the power to create an agency to enforce these laws" (IRS, 2014a). The IRS is supervised by a commissioner who is appointed through the Internal Revenue Code.

Centers for Medicare and Medicaid Services

Medicare was established as a result of Title XVIII of the Social Security Act. This was designated as being "Health Insurance for the Aged and Disabled" (CMS, 2012), which is commonly known as Medicare. The Medicare legislation started a program that provided health insurance for persons over the age of 65 to complement other insurances a person may have, such as retirement benefits, survivor's benefits, and disability insurance benefits (Klees, 2009a). According to Centers for Medicare and Medicaid Services (CMS), the Health Insurance for the Aged and Disabled Act (title XVIII of the Social Security Act), or as we know it to be Medicare, has made this coverage available to almost every American over the age of 65 years old. In addition, this broad program is designed to assist the nation's elderly to meet hospital, medical, and other covered healthcare costs. The program includes two related health insurance programs called Hospital Insurance (HI) and a Supplementary Medical Insurance (SMI), which is under Part B (CMS, 2012). CMS will be covered in greater detail in later parts of this text.

■ Objectives for Financial Reporting

The objective of effective financial reporting is to provide information in a timely and efficient manner that will assist in the making of decisions regarding the allocation of resources for the organization. Managers need financial reports so the information about the organization makes sense in a way that will assist them in predicting future cash flows of the organization. This cash flow affects an organization's ability to meet its obligations, such as accounts payable, payroll, and loans, along with paying dividends to the shareholders. There are several information categories that provide information such as economic resources, claims against the entity, and owners' **equity,** which is where the financial reporting illustrates the organization's cash flows and identifies its strength, weaknesses, and solvency. Next, there is economic performance and earnings, which is where the organization looks at past performance to predict its future performance. According to GAAP, "in this instance, when an organization uses the accrual accounting method, it will be a better indicator of future cash flows and overall performance than using current cash receipts and disbursements" (Flood, 2014b, p. 18). The liquidity, solvency, and funds flows is information about cash and other funds from borrowing, expenditures, capital transactions, obligations, owners' equity, and earnings that an organization may experience. The management stewardship and performance is an assessment of an organization's management, measuring how effective they are with regards to managing the organization and the earnings that they report. Finally, management explanations and interpretations covers managers' responsibility to be efficient with regard to the use of the organization's resources.

Usefulness of Financial Information

Financial reporting is a tool for providing information to decision makers that will influence and support the decision-making process. Information for the purposes of decision making need to have the following traits, including usefulness for the decision, relevance, faithful representation, comparability, verifiability, timeliness, understandability, trade-offs, and cost constraint.

The first area is *usefulness for decision-making*. According to GAAP, this "is considered to be the most important characteristic of information for the organization and the information must be useful and have benefit to the user and the accounting information must be relevant and faithfully represent what it claims to represent" (Flood, 2014c, p. 20). These two characteristics are impacted by the overall completeness of the information reported.

Relevance of information is determined by whether the data provided can impact the individual's decision-making process, as it can influence the ability of the person to effectively predict **events** or to accurately authenticate expectations. Even though the information provided may not ultimately change the person's decision process, it can reduce the level of uncertainty of the outcome of the decision. Information is necessary and relevant if it provides understanding surrounding past and future events, and if it is timely. In addition, based on the materiality of the information to the organization, information should be reported if it has value to the organization.

Faithful representation is where financial statements demonstrate the important financial relationships of the organization itself. For information to be considered faithfully representative, it must be complete, neutral, and free from errors (Flood, 2014d, p. 20). A *complete representation* contains all information, such as quantitative and descriptive information, that can be used in a decision-making process. Another area related to faithful representation is *neutrality*. This is where accounting information is a tool to communicate without providing any influence that would sway a decision in a particular direction that would favor a particular interest group. The term *free-from-error* is not meant to identify the information provided as being perfectly accurate, but it does mean that the information or description is accurately described and there is an explanation of any unusual occurrences.

Another feature that will generally enhance the information is *comparability*, which means that, at the time that information is relevant and faithfully represented, it can be used to assess the similarities or differences of like organizations during the same time period. *Verifiability* is where a measure, such as an accounting measure, may be repeated with the same result each time. *Timeliness* means that all information needs to be presented or reported in a timely manner to be useful. *Understandability* of information or reports means that the person reading the report—someone who has sufficient experience or knowledge of the business and activities to be able to analyze the data provided in the reports—will be able to understand the information presented. A *trade-off* is a situation where there may be a characteristic that is obtained from the information; however, accomplishing this will come at the expense of eliminating another characteristic. Finally, there is a characteristic called a *cost constraint*. This is where information should only be presented if the benefit of the information outweighs the cost of obtaining the information.

EXHIBIT 1-1   TRAITS OF USEFUL INFORMATION

- Usefulness for decision making
- Relevance
- Faithful representation
- Comparability
- Verifiability
- Timeliness
- Understandability
- Trade-offs
- Cost constraint

Recognition and Measurement in Financial Statements

Financial statements are considered to be the principal means of communicating useful financial information. The data that are included cover the financial position of the organization at the end of the period, the earnings of the period, overall income for the period, the cash flows during the period, and the investments by and distributions to the owners (Flood, 2014d, p. 21).

Financial statements are a result of taking transactions of the organization, simplifying and condensing them, and aggregating them, into one financial report. A financial report or statement of financial position can provide information about an organization's **assets**, liabilities, and equity. An effective measure of an organization's performance during a period is when, at the end of the period, there are earnings that are realized. *Earnings* are similar to *net income* but do not include any accounting adjustments. Comprehensive income takes into account all changes in equity outside of any investments or distributions involving the owners. A statement of cash flows reflects payments made to the company in cash that are derived from operations, financing, and any investment activities. Any investments by the owners or distributions to the owners during the period will be considered capital transactions during the same period.

Income, or a profit, is when the money amount increases during a period. This includes all sales transactions collections during a period; if this value is greater than the expenses of the period and the net assets have increased, then there is a profit.

Elements of Financial Statements

The following are some of the elements that comprise various financial statements:

- Assets–as a result of past transactions, a positive economic benefit is realized by the organization, such as an increase in accounts receivable, cash, or inventory.

- Liabilities–as a result of a past transaction, a negative economic benefit is realized by the organization, such as accounts payable, loans payable, and variable expenses.

- Equity–this amount is what is left in an asset after removing any liability from its value. For example, in a **partnership** equity is considered to be the owner's interest.

- **Revenues**–this is where an organization increases accounts receivable or cash in exchange for products or services provided by the organization.

- Expenses–these are items that are satisfied by the discharge of assets, such as cash, to the organization or entity that supplied the items to the company.

- **Gains**–are increases in equity, or net assets, from the process of completing transactions to external customers.

- **Losses**–are a negative impact on an owner's equity in the organization. In addition, this is defined by situations where the liabilities are greater than the increases in assets during a period.

- Event–the use of raw materials by a company to be provided to a customer and in exchange is made.

- **Transaction**–is an external event that involves transferring something of value such as services or products to another company and in exchange the company will receive payment.

Financial Organizations

There are three types of organizations that will be discussed here: sole proprietorships, partnerships, and corporations. Organizations will be structured based on their financing, leadership, and tax status. In addition, two characteristics that define the type of organizations are for-profit organizations and not-for-profit organizations.

The first type of organization is a **sole proprietorship**. This type of organization it consists of one person who owns the company. The owner may be considered a proprietor who leads the organization and is responsible for all aspects of managing this business. All revenues are realized by the owner on his or her individual tax return. The structure of the organization can change with regards to adding consultants, independent contractors, or employees.

The next type of organization is a **partnership**. This is where two or more people get together to form what would be considered a partnership. The partners will share duties and responsibilities for running the company, and all revenues will be distributed to the partners, who will pay taxes on the money through the reporting of their individual tax returns. In some cases, the partnership can be required to file its own tax return that will show in detail the income distributed to the partners of the company. If there is any change in ownership, it will dissolve the original partnership that was formed.

Finally, a **corporation** is a legal entity that exists separately from the owners. A corporation will pay its own taxes and is subject to its own legal rights and responsibilities (LaTour & Eichenwald Maki, 2014b, p. 767). In this situation, the owners of a corporation can operate as not having anything to do with the day-to-day operations or have different levels of responsibility. The corporation may be governed by a board of directors or trustees. The administrator, CEO, or president will report directly to the board of directors. If there is money left over at the end of the period or year, this income can be distributed to the shareholders or held for future projects. The corporation's income is taxed and then when there are distributions to shareholders, they are taxed at a personal level. This is considered a two-tiered taxation occurrence or double taxation and can make this type of structure less appealing to individuals.

The status of sole proprietorships, partnerships, or corporations can be categorized as either a for-profit or not-for-profit entity. For-profit is where the organization realizes the profit after all obligations have been discharged, from accounts payable to taxes. These profits will increase the wealth of the owners or the company itself, as the profits can be distributed to the shareholders or held onto for future projects. A for-profit company can be held privately or publicly with regards to ownership. In a private ownership, the owner(s) can be an individual or group of people that join together to form the organization. In a public organization, the ownership of the company can be bought or sold on the open stock market. In a publicly held company, the board of directors will be the deciding factor on the distribution of profits and satisfaction of liabilities such as mortgages.

Not-for-profit organizations are held in trust rather than owned as in the for-profit-organizations. There are many hospitals that fit into this tax status. There are also other organizations that fall into this category, such as professional associations like the American Red Cross. To set these organizations apart, the IRS has established two categories for not-for-profit organizations: 501(c)(6) and 501(c)(3).

The 501(c)(6) consists of professional organizations that may buy and sell goods and services but are doing so with the intent of benefiting a major interest group. These organizations are subject to state sales tax.

The 501(c)(3) organizations are, for the most part, exempt from federal taxes. However, they must limit their activities to those that are in the public interest. Any donations to this type of organization will be tax deductible for the person making the donation. Charities or charitable components make up the vast majority of organizations in this category.

EXHIBIT 1-2   TYPES OF ORGANIZATIONS

For-Profit Organizations
    Sole proprietor
    Partnership
    Corporation
Not-For-Profit Organizations – Voluntary
    Church-related
    Private schools
    Foundations
Not-For-Profit – Government
    Federal
    State
    County
    City
    Hospital
    State universities

■ Sources of Financial Data

Transactions in a Healthcare Facility

Typically there are three vital components that comprise the financial transactions: goods or services are provided, a transaction is recorded, and compensation is exchanged (LaTour & Eichenwald Maki, 2014c, p. 768).

In a healthcare setting, there are many services that are performed and four areas that are of particular importance, the first of which is clinical services. This is where all clinical documentation is completed, and these services, as long as they are documented, will assist the facility in validating that the services were actually rendered to the patient. This clinical documentation will show who was in contact with the patient, what services were delivered, and any other clinical information that can help in the decision-making process for the patient while he or she is in the facility.

The next area is the patient accounts department, which is responsible for gathering all the transactions that are recorded in the patient account through the charge master, producing a bill for the payer, and sending it to them either on paper or via electronic transmission. The overall success of this department is predicated on how accurate the charge description master is and the accuracy of the clinical staff who are recording the transactions in the patient's account.

Health Information Management is the next area. This department is fully responsible for the soft coding of the inpatient medical records. This soft coding process is where the Coding Department, which consists of coding professionals who usually carry the credential of Certified Coding Specialists (CCS), assign diagnosis codes, procedure codes, and query the physician with any questions regarding documentation of the patient's illness and treatment. Once complete, the chart is finalized, and the bill is dropped and sent to the Patient Accounts Department for processing to the payer.

Administration is the last area that we are going to look at for financial transactions. These transactions take place throughout the facility and include employee compensation, purchasing of equipment and supplies, and services performed by some departments for other departments. At this level, the entire management team will review all transactions for the entire facility that impact the financials in the clinical and support areas.

■ Uses of Financial Data

Reimbursement

A healthcare facility will realize most of their revenue, or income, from clinical activities that surround patient care. So the key here is to track all financial data and make sure that it is accurate, timely, and documented. Typically, a good Revenue Cycle

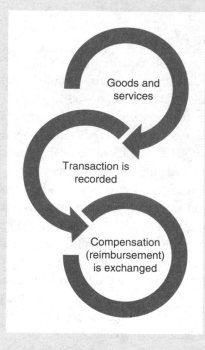

FIGURE 1.1   Components of a healthcare transaction.

Management Team will put a process in place to ensure timely capturing of all data necessary to support the charges to the various payers.

Cost Control

The idea of cost control is best suited at the individual department level. There are many layers in a healthcare facility, and attempting to manage costs across the various departments would create room for error. When the costs are controlled at the individual department level, it makes it possible to manage costs more effectively since the costs are generally associated closely with the day-to-day flow of patient activity.

Planning and Forecasting

Planning and forecasting fall in the administrative area of the facility. **Planning** is something that reflects what the organization is going to do based on its mission statement. In the mission statement are goals and objectives that support the vision of the organization and how it will service the population for which it was established. Planning is an excellent tool for the healthcare administrator; however, this can't be effectively done on historical data alone. This is due to the constant industry changes that have been occurring and will continue to occur as time goes on. With that said,

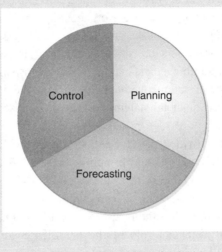

FIGURE 1.2   Use of financial data.

healthcare administrators will need to plan multiple scenarios in the future and track them with current results and make the necessary changes to the plan to reflect the changing environment going forward.

Forecasting goes hand in hand with planning, as this too looks at future trends based on historical data. Organizations can predict revenues, profits, costs, staffing levels, profitability of contracts over the life of the agreement, and can also predict things like consumer behavior with the use of predictive models that will give the healthcare administrator the ability to look forward based on historical results to stay ahead in this prospective environment.

■ Conclusion

Although health care seems to be as simple as providing a service and getting paid for it, this chapter demonstrates that there are many components that go into the generating of the financial statements that support the results of the organization's efforts. Not only are there different categories of organizations, such as for-profit and not-for-profit, there are also different types of organizations such as a sole proprietorship, partnership, and a corporation where the accounting and financial functions are governed by different authorities. In the healthcare arena, organizations are overseen by the Federal Accounting Standards Advisory Board and operate under Generally Accepted Accounting Principles. This structure is a result of Title XVIII of the Social Security Act that provided health insurance and supplementary medical insurance for those beneficiaries who are

65 and older or have certain disabilities that would make them eligible for Medicare. The financial components of a healthcare organization are defined by the financial data and transactions that take place in the day-to-day operations. The result of the transactions come in the form or reimbursement, or lack thereof, for services rendered to the patients they serve. These reimbursements, along with the costs of operating a facility, make up the different financial statements that help to guide the decision-making process for the organization. These financial statements consist of assets, liabilities, equity, revenues, expenses, and profit or loss.

This chapter provides the student, or future healthcare administrator, with an introduction to the concepts and principles of the basics with regards to accounting and the information related to the sources and uses of financial data. A good understanding of financial statements is a foundation for the successful evaluation and use of the financial data within the healthcare organization that will enhance the overall foundation of the financial role of the healthcare administrator in this constantly changing and challenging environment.

References

Casto, A.B., & Forrestal, E. (2013a). *Principles of healthcare reimbursement* (4th ed.). Chicago: AHIMA.

Centers for Medicare and Medicaid Services. (2012, June 1a). *Medicare benefit policy manual: Coverage of hospice services under hospital insurance* (p. 3). Retrieved from http://www.cms.gov/Regulations-and-Guidance/Guidance/Manuals/Downloads/bp102c09.pdf

Cleverley, W., & Cameron, A. (2012). *Essentials of health care finance* (7th ed.). Sudbury, MA: Jones & Bartlett Learning.

Federal Accounting Standards Advisory Board. (2014). Our mission. Retrieved from http://www.fasab.gov/about/mission-objectives/

Flood, M. J. (2014a). *GAAP 2014: Interpretation and application of generally accepted accounting principles*. Somerset, NJ: Wiley.

Flood, M. J. (2014b). *GAAP 2014: Interpretation and application of generally accepted accounting principles*. Somerset, NJ: Wiley.

Flood, M. J. (2014c). *GAAP 2014: Interpretation and application of generally accepted accounting principles*. Somerset, NJ: Wiley.

Flood, M. J. (2014d). *GAAP 2014: Interpretation and application of generally accepted accounting principles*. Somerset, NJ: Wiley.

Klees, B. S. (2009a). Brief summaries of Medicare & Medicaid: Title XVIII and Title XIX of The Social Security Act. (p 6). Retrieved from http://www.cms.gov/Research-Statistics-Data-and-Systems/Statistics-Trends-and-Reports/MedicareProgramRatesStats/downloads/MedicareMedicaidSummaries2009.pdf

LaTour, K.M., & Eichenwald Maki, S. (2013a). *Health information management: Concepts, principles, and practice* (4th ed.). Chicago: AHIMA.

LaTour, K.M., & Eichenwald Maki, S. (2013b). *Health information management: Concepts, principles, and practice* (4th ed.). Chicago: AHIMA.

LaTour, K.M., & Eichenwald Maki, S. (2013b). *Health information management: Concepts, principles, and practice* (4th ed.). Chicago: AHIMA.

Securities and Exchange Commission. (2014a). Retrieved from http://www.sec.gov/about/whatwedo.shtml

Securities and Exchange Commission. (2014b). Retrieved from http://www.sec.gov/about/whatwedo.shtml

United States Treasury. (2014). Internal Revenue Service: The agency, its mission and statutory authority. Retrieved from http://www.irs.gov/uac/The-Agency,-its-Mission-and-Statutory-Authority

Financial Management

Learning Outcomes

After reading this chapter, the student will be able to:

- Recognize the importance of the accounting function, reporting, analyzing, and planning for the nonfinancial manager.
- Understand the differences between financial accounting and managerial accounting for the nonfinancial manager.
- Interpret the basic financial reports such as income statements, cash flow statements, and balance sheets.
- Identify and explain the different components of financial statements such as revenue, expenses, and owner's equity.
- Understand the impact of net income financial statements and what it means to the organization with regards to planning and budgeting process.
- Explain the use of the general ledger in the financial management process.
- Identify, interpret, and respond to variances in the financial reporting process in both the immediate and long-range planning process of an organization.
- Classify the different costs, both direct and indirect, of an organization and the proper allocation of these costs throughout the organization.
- Compile the necessary data to calculate and analyze the basic financial ratios for an organization.
- Categorize the revenue and expenses of an organization to effectively select and construct the appropriate type of budget for the organization.

■ Introduction

This chapter, Financial Management, is geared towards assisting the healthcare manager with some level of accounting background, either basic or somewhat more advanced through experience or education, to better understand the tools that come along with the financial reporting side of the operation. This chapter will introduce the student to financial accounting and the importance that this has on the organization's decision-making process. Inside these reports reside the main components of the financial report. First, there are assets, which are things or items that are owned by the company that have value. Second, there are liabilities, which represent amounts owed by the company for services or items purchased to run the daily operations or to help build what the company sells to their clients. Third, income or revenues that the company generates to increase cash and accounts receivable through selling an item or service to another company that will increase cash or accounts receivable. Fourth, owner's equity, which represents the difference between the assets that the company has accumulated and liabilities, or bills, that the company has incurred as a result of generating sales for the company. This chapter will also explore general ledger and journal entries that help to track and categorize various revenues and expenses into similar groups and accounts.

The next part of the chapter will focus on budgets and financial statements. These two tools are frequently used in making short-term and long-term decisions for the company. The different types of budgets, such as fixed or flexible, and the variances that occur during the budget period will help to guide the company on the path, or plan, that the management team has outlined in their strategic planning. The financial statements will identify, in real time, where the organization is performing at a variety of levels.

Inside these financial statements are tools that measure information in a snapshot or over a period of time. You will see that you can use this information to develop key indicators, or ratios, that help to identify current trends with a short-term approach. These indicators, or ratios, will assist the managerial staff in assessing and developing various strategies to keep the company moving in the right direction. Finally, this chapter will cover managerial accounting and the purposes for the reporting, current vs. future, and the necessary levels of consistency that come along with managerial accounting.

■ Financial Accounting

Financial accounting is defined as "the branch of accounting that provides general-purpose financial statements or reports to aid many decision-making groups, internal and external to the organization, in making a variety of decisions" (Cleverley & Cameron, 2012, p. 182). There are four main reports that are outputs of financial accounting: the balance sheet, the statement of operations, the statement of cash flows, and the statement of changes in net assets. These four statements are not the only statements that are produced in financial accounting. There are also reports required for decision-making purposes such as cost reports and financial projections. All of the reports are utilized based on the reporting needs of the industry and the information available to create the reports. In addition, these reports are not generally audited by independent Certified Public Accountants (CPAs), but are created based on GAAP.

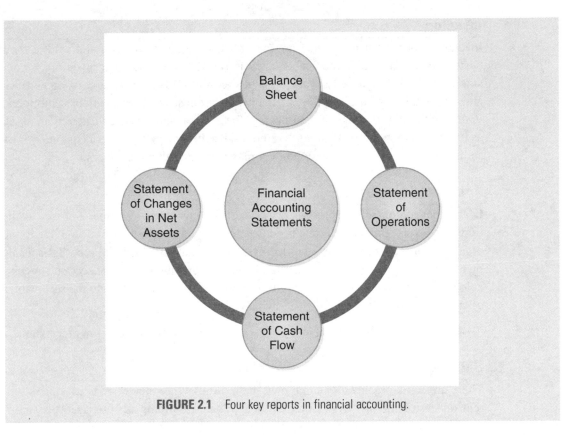

FIGURE 2.1 Four key reports in financial accounting.

■ Assets

An asset is something that is owned by the company. This can be something that is owned and in possession of the company, although assets also can be items that are due to be received. An example of this is accounts receivable, where an organization provides a service to a customer and this customer agrees to pay for the services after they are completed. Some examples of an asset are cash, accounts receivable, inventory, equipment, and buildings.

Cash

Cash assets are considered to be cash on-hand or items that can be converted into cash easily and in a short period of time. Items that are included are cash in bank accounts and cash that is part of a wire transfer. An example of a wire transfer, or electronic funds transfer (EFT), is when an insurance company pays a provider for services rendered to one of their members through an EFT. This wire transaction is considered to be the same as if you walked up to the bank teller and handed cash over for the deposit.

Inventory

Inventory consists of goods that are purchased by the organization and sold to their customers. For a durable medical equipment (DME) company, their inventory is considered to be hospital beds, walkers, canes, commodes, wheelchairs, oxygen tanks, and ventilators. For a pharmacy, their inventory consists of medications, compound items, and blood products, just to name a few. This inventory is considered an asset, as it can usually be turned into cash rather easily through selling it to a customer or by selling it to a vendor for cash, who then may sell it to other customers.

Accounts Receivable

If an organization sells a product or service to a customer who does not pay at the time of delivery, this sale amount is considered to be an accounts receivable due to the organization. This revenue is recorded in the organization's financial records as a sale by reducing any inventory that may have been sold and increasing the accounts receivable account by the amount of the sale. A simple formula to calculate the receivables of an organization is to take the following:

beginning accounts receivable + sales − collections = ending accounts receivable

Building

There are some organizations that own the buildings that they operate in; others will rent or lease buildings from other entities. When a building is purchased, it is considered an asset, as it is owned by the company. When a building is leased, it is not considered to be an asset, as the company does not own the building. When a company purchases a building, it often will put a down payment on the building and finance the balance in the form of a mortgage. The difference between the amount owed on the mortgage and the value of the building is considered to be equity.

Equipment

When an organization purchases a piece of equipment for use or for resale, the value is recorded in the records as the amount of the purchase price for the equipment. Equipment is considered to be a long-term asset and, with some equipment being at a lower price, it is up to the individual organization as to how they record the equipment. It can be recorded as a long-term asset, where the cost of the equipment is spread out over a few years, or else a purchase of equipment is paid for and the expense is recorded in the current period such that the entire value paid will be part of the financial reporting for that period.

A piece of equipment has a purchase price, and this number is used to determine the value that is recorded. For example, a DME provider purchases a hospital bed for $1,000 from the manufacturer. Now the DME company has an asset with a value of $1,000, and this asset can now be depreciated based on the individual company's

Assets	Liabilities
Cash	Accounts Payable
Inventory	Loans (Short and Long Term)
Accounts Receivable	Mortgage
Building	Payroll Taxes
Equipment	Income Taxes

FIGURE 2.2   Examples of assets and liabilities.

policies. Regardless, at this point the company has an asset that will have a life of several years.

With regards to **depreciation**, this is where the company takes the value of the asset and spreads out the cost over a period of time that is consistent with the accounting practices of the company. In the example of the DME company where they purchased a hospital bed for $1,000, the company will now record the asset and take the value of the equipment each year over the expected life of the asset. For example, the hospital bed should last at least 5 years, and the purchase price was $1,000. Now if the company is taking assets of this value and depreciating it over the five years of the expected life of the unit, it will take $200 for each year over the next 5 years as a depreciation expense until it has a zero value.

■ Liabilities

Liabilities are basically debts of the company. These amounts that are part of the liabilities of the company represent items purchased, services utilized, or money spent purchasing items that turn into inventory for resale. The amount that is due to the company that the item was purchased from will be considered a debt, and the inventory will be recorded in the books for the company as an asset.

Accounts Payable

An accounts payable is an amount due to an outside vendor for the purchase of supplies, equipment, or services. The recording of an accounts payable is considered a liability to the company and will need to be paid to the company that is owed the money. For example, the DME company purchased the hospital bed for $1,000; now they have the asset but there is a corresponding liability for the purchase of this bed. The amount due to the vendor of $1,000 is considered to be an accounts payable that will be scheduled to be paid based on the terms and conditions of the company that they purchased the equipment from originally.

Notes Payable

A notes payable is considered to be a financial obligation that is supported by a contract and has a time frame for repayment. A note may be associated with a large purchase or a loan, when an organization uses some of their assets as collateral.

■ Net Assets and Equity

The difference between what is owed versus assets is considered equity. According to LaTour, "equity (or owner's equity) is the arithmetic difference between assets and liabilities" (LaTour & Eichenwald Maki, 2013, p. 772). Simply put, the equation is as follows:

$$\text{Assets} - \text{Liabilities} = \text{Net Assets (or owner's equity)}$$

Another way of defining this equation is as follows:

$$\text{Assets} = \text{Liabilities} + \text{Net Assets (owner's equity)}$$

All of these parts, assets, liabilities, and owner's equity are part of the organization's balance sheet. The balance sheet will be discussed later in this chapter.

■ Revenue

Revenue is the income that is produced through the sales function of an organization to sell products and/or services to customers. The amount that the customers will pay for these products and/or services will be revenue. In a healthcare facility, the main source of revenue is driven by patient services. This can include outpatient services such as lab and x-ray, inpatient services such as surgical and medical care along with other services such as OB-GYN, rehabilitation, dialysis, homecare, and physician services.

Revenue Categories

The categories of revenue are broken down into operating and nonoperating revenue. An example of operating revenue is patient services revenue, which is generated by

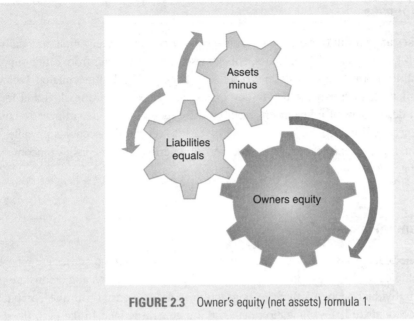

FIGURE 2.3   Owner's equity (net assets) formula 1.

daily operations. And an example of nonoperating revenue is investment income and the money generated from the gift shop that is run by the volunteer organization in the hospital, which are only indirectly related to daily operations.

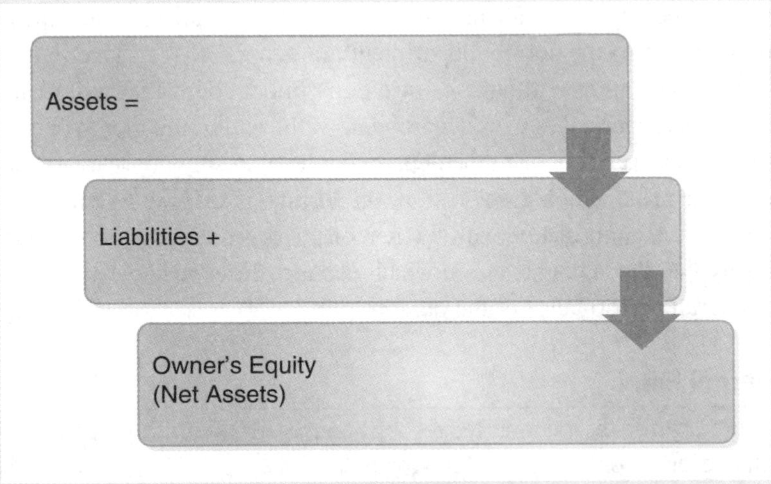

Assets =

Liabilities +

Owner's Equity (Net Assets)

FIGURE 2.4   Assets formula 2.

◼ Expenses

Expenses are a result of expending resources to operate the organization on a daily basis that will lead to generating revenues. An expense can be anything from office supplies in the Health Information Department to software expenses in the Information Technology Department that support the day-to-day operations. Expenses are tracked and recorded in each department of a healthcare facility. The expense that a department or company experiences will reduce the asset account of cash to relieve the accounts payable. In the long run, if the revenue exceeds the expenses for a period, there is positive income for the organization.

◼ General Ledger

The general ledger is part of the accounting system where all the entries are recorded in chronological order. Once posted to the general ledger, the debits and credits are posted to the individual accounts that the transaction is associated with in the company. All of the accounts in the organization make up the general ledger. In the past, the general ledger was on paper, but with the evolving technology, most accounting systems are computerized. This allows the reporting to be more streamlined and more readily available to the departments and managers for review. The individual department does not make the entries in the general ledger, but it will sign off on expenses that are related to the individual department and forward them to accounting so an invoice can be processed for posting to the general ledger and the particular account, along with processing payment to the vendor for the product or services that the organization purchased.

Another layer of information that will help to make sure all expenses and revenues are allocated to the correct department are general ledger accounts. Each department in the organization will have its own department codes that will identify the expenses and revenue accrued to their department. At the end of the month or period, the accounting team can run reports at the department level to show only that department's activity and at the management level to show the facility as a whole. When there are things in the report that are out of line with the rest of the organization, the manager can look more closely into the accounts to see which department is negatively or positively impacting the overall performance of the organization.

Journal Entry

Each entry for the general ledger will consist of a debit and a credit—and they must balance out. For example, suppose there was a purchase of supplies in the amount of $500 from a local vendor. The supplies have arrived, and the vendor has sent an invoice for payment to the organization. The individual department will verify that the items on the invoice were received and approve for payment. The invoice will be sent to the accounting department for posting and payment. The accounting office will make a debit entry in the general ledger for office supplies expense and a credit for $500 in accounts payable. Then when the invoice is paid, the entries will be a debit to accounts payable in the amount of $500 and a credit (reduction) in the amount of $500 to the cash account. All entries must balance out, in that if you have $500 in debits, you need to have $500 in credits to balance out.

■ Managerial Accounting

Managerial accounting focuses on the needs of the internal customer or user. Since the information is generally used for internal purposes, it does not come under the same requirements that are expected of for external reporting. With this in mind, there still needs to be a level of consistency in the preparation of information delivered to the internal customer. The difference between managerial accounting and financial accounting is that managerial accounting focuses more on the future planning of the organization, where financial accounting focuses more on recording transactions that cover historical financial transactions.

Definition of Costs

The utilization of resources in the manufacturing of product, distribution of product, or providing services to a customer is important to the overall management of the operation with regards managing costs and profitability. The ability for an organization to measure costs throughout the manufacturing and sales cycle is done through the appropriate classification of costs. Moreover, the use of this data, from an internal perspective, will provide a variety of additional data for the management team.

Direct Costs

A direct cost is one that is able to be tracked back to a specific service provided or a product that was manufactured. For example, a medication was provided to a patient by the pharmacy. This type of transaction can be traced directly back to the patient, as it is associated with patient care. Another direct cost example is where a homecare company purchases liquid oxygen to fill portable oxygen tanks for patients to use when outside the home. This cost for product can be captured and associated directly with the tanks that are delivered to the patient each week.

Indirect Costs

An indirect cost is a cost that is incurred in the organization as they provide products or services to a customer, but the cost is not directly related to the manufacturing of goods

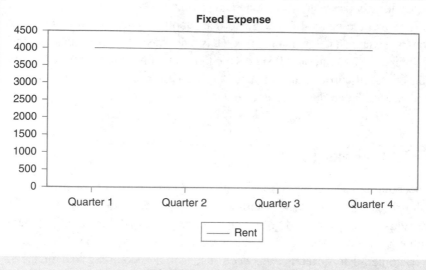

FIGURE 2.5 Fixed expense.

or services provided by the organization. Some examples of indirect costs in a hospital are security and housekeeping. The payroll cost for security and housekeeping is considered to be indirect, or not related to providing clinical care or services, and these costs are distributed to all the departments that they serve in the hospital. The costs are allocated to the departments through the hospital based on the percentage of revenue a particular department has in comparison to the total revenue of the facility. Or it is distributed based on the square footage a department in relation to the total square footage of the facility.

Fixed Costs

The costs in a facility can be fixed or variable. The classification of a fixed cost is one that will remain constant and will not be influenced by volume. An example of a fixed cost is a mortgage payment, as it is the same each month for the term of the loan. Another example of a fixed cost is the salary of a manager in a department. Regardless of the amount of hours this manager works, the salary remains the same.

Variable Costs

Variable costs, on the other hand, are influenced by volume and can change each month based on those changes in volume. For example, the Health Information Management (HIM) department uses office supplies to complete their work such as file folders. If the hospital has only 50 percent occupancy one month and then the next month there is 90 percent occupancy the variable cost of file folders will increase based on volume.

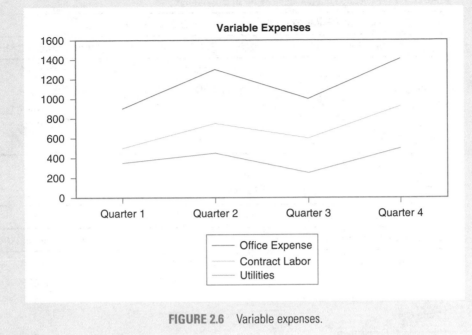

FIGURE 2.6   Variable expenses.

Semi-fixed Costs

There are some costs that are impacted by volume, but are not extremely sensitive to volume changes. For example, you have a coding staff in the HIM department and they currently handle 1,800 charts per month, but the capacity of the current staff is 2,000 charts per month. If the hospital increases discharges to 1,950 the next month the staffing will not need to be adjusted. On the other hand, if the hospital increases discharges to 2,250 per month the department will need to hire another coder or utilize an outside coding service. This makes the coding payroll a semifixed cost based on the volume that the department realizes, but it is not sensitive to every change in volume.

Allocation of Overhead

As mentioned earlier in the direct and indirect costs for a facility there are costs that will need to be allocated to the entire facility. These indirect costs can be distributed through several methods that include direct method, step-down allocation, double distribution, and simultaneous equations method.

The direct method of allocating costs will allocate the costs involved with overhead to the departments that are revenue producing. These costs will be distributed to the individual revenue-generating departments based on a percentage of revenue that they produce compared to the entire facility or the square footage that they occupy in comparison to the entire facility's square footage. For example, the radiology

TABLE 2.1   Allocation of indirect costs by square footage.

Springfield Medical Center Total Square Footage 250,000 sq. ft.

Square Footage by Cost Center	Total	Percentage of Allocation
Dietary	4,500	1.8%
Laundry	3,800	1.5%
Housekeeping	1,250	0.5%
Security	1,000	0.4%
Health Information Management	4,950	1.98%

TABLE 2.2   Allocation of indirect costs by revenue.

Springfield Medical Center Total Revenue $227,500,000

Revenue by Department	Total	Percentage of Allocation
Radiology	$24,500,000	10.76%
Laboratory	$8,257,500	3.62%
Surgery	$133,250,500	58.57%
Home Care	$8,000,000	3.51%
Emergency Department	$36,400,950	16.00%

department produces 3 percent of the facility's total square footage. Therefore, the radiology department will be allocated 3 percent of the facility's total indirect costs.

The step-down allocation method is designed to distribute the indirect costs, starting with the department that provides the least amount of revenue-generating services. The next method is double distribution, a process that allocates costs associated with overhead two times such that costs will be distributed to some overhead departments that provide services to each other. And finally, the simultaneous equations method is one that allocates overhead through multiple scenarios ensuring the maximum allocation of interdepartmental costs to the overhead areas.

■ Budgets

Managers not only oversee the financial reports, they manage the process that feeds the financial reporting process—and this starts with the budget. It is important for a manager to understand basic accounting to properly read financials and check for appropriate allocation of revenue and expenses, but it is equally as important to have the ability to forecast revenue and expenses for the department or organization to meet the mission and vision of the organization through the budget process.

Fixed Budget

This type of budget is designed to account for expected activity in the upcoming year based on historical data. The budget will not change during the year even if the volume of business changes over the year. If there are changes in volume, this will create variances that are either positive or negative. For example, if the hospital increases the volume of patients over the year, then the amount of discharges that the coding department will have to code increases as well. If the HIM department has to hire another coder to handle the increased volume or increase the amount of outside services used, there will be a negative variance, where the budgeted salaries will be lower than the actual salaries paid in the department. For the most part, variances, either positive or negative, that exceed a percentage set by the organization will need to be explained by the manager.

Flexible Budget

A flexible budget is one that is created based on productivity that is projected based on historical data. In the example with the HIM department and the increase in discharges through the year, the department will have a budget based on levels of volume, and the department will need to manage to the level of activity and balance this with the actual levels of staffing.

Activity-based Budget

These budgets are based on projects instead of departments. Activity-based budgets are typically used for projects, for example in construction or in an IT department, that will be running over the course of a year or longer.

Zero-based Budget

This type of budget is where an organization will decide to continue or discontinue a service based on each department justifying and prioritizing activities each year. The use of zero-based budgeting is commonly used in professional associations and charitable foundations.

Budget Cycles

The budget cycle is generally related to a **fiscal year** of a company. The process takes into account the projected revenues generated from sales by the organization and expenses for the organization to manufacture product or deliver these services. The budget process will start three to four months prior to the next fiscal year. This will give ample time for the management team to gather historical data and forecast the activity for the upcoming fiscal year.

TABLE 2.3   Budget variance.

Category	Budget	Actual	Variance	Percentage
Office Supplies	$1,500.00	$1,670.00	$170.00	10.2%
Outside Coding Service	$7,500.00	$7,525.00	$ 25.00	0.4%
File Room Labor	$8,000.00	$7,100.00	$(900.00)	(11.25%)

Budget Components

The components of the budget consist of revenues and expenses. The revenue will be any amount that is related to the sale of products or services to customers that are associated with a particular department. In the HIM department, there are few revenues generated, so their budget will consist mainly of expenses. The manager will need to look at historical costs and trends to come up with a budget that will appropriately reflect the anticipated costs associated with operating the HIM department over the next fiscal year.

Budget Variances

A budget variance is the mathematical difference between what was budgeted versus what actually happens. This variance will be the responsibility of the manager to explain and to manage. These variances are often calculated by looking at the actual results from the financial reports for the month and compare it to what was budgeted. The variance will be reported on the financial report and it can be a positive or negative variance.

A variance can also be classified as a temporary variance or a permanent variance. The temporary variance can be one that a department incurred to cover vacations during the summer by bringing in contract labor. The variance that this creates will be a temporary one as it is only happening based on the staff taking vacations. A permanent variance will be one that will not change in the near future or current fiscal year. For example, if the hospital occupancy rate is increasing due to added services such that the HIM department coder's volume increases, and they hire an additional coder to cover the volume, this will be considered a permanent variance, as it will not be rectified during the current fiscal year.

Explanation of Variances

A variance is something that will need to be explained by the manager supervising the department where the variance occurred. The information that the manager needs to communicate is the nature of the variance—is it temporary or permanent?—the exact dollar amount and percentage of variance, the issue or issues that caused the variance, and any explanations that can justify the variance or show an offset in another area.

The reporting of a variance can be based on dollar amount of variance or percentage of variance. The idea is to have only variances explained that are of certain value and impact on the overall performance of the organization. A small variance of

$100 or a 1 percent variance may not have the impact on the organization that needs to be explained in detail. The administrator should look at managing this variance throughout the fiscal period so as to maintain control of costs over the year. There may be reasons for the variance, such as an increase in contract labor expense for which not enough money was budgeted, which may be balanced by a decrease in payroll for the department related to two vacancies. This offset is good to explain, but it needs to be managed appropriately; once the positions are filled, the use of contract labor should go back to the budgeted amount.

■ Capital Budgets

A capital budget is one that looks mainly at large purchases in the upcoming year. These can consist of capital investments, which are of a large value and can be a long-term investment. These capital budgets are sometimes associated with capital improvements or expansion of services. This capital budget will direct resources to support the organization's plan that will be over and above the operating budget for the organization.

■ Financial Statements

Balance Sheet

The statements of financial positions, otherwise known as the balance sheet, display information about the organization's assets and owner's equity along with the financing structure of liabilities and equity in accordance with GAAP. The balance sheet shows, at a certain point in time, the impact that all the transactions organization have had on the assets, liabilities, and owner's equity of the organization (Flood, 2014, p. 43).

In addition, the report looks at the following items to assess the financial position of the organization, including liquidity of the organization or the level of cash in the operating system, financial flexibility or the organization's ability to respond to unexpected turns in the financial position of the operations, the organization's ability to pay its debts when they come due, and the ability to distribute cash to the owners or the shareholders.

The report also breaks up the assets into current assets, such as cash and accounts receivables, and long-term assets, such as buildings and equipment. The liabilities are also treated the same way, in that there are current liabilities, such as accounts payable, and long-term liabilities, such as notes or mortgages. The calculation of assets minus liabilities will result in the determination of owner's equity. If the owner's equity is positive, then the organization is somewhat liquid, but if the owner's equity account is negative, then the organization is not as liquid and may lack the working capital to handle any unexpected event that could impact the organization.

EXHIBIT 2-1   BALANCE SHEET

Springfield Medical Center
Balance Sheet
as of December 31, 2014

Assets
Current Assets

Cash	$165,000
Accounts Receivable	$725,000
Inventory	$87,500
Total Current Assets	$977,500

Property, Plant, and Equipment

Land	$85,000
Building	$2,500,000
Equipment	$450,000
Total Property, Plant, and Equipment	$3,035,000
Total Assets	$4,012,500

Liabilities
Current Liabilities

Accounts Payable	$287,500
Other	$56,000
Total Current Liabilities	$287,500

Long-Term Debt

Mortgage	$2,400,000
Total Liabilities	$2,687,500

Fund Balance

Restricted Funds	$0
Unrestricted Funds	$1,325,000
Total Fund Balance	$1,325,000
Total Liabilities and Fund Balance	$4,012,500

Income Statement

The income statement is also known as the profit and loss statement. The profit and loss statement is intended to demonstrate how much money a company is making or losing, and it accomplishes this "by subtracting all of the costs of production of goods that have been sold during the period and other expenses of running the company from the revenues generated from sales of products or from services provided" (Bandler, 1994, p. 34).

The statement consists of revenues, which represent actual or expected cash inflows that result from an organization's operations. According to GAAP, "revenues are generally recognized at the culmination of the earnings process-when the entity has substantially completed all it must do to be entitled to future cash inflows" (Flood, 2014, p. 72). For the most part, once a transaction has been completed, the organization has realized revenues that have been earned.

EXHIBIT 2-2   STATEMENT OF REVENUE AND EXPENSES

Springfield Medical Center
Statement of Revenue and Expenses

	12/31/2013	12/31/2014
Revenues		
Net Patient Services Revenue	$8,300,000	$9,250,000
Total Operating Revenue	$4,300,000	$5,015,000
Operating Expenses		
Med/Surg Services	$2,450,000	$2,750,000
Homecare Services	$845,000	$917,000
Infusion Services	$218,000	$245,000
Support Services	$78,000	$86,500
Depreciation	$32,000	$32,000
Interest	$15,000	$18,000
Total Operating Expenses	$3,638,000	$4,048,500
Income from Operations	$662,000	$966,500
Interest Income	$3,200	$4,000
Nonoperating Gains	$3,200	$4,000
Increase in Unrestricted Fund Balance	$665,200	$970,500

Cost of Goods Sold and Gross Profit

Cost of goods is defined as "made up of all costs allocated to inventory sold during the period, including labor, materials, and overhead" (Bandler, 1994, p. 35). For a hospital, cost of goods can consist of supplies, equipment, salaries, and other overhead.

The difference between the sales of an organization and the cost of goods sold will be the gross profit. This is referred to as gross profit as there are still other expenses that need to be factored into the operations to come to the net profit of a particular time period for the organization. The net profit, or net income, is the amount of money that is left over after all revenues are accounted for and all expenses, or costs of doing business in that time period, are deducted from the revenue; the difference (positive or negative) is the net income for the organization.

The profits or losses are added to the balance sheet in the owner's equity account. The impact on the balance sheet is that when there is a profit, the owner's equity account is increased by that amount. When the organization realizes a loss, the owner's equity account is impacted in a negative way.

Cash Flow Statement

The statement of cash flows "is a required part of a complete set of financial statements for business enterprises and not-for-profit organizations" (Flood, 2014, p. 85). The primary function of the cash flow statement is to provide the organization with the amount of cash receipts during a particular period. Another purpose for this statement is to identify the investing and financing activity during the statement period. The cash flow statement will only track cash in and cash out, including cash equivalents such as investments that are considered to be liquid, or easily turned into cash.

The cash flow statement will help the organization to determine its ability to generate positive cash flows in the future, the ability to meet obligations of the organization with regards to payments for accounts payable and distributions to shareholders or owners, to identify variances in net income and cash in and cash out, and the impact of investing and financing on the organization's financial position.

■ Who Uses Financial Statements

Financial statements can be viewed as boring and uninviting documents that can induce long naps at work or the occasional mental vacation where you are looking at a piece of paper, but your mind is in a beach scene where the conditions are absolutely perfect, but then you come back to reality. Financial statements can be very interesting if one can just get to know their value, and the financial picture that they can paint that will be much more interesting than the nicest beach that you can dream up while at work.

The financial reports tell a story of every employee and vendor, sales representative and customer, and every regulatory agent and surveyor's impact on the financial picture of the company. These reports allow you to look into the future and forecast what it may be like in 30, 60, 90, or 120 days—or for that matter, a year or two from the present time. By using historical data, a manager can easily take the reports and extrapolate data that can show what the trends are showing for growth, or lack of growth, for the organization over a specified time period. Once the healthcare manager experiences the power of a financial report and the forward vision it provides to both the manager and the organization as a whole, the manager will use these reports on a regular basis.

Now, for the owners of a company, financial reports are critical to them as they need to report to the bank or lenders on the financial position of their company. If they are using the accounts receivable for leverage or collateral for a line of credit, the balance sheet and income statement are key to painting a complete and timely picture of where the company is at and where it is going. The balance sheet is used to see the owner's equity in the company and it is used to calculate ratios such as debt to equity and alike.

Lenders will look at the profitability of the company, and this will determine how much the company may be able to borrow. Moreover, if the balance sheet is strong and shows that the company can withstand a bad month or two and still be strong and liquid, the lender may feel more comfortable in the lending relationship that they and the company are engaged in currently.

Suppliers will sell to their customers on credit, and the use of financial statements will assist them in determining what levels of credit they can give to their customer. In addition, the reports show how the company they are dealing with can pay their bills and continue to operate and not have a negative impact on the supplier. In addition, the supplier can see if the customer is growing and may be relying on them more and more for product that will in turn have an impact on the supplier's daily operations.

Current employees and individuals seeking to gain employment at an organization should look at the financials of the organization that they are thinking about going to work for. The reason is simple: as an employee, you will be relying heavily on the financial viability of the company that you will be working for so you get a regular paycheck and can continue the lifestyle that you have become accustomed to living. So, if an organization had a poor financial position, then the likelihood that a person will look to gain employment or a current employee remain employed at the organization is not good. The financial statements can show the cash flow of the organization, how they pay their bills, are they in a positive or negative situation with regards to the balance sheet, or are they struggling based on their income statements. Keep in mind that the financial statements need to be accurate and timely to help the current or prospective employee make an educated decision as to whether or not to join an organization.

■ Accrual Accounting Method

There is an important factor in the accrual accounting method for the healthcare administrator to understand. In the accrual concept, the organization will account for revenue in the period it was realized even though it may not have received payment yet. Moreover, for the expense part of the equation, if there are expenses realized during a period but not paid for as of yet, they too will be accounted for in the accrual method.

The goal is to have all revenue and related expenses accounted for in the same accounting period. This way, the utilization of assets to produce the revenue, and the expenses or obligations associated with the generating of revenue, are all captured in the same period. This will bring consistency to the financial reporting, keeping in mind that it is a complicated system, and will give the individuals using the reports sound and consistent information to base their decisions on with regards to running the department or company on a daily basis.

Overall, accrual accounting focuses on the transactions that move the company and not just the cash in or cash out. Accrual accounting recognizes that revenues can be earned even before the customer pays their bill. Moreover, the organization that utilizes the accrual basis will treat the company's expenses in the same way. If an expense, or invoice, comes in but is not paid in the period, the company still recognizes the expense in the same period it recognized the revenue. This level of consistency will allow for more accurate financial planning by all levels of management.

■ Ratio Analysis

Once all the financial statements are completed, they are ready to be used to calculate ratio analyses to assist in further detailing the organization's results based on these ratios. Another reason to look at ratios is that for an organization that is doing any financing, the lenders will look at not only the financial report results, but the ratios of certain parts of the financial reports. A review of the ratios and comparison of like organizations in the same industry, or checking the organization's assets versus their liabilities based on the ratio analysis that can be performed, will assist a lender in the decision process of whether or not to participate in the financing of an organization.

Any changes in an organization's ratio analysis is of great interest to the organization and the lender. This comparative tool, when used within the organization's industry, will be of great help in comparing the performance of one organization against another to see if the results are consistent and if they are good in comparison to like organizations or if they are on the decline such that practices need to be looked at immediately to address the problem.

Current Ratio

This ratio determines the ability of the organization to pay their current liabilities with the use of their current assets. This is a very important ratio for lenders today. This ratio looks at current assets that include cash-on-hand, the company's short-term investments, accounts receivable generated through sales, and inventory that the organization has at present. The category of current assets means that an organization can take these assets and turn them into cash rather quickly if needed, or during the course of the **calendar year** or fiscal year the organization will use up these current assets in the normal course of doing business. The current liabilities are similar in nature to the current assets in that the liabilities that are considered to be current are accounts payable and any current portion of a loan or obligation. The current ratio is calculated as follows:

$$\frac{\text{Total current assets of the organization}}{\text{Total current liabilities of the organization}}$$

The current ratio of 2.0 simply means that for every $1.00 of current liabilities, the organization has $2.00 of current assets to satisfy the liability.

Acid-Test Ratio

The acid-test ratio takes it a step further, as it measures current assets versus current liabilities, but with a different approach. The current assets that are measured are only those that are considered truly liquid, meaning they can be turned into cash very quickly. Inventory is used in the current ratio, but even though it may be a current asset, it is not one that can be turned into cash quickly. With that said, the acid-test ratio will take into account cash, short-term investments, and net current receivables and divide by total current liabilities. The example is as follows:

$$\frac{(\text{Cash + short-term investments + net current receivables})}{\text{Total current liabilities}}$$

In this example, the acid-test ratio came up to be 1.75; this would mean that for every $1.00 of current liabilities, the company has $1.75 of current, liquid assets to discharge this debt.

Debt Ratio

In the debt ratio, the lender will take a look at the total assets and the total liabilities that an organization may have on their balance sheet. The total assets of the organization are divided by the total liabilities of the organization. The result, or findings, can be used to measure up like organizations to compare operating results between them to help manage the organization.

EXHIBIT 2-3   EIGHT BASIC RATIOS USED IN HEALTH CARE

Liquidity Ratios

1. Current Ratio

Current Assets
Current Liabilities

2. Quick Ratio

Cash and Cash Equivalents + Net Receivables
Current Liabilities

3. Days Cash on Hand (DCOH)

Unrestricted Cash and Cash Equivalents
Cash Operation Expenses ÷ No. of Days in Period (365)

4. Days Receivables

Net Receivables
Net Credit Revenues ÷ No. of Days in Period (365)

Solvency Ratios

5. Debt Service Coverage Ratio (DSCR)

Change in Unrestricted Net Assets (net income)
+ Interest, Depreciation, Amortization
Maximum Annual Debt Service

6. Liabilities to Fund Balance

Total Liabilities
Unrestricted Fund Balances

Profitability Ratios

7. Operating Margin (%)

Operating Income (Loss)
Total Operating Revenues

8. Return on Total Assets (%)

EBIT (Earnings Before Interest and Taxes)
Total Assets

Courtesy of Research Group Limited.

■ Conclusion

The importance of financial management in the healthcare organization cannot be emphasized enough. Leadership needs to understand the difference between financial and managerial accounting and the best way to use these methods to better manage the operations more efficiently. More importantly, the leader needs to understand the data collected in the reporting process related to each type of accounting. The data is used to manage variances, evaluate processes impacting results, manage assets and liabilities, complete the budget process, plan for the future, and maintain the financial health of the organization. Basically, the income statement, balance sheet, general ledger, and budgets are vital tools to determine the current and long-term effectiveness of the operation. If you can imagine working as hard as you can, but without direction and any measures of how you are doing, you will feel puzzled as to why the operation is not doing as well as it can or why it is failing, you can usually trace these issues back to an uninformed manager or leader. It is hard to imagine, but if you are managing a facility and you do not know the flow of financial information and the reports that reflect your operations, it should be no surprise that you are failing. Even more of a surprise is that all of the information is right in front of you in your financial statements, budgets, and ratios. This information will be very helpful to assess where you are at currently in your operations and what you need to do to achieve your financial and operational goals for the future.

References

Bandler, J. (1994). *How to use financial statements: A guide to understanding the numbers.* New York, New York: McGraw-Hill.

Cleverley, W., & Cameron, A. (2012). *Essentials of health care finance* (7th ed.). Sudbury, MA: Jones & Bartlett Learning.

Flood, M. J. (2014). *GAAP 2014: Interpretation and application of generally accepted accounting principles.* Somerset, NJ: Wiley.

LaTour, K.M., & Eichenwald Maki, S. (2013). *Health information management: Concepts, principles, and practice* (4th ed.). Chicago: AHIMA.

Part II

3 Introduction to Claims Processing

◼ Introduction

The United States healthcare sector accounted for $2.5 trillion, which translates to 17.6 percent of the nation's gross domestic product. To better understand this amount in a smaller number, this equates to the United States spending $8,086 on each person. Moreover, with the United States spending $2.5 trillion, this makes the United States healthcare sector larger than the entire economy of France (Casto & Forrestal, 2013, p. 3).

In addition to being the largest, the United States healthcare system is very complex in that it is very competitive, and at the same time, it is fragmented. The healthcare delivery model has many different, fragmented sources of healthcare providers such as physicians, large and small hospitals, rehabilitation companies, various homecare companies, chiropractors, durable medical equipment companies, and other healthcare providers, just to name a few (Casto & Forrestal, 2013, p. 3). This chapter will help you understand the complex nature of claims processing and all the components associated with this process such as all of the compliance requirements and the elements included in a clean claim. This valuable information will help the healthcare administrator to be more successful in maintaining the financial health of the organization.

History of Reimbursement

There are **fee-for-service** and **reimbursement** methodologies in our healthcare system that issue payments to providers based on the charges assigned to each individual service that were provided to the patient. Before the Medicare and Medicaid programs were developed in the 1960s providers sent their bills directly to the patient for services provided. The patient or responsible party in the family were responsible to the provider for payment for the services rendered. Upon the implementation of the prepaid health insurance plans and Medicare and Medicaid, they kept the format of billing by allowing the providers to bill for all itemized services provided to the patient.

The typical fee-for-service payment structure is where a provider will bill for all services rendered to the third-party payer after the services have been provided and then the third-party payer, retrospectively, will pay the provider. These payments were based on the usual, customary, and reasonable (UCR). Some third-party payers would negotiate a discounted rate to pay their providers, through a contract, that established a cost-sharing environment between the payer and provider. In the beginning, the cost sharing was 80 percent third-party payer and 20 percent patient. The provider would send a claim to the third-party payer and receive payment of 80 percent of the contracted amount, and then send a bill to the patient for the balance of their 20 percent.

Currently, we are in a prospective payment environment and have various forms of payment such as managed care, episode-of-care, capitation, and **global payment**. This prospective form of payment allows the third party to know what they will be spending, in advance, for services provided to their members by healthcare providers. Moreover, prospective payment allows the third-party payers, including Medicare and Medicaid, to reduce costs in comparison to the former fee-for-service environment, to better plan for healthcare expenditures, to implement a cost-sharing environment where the provider is responsible for their profit or loss, and to standardize the cost for health care that will make the patient's out-of-pocket costs for co-pays and coinsurances consistent for the same procedures from different providers.

■ Providers, Suppliers, and Claims

Providers Defined

A provider is a hospital, a Critical Access Hospital (CAH), a skilled nursing facility, a comprehensive outpatient rehabilitation facility, home health agency, hospice agency that has agreed to participate in Medicare, clinic, rehabilitation agency or public health agency that has a similar agreement to provide outpatient physical therapy or speech-language pathology services, or community mental health agency that has a similar agreement but will only furnish partial hospitalization services (CMS, 2013a, p. 11).

Suppliers Defined

A **supplier** is a physician or other practitioner, or an entity other than a provider that furnishes healthcare services under Medicare. A supplier must meet certain requirements as outlined in the Medicare Program Integrity Manual. A provider may also enroll as a supplier if they meet applicable conditions and bill separately for that service where Medicare payment policy allows for these separate payments (CMS, 2013a, p. 11).

EXHIBIT 3-1   TYPES OF HEALTHCARE PROVIDERS

Healthcare Provider Types

- Acute Care Hospital
- Critical Access Hospital
- Skilled Nursing Facility
- Inpatient Rehab Facility
- Outpatient Rehab Facility
- Home Health Agency
- Hospice Agency
- Home Infusion
- Durable Medical Equipment

Types of Claims

There are two types of claims: institutional and professional. An **institutional claim** is any claim that is submitted using the Health Insurance Portability and Accountability Act (HIPAA) mandated transaction ASC X12N 837 – Health Care Claim: Institutional or the UB-04 paper claim form. A **professional claim** is any claim submitted using the HIPAA mandated transaction ASC X12N 837 – Health Care Claim: Professional or the CMS-1500 paper claim form (CMS, 2013a, p. 11).

A UB-04 claim form consists of 81 sections that include:

- Patient demographics – patient name, address, date of birth, sex, admission or date of service, social security number or identification number.
- Provider information – name, location of provider, federal tax identification number, and National Provider Identifier (NPI) number.
- Services provided – revenue code and description of services, HCPCS and/or HIPPS code, service date, number of units, total charges, and noncovered items.
- Payer information – insurance carrier, health plan identification number, insured's name, insured's unique identification number, group name, treatment authorization codes, and employer name.
- Diagnosis codes – admitting diagnosis, reason for admission diagnosis, PPS code, principal procedure, and other procedures.
- Physician information – attending physician name and NPI number, operating physician name and NPI number, and other treating physicians and their NPI number.

A CMS-1500 form contains the following:

- Check box for insurance carrier – Medicare, Medicaid, TRICARE/CHAMPUS, CHAMPVA, Group Health Plan, FECA Black Lung, and Other.
- Patient demographics – patient name, address, date of birth, social security number or insurance identification number.
- Insurance information – patient relationship to insured, marital status, employment status/student status, is admission related to a work accident or auto accident.
- Physician information – name of referring provider or physician, NPI, work accident related dates, hospitalization dates, diagnosis, and **prior authorization** number.
- Dates of service and charge information – dates from and dates to, place of service, procedure CPT/HCPCS, modifiers, charges, days or units, rendering provider NPI, provider federal tax identification number (social security number or employer identification number), total charges, amounts paid, balance due, and service facility location and NPI along with billing provider information and NPI.

For pricing purposes, the ANSI X12N 837 P (837P) Electronic Claim Form when the Place of Service (POS) is listed as 12, the pricing will be based on where the beneficiary's home is located. When not using the POS 12, the claim processing and pricing calculations will be based on the service location. For pricing when using

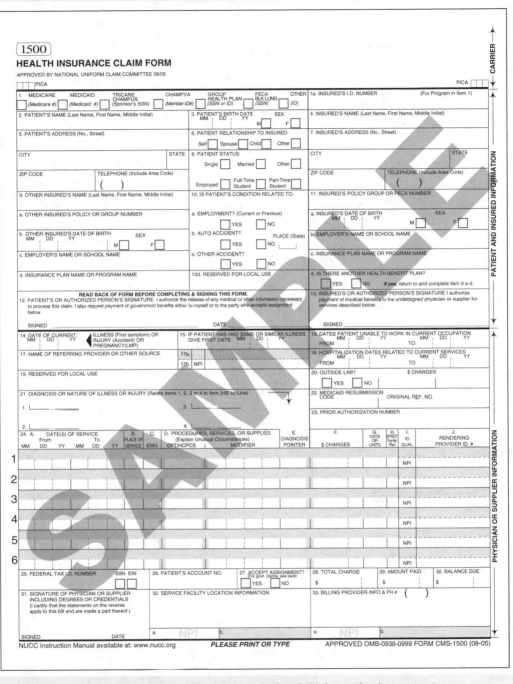

FIGURE 3.1 CMS 1500 claim form (with instructions). (*continued*)

Courtesy of Center for Medicare & Medicaid Services.

BECAUSE THIS FORM IS USED BY VARIOUS GOVERNMENT AND PRIVATE HEALTH PROGRAMS, SEE SEPARATE INSTRUCTIONS ISSUED BY APPLICABLE PROGRAMS.

NOTICE: Any person who knowingly files a statement of claim containing any misrepresentation or any false, incomplete or misleading information may be guilty of a criminal act punishable under law and may be subject to civil penalties.

REFERS TO GOVERNMENT PROGRAMS ONLY

MEDICARE AND CHAMPUS PAYMENTS: A patient's signature requests that payment be made and authorizes release of any information necessary to process the claim and certifies that the information provided in Blocks 1 through 12 is true, accurate and complete. In the case of a Medicare claim, the patient's signature authorizes any entity to release to Medicare medical and nonmedical information, including employment status, and whether the person has employer group health insurance, liability, no-fault, worker's compensation or other insurance which is responsible to pay for the services for which the Medicare claim is made. See 42 CFR 411.24(a). If item 9 is completed, the patient's signature authorizes release of the information to the health plan or agency shown. In Medicare assigned or CHAMPUS participation cases, the physician agrees to accept the charge determination of the Medicare carrier or CHAMPUS fiscal intermediary as the full charge, and the patient is responsible for the deductible, coinsurance and noncovered services. Coinsurance and the deductible are based upon the charge determination of the Medicare carrier or CHAMPUS fiscal intermediary if this is less than the charge submitted. CHAMPUS is not a health insurance program but makes payment for health benefits provided through certain affiliations with the Uniformed Services. Information on the patient's sponsor should be provided in those items captioned in "Insured"; i.e., items 1a, 4, 6, 7, 9, and 11.

BLACK LUNG AND FECA CLAIMS

The provider agrees to accept the amount paid by the Government as payment in full. See Black Lung and FECA instructions regarding required procedure and diagnosis coding systems.

SIGNATURE OF PHYSICIAN OR SUPPLIER (MEDICARE, CHAMPUS, FECA AND BLACK LUNG)

I certify that the services shown on this form were medically indicated and necessary for the health of the patient and were personally furnished by me or were furnished incident to my professional service by my employee under my immediate personal supervision, except as otherwise expressly permitted by Medicare or CHAMPUS regulations.

For services to be considered as "incident" to a physician's professional service, 1) they must be rendered under the physician's immediate personal supervision by his/her employee, 2) they must be an integral, although incidental part of a covered physician's service, 3) they must be of kinds commonly furnished in physician's offices, and 4) the services of nonphysicians must be included on the physician's bills.

For CHAMPUS claims, I further certify that I (or any employee) who rendered services am not an active duty member of the Uniformed Services or a civilian employee of the United States Government or a contract employee of the United States Government, either civilian or military (refer to 5 USC 5536). For Black-Lung claims, I further certify that the services performed were for a Black Lung-related disorder.

No Part B Medicare benefits may be paid unless this form is received as required by existing law and regulations (42 CFR 424.32).

NOTICE: Any one who misrepresents or falsifies essential information to receive payment from Federal funds requested by this form may upon conviction be subject to fine and imprisonment under applicable Federal laws.

NOTICE TO PATIENT ABOUT THE COLLECTION AND USE OF MEDICARE, CHAMPUS, FECA, AND BLACK LUNG INFORMATION
(PRIVACY ACT STATEMENT)

We are authorized by CMS, CHAMPUS and OWCP to ask you for information needed in the administration of the Medicare, CHAMPUS, FECA, and Black Lung programs. Authority to collect information is in section 205(a), 1862, 1872 and 1874 of the Social Security Act as amended, 42 CFR 411.24(a) and 424.5(a) (6), and 44 USC 3101;41 CFR 101 et seq and 10 USC 1079 and 1086; 5 USC 8101 et seq; and 30 USC 901 et seq; 38 USC 613; E.O. 9397.

The information we obtain to complete claims under these programs is used to identify you and to determine your eligibility. It is also used to decide if the services and supplies you received are covered by these programs and to insure that proper payment is made.

The information may also be given to other providers of services, carriers, intermediaries, medical review boards, health plans, and other organizations or Federal agencies, for the effective administration of Federal provisions that require other third parties payers to pay primary to Federal program, and as otherwise necessary to administer these programs. For example, it may be necessary to disclose information about the benefits you have used to a hospital or doctor. Additional disclosures are made through routine uses for information contained in systems of records.

FOR MEDICARE CLAIMS: See the notice modifying system No. 09-70-0501, titled, 'Carrier Medicare Claims Record,' published in the Federal Register, Vol. 55 No. 177, page 37549, Wed. Sept. 12, 1990, or as updated and republished.

FOR OWCP CLAIMS: Department of Labor, Privacy Act of 1974, "Republication of Notice of Systems of Records," Federal Register Vol. 55 No. 40, Wed Feb. 28, 1990, See ESA-5, ESA-6, ESA-12, ESA-13, ESA-30, or as updated and republished.

FOR CHAMPUS CLAIMS: PRINCIPLE PURPOSE(S): To evaluate eligibility for medical care provided by civilian sources and to issue payment upon establishment of eligibility and determination that the services/supplies received are authorized by law.

ROUTINE USE(S): Information from claims and related documents may be given to the Dept. of Veterans Affairs, the Dept. of Health and Human Services and/or the Dept. of Transportation consistent with their statutory administrative responsibilities under CHAMPUS/CHAMPVA; to the Dept. of Justice for representation of the Secretary of Defense in civil actions; to the Internal Revenue Service, private collection agencies, and consumer reporting agencies in connection with recoupment claims; and to Congressional Offices in response to inquiries made at the request of the person to whom a record pertains. Appropriate disclosures may be made to other federal, state, local, foreign government agencies, private business entities, and individual providers of care, on matters relating to entitlement, claims adjudication, fraud, program abuse, utilization review, quality assurance, peer review, program integrity, third-party liability, coordination of benefits, and civil and criminal litigation related to the operation of CHAMPUS.

DISCLOSURES: Voluntary; however, failure to provide information will result in delay in payment or may result in denial of claim. With the one exception discussed below, there are no penalties under these programs for refusing to supply information. However, failure to furnish information regarding the medical services rendered or the amount charged would prevent payment of claims under these programs. Failure to furnish any other information, such as name or claim number, would delay payment of the claim. Failure to provide medical information under FECA could be deemed an obstruction.

It is mandatory that you tell us if you know that another party is responsible for paying for your treatment. Section 1128B of the Social Security Act and 31 USC 3801-3812 provide penalties for withholding this information.

You should be aware that P.L. 100-503, the "Computer Matching and Privacy Protection Act of 1988", permits the government to verify information by way of computer matches.

MEDICAID PAYMENTS (PROVIDER CERTIFICATION)

I hereby agree to keep such records as are necessary to disclose fully the extent of services provided to individuals under the State's Title XIX plan and to furnish information regarding any payments claimed for providing such services as the State Agency or Dept. of Health and Human Services may request.

I further agree to accept, as payment in full, the amount paid by the Medicaid program for those claims submitted for payment under that program, with the exception of authorized deductible, coinsurance, co-payment or similar cost-sharing charge.

SIGNATURE OF PHYSICIAN (OR SUPPLIER): I certify that the services listed above were medically indicated and necessary to the health of this patient and were personally furnished by me or my employee under my personal direction.

NOTICE: This is to certify that the foregoing information is true, accurate and complete. I understand that payment and satisfaction of this claim will be from Federal and State funds, and that any false claims, statements, or documents, or concealment of a material fact, may be prosecuted under applicable Federal or State laws.

According to the Paperwork Reduction Act of 1995, no persons are required to respond to a collection of information unless it displays a valid OMB control number. The valid OMB control number for this information collection is 0938-0999. The time required to complete this information collection is estimated to average 10 minutes per response, including the time to review instructions, search existing data resources, gather the data needed, and complete and review the information collection. If you have any comments concerning the accuracy of the time estimate(s) or suggestions for improving this form, please write to: CMS, Attn: PRA Reports Clearance Officer, 7500 Security Boulevard, Baltimore, Maryland 21244-1850. This address is for comments and/or suggestions only. DO NOT MAIL COMPLETED CLAIM FORMS TO THIS ADDRESS.

FIGURE 3.1   CMS 1500 claim form (with instructions).
Courtesy of Center for Medicare & Medicaid Services.

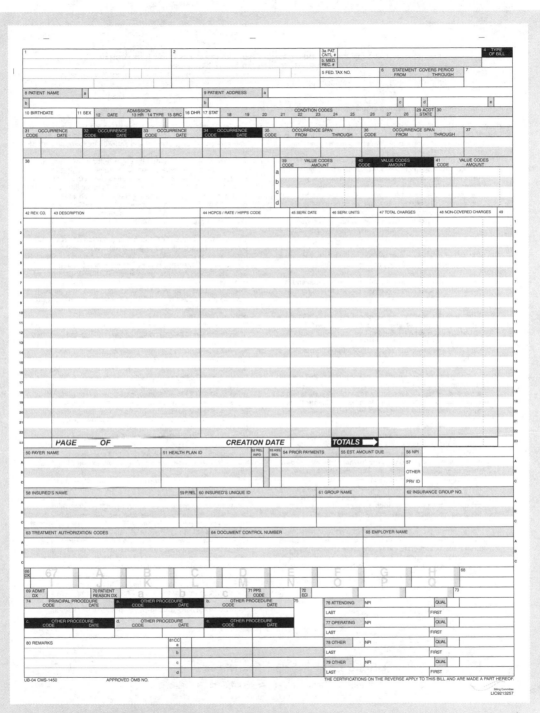

FIGURE 3.2   UB-04 claim form (with instructions). (*continued*)

Courtesy of Center for Medicare & Medicaid Services.

UB-04 NOTICE: THE SUBMITTER OF THIS FORM UNDERSTANDS THAT MISREPRESENTATION OR FALSIFICATION OF ESSENTIAL INFORMATION AS REQUESTED BY THIS FORM, MAY SERVE AS THE BASIS FOR CIVIL MONETARY PENALTIES AND ASSESSMENTS AND MAY UPON CONVICTION INCLUDE FINES AND/OR IMPRISONMENT UNDER FEDERAL AND/OR STATE LAW(S).

Submission of this claim constitutes certification that the billing information as shown on the face hereof is true, accurate and complete. That the submitter did not knowingly or recklessly disregard or misrepresent or conceal material facts. The following certifications or verifications apply where pertinent to this Bill:

1. If third party benefits are indicated, the appropriate assignments by the insured /beneficiary and signature of the patient or parent or a legal guardian covering authorization to release information are on file. Determinations as to the release of medical and financial information should be guided by the patient or the patient's legal representative.
2. If patient occupied a private room or required private nursing for medical necessity, any required certifications are on file.
3. Physician's certifications and re-certifications, if required by contract or Federal regulations, are on file.
4. For Religious Non-Medical facilities, verifications and if necessary re-certifications of the patient's need for services are on file.
5. Signature of patient or his representative on certifications, authorization to release information, and payment request, as required by Federal Law and Regulations (42 USC 1935f, 42 CFR 424.36, 10 USC 1071 through 1086, 32 CFR 199) and any other applicable contract regulations, is on file.
6. The provider of care submitter acknowledges that the bill is in conformance with the Civil Rights Act of 1964 as amended. Records adequately describing services will be maintained and necessary information will be furnished to such governmental agencies as required by applicable law.
7. For Medicare Purposes: If the patient has indicated that other health insurance or a state medical assistance agency will pay part of his/her medical expenses and he/she wants information about his/her claim released to them upon request, necessary authorization is on file. The patient's signature on the provider's request to bill Medicare medical and non-medical information, including employment status, and whether the person has employer group health insurance which is responsible to pay for the services for which this Medicare claim is made.
8. For Medicaid purposes: The submitter understands that because payment and satisfaction of this claim will be from Federal and State funds, any false statements, documents, or concealment of a material fact are subject to prosecution under applicable Federal or State Laws.

9. For TRICARE Purposes:

(a) The information on the face of this claim is true, accurate and complete to the best of the submitter's knowledge and belief, and services were medically and appropriate for the health of the patient;
(b) The patient has represented that by a reported residential address outside a military medical treatment facility catchment area he or she does not live within the catchment area of a U.S. Public Health Service medical facility, or if the patient resides within a catchment area of such a facility, a copy of Non-Availability Statement (DD Form 1251) is on file, or the physician has certified to a medical emergency in any instance where a copy of a Non-Availability Statement is not on file;
(c) The patient or the patient's parent or guardian has responded directly to the provider's request to identify all health insurance coverage, and that all such coverage is identified on the face of the claim except that coverage which is exclusively supplemental payments to TRICARE-determined benefits;
(d) The amount billed to TRICARE has been billed after all such coverage have been billed and paid excluding Medicaid, and the amount billed to TRICARE is that remaining claimed against TRICARE benefits;
(e) The beneficiary's cost share has not been waived by consent or failure to exercise generally accepted billing and collection efforts; and,
(f) Any hospital-based physician under contract, the cost of whose services are allocated in the charges included in this bill, is not an employee or member of the Uniformed Services. For purposes of this certification, an employee of the Uniformed Services is an employee, appointed in civil service (refer to 5 USC 2105), including part-time or intermittent employees, but excluding contract surgeons or other personal service contracts. Similarly, member of the Uniformed Services does not apply to reserve members of the Uniformed Services not on active duty.
(g) Based on 42 United States Code 1395cc(a)(1)(j) all providers participating in Medicare must also participate in TRICARE for inpatient hospital services provided pursuant to admissions to hospitals occurring on or after January 1, 1987; and
(h) If TRICARE benefits are to be paid in a participating status, the submitter of this claim agrees to submit this claim to the appropriate TRICARE claims processor. The provider of care submitter also agrees to accept the TRICARE determined reasonable charge as the total charge for the medical services or supplies listed on the claim form. The provider of care will accept the TRICARE-determined reasonable charge even if it is less than the billed amount, and also agrees to accept the amount paid by TRICARE combined with the cost-share amount and deductible amount, if any, paid by or on behalf of the patient as full payment for the listed medical services or supplies. The provider of care submitter will not attempt to collect from the patient (or his or her parent or guardian) amounts over the TRICARE determined reasonable charge. TRICARE will make any benefits payable directly to the provider of care, if the provider of care a participating provider.

FIGURE 3.2 UB-04 claim form (with instructions).
Courtesy of Center for Medicare & Medicaid Services.

the CMS-1500 claim form and the POS is 12, the pricing address will be drawn from the beneficiary address. If the bill contains both POS home and another site, the POS home address does not need to be entered, as it will default to the beneficiary and the other POS will be pulled from the claim. Except for the situation above, when using the POS 12 (home) and another service location on the CMS-1500, the provider will submit separate claims for each POS that the beneficiary received services (CMS, 2013a, p. 17).

If multiple POS are submitted on a claim form, the message will read as follows, Adjustment Reason Code 16 – "Claim/Service lacks information which is needed for adjudication." And Remark Code – M77 – "Missing/incomplete/invalid place of service," or MSN – 9.2 – "This item or service was denied because information required to make payment was missing" (CMS, 2013a, p. 17).

Claims for Medicare Services Furnished to Patients Not Lawfully Present in the United States

Medicare will not make payments for services that are furnished to alien beneficiaries that are not lawfully present in the United States on the date the services were rendered. The Common Working File must establish an auxiliary file based on enrollment data contained in the Enrollment DataBase maintained by the Social Security Administration in order to appropriately edit the claims specifically associated with alien beneficiaries. The auxiliary file will be the basis for an edit that rejects the claims for a beneficiary that was not lawfully present in the United States on the date of service. The denial that the provider will receive is MSN message 5.7 that states, "Medicare payment may not be made for the item or service because, on the date of service, the patient was not lawfully present in the United States (CMS, 2013a, p. 29).

At the point of denial, the provider's only recourse is an appeal to the denial if, and only if, the provider can prove that the beneficiary was lawfully present in the United States at the time that the services were rendered to the beneficiary.

Domestic Claims Processing Jurisdiction

Suppliers of Durable Medical Equipment, Prosthetics, Orthotics, Supplies, Parental and Enteral Nutrition (PEN), or otherwise known as DMEPOS, submit their claims to Durable Medical Equipment Medicare Administrative Contractors (DME MACs). There are special codes and services that are classified by HCPCS codes that will determine who will bill for services. There are certain surgical procedures that will fall under the **Diagnosis Related Group (DRG)** or Ambulatory Payment Classification (APC), and there are some devices that will be eligible for separate pass-through under the Outpatient Prospective Payment System (OPPS). DME MACs will not process a claim for DMEPOS items that are subject to consolidated billing or bundled payment under Prospective Payment System (PPS) or in a DRG (CMS, 2013a, p. 30).

The claims processing jurisdiction among the DME MACs is determined by the beneficiary's permanent address. This permanent address is determined by where the beneficiary resides for more than 6 months a year (CMS, 2013a, p. 30).

Portable X-Ray and Other Portable Services

If a supplier operates mobile units for x-ray and/or other portable services and the supplier deliveries services in multiple MAC DMEs, then the permanent address for where the beneficiary received services will determine which carrier will process the claim (CMS, 2013a, p. 31).

Ambulance Services

The first determining factor on the jurisdiction of where the claim is processed is whether one or more ambulances were used in the transportation of the beneficiary. If only one ambulance was used to transport the patient from the initial pick-up location to the final destination, the jurisdiction is with the carrier that is for the point of origin of the ambulance. If two or more ambulances were used in the delivery of a patient, the carrier that will have jurisdiction over the claim will be the carrier that services the final location or leg of the trip for the beneficiary.

Laboratory Services

If a laboratory services a beneficiary the carrier that has jurisdiction over the claim is the carrier that handles the service area of the laboratory. If the laboratory performs a test and then submits the test/specimen to another laboratory that is outside the carrier for the primary laboratory, the carrier for the referring laboratory retains jurisdiction over the claim (CMS, 2013a, p. 32).

Railroad Retirement Beneficiary Carrier

Carrier jurisdiction for claims involving individuals that are part of the Railroad Retirement Beneficiary includes those who are entitled to both social security and railroad retirement benefits are handled by the Palmetto Government Benefits Administrators (GBA) LLC, a subsidiary of Blue Cross and Blue Shield of South Carolina. The exceptions that apply are if the services are furnished by an organization that deals directly with CMS on a cost basis, the beneficiary is enrolled under a buy-in agreement involving a state agency that has entered into an agreement to act as a carrier with respect to the individual, or if the medical services were supplied outside the United States. In the case where the beneficiary receives care outside the United States, the Railroad Retirement Board will handle the claim (CMS, 2013a, p. 33).

Misdirected Claims to Carrier for Payment

A misdirected claim is one that has been submitted to the wrong carrier. This will be determined by the address of the servicing provider or permanent address of the beneficiary, in the case of mobile or homecare services.

Misdirected claims include some of the following (CMS, 2013a, p. 35–38):

- If a CMS-1500 claim form was sent in via paper or electronic and was sent to the wrong carrier the receiving carrier must return the claim as unprocessable.

- If a local carrier receives a CMS-1500 claim that was to go to a DME MAC for payment, it will be returned as unprocessable.

- If a local DME MAC receives a CMS-1500 claim form or electronic claim for processing that covers a Part B MAC, the claim will be returned as unprocessable.

- If a local carrier receives a CMS-1500 claim form or electronic claim that is for a RRB claim, the claim will be returned as unprocessable as it is not processed by the local carrier as the RRB claims are processed by Palmetto GBA.

- If a local carrier receives a CMS-1500 claim form or electronic claim for a United Mine Workers of America (UMWA) beneficiary the claim must be processed by UMWA and will be returned as unprocessable.

- If a local carrier for DME MAC receives a claim for a beneficiary not in their jurisdiction the claim will be returned as unprocessable.

Claims for Payment When Items/Services Are Part of PPS

When a patient is a client of a homecare agency, skilled nursing facility (SNF), hospital inpatient, or part of a rural health clinic or federally funded health clinic services that are provided to the beneficiary that fall under Part B, coverage will not be the responsibility of the carrier. The agency or facility providing the care to the patient will be responsible for payment of the supplies that are covered under Part B, as they are covered under the payment for PPS. In this instance, the provider of the services/supplies will bill the agency/facility directly.

Provider Charges to Beneficiaries

In the agreement/attestation statement signed by a provider, it agrees not to **charge** Medicare beneficiaries (or any other person acting on a beneficiary's behalf) for any services which Medicare beneficiaries are entitled to have payment made on their behalf by the Medicare program. The provider may bill the beneficiary for Part A deductible, Part B deductible, first 3 pints of blood (blood deductible), Part B coinsurance, Part A coinsurance, or services that are not covered by Medicare (CMS, 2013a, p. 54).

Skilled Nursing Facilities (SNF) may not request, require, or accept a deposit or other payment from a Medicare beneficiary as a condition for admission, continued care, or other provision of services, except in the following circumstances (CMS, 2013a, p. 55):

- A SNF may request and accept payment for a Part A deductible and coinsurance amount on or after the day to which it applies.

- A SNF may request and accept payment for a Part B deductible and coinsurance amount at the time of or after the provision of the service to which it applies.

- A SNF may not request or accept advance payment of Medicare deductible and coinsurance amounts.

- A SNF may require, request, or accept a deposit or other payment for services if it is clear that the services are not covered by Medicare and proper notice is provided. (See **Advance Beneficiary Notice (ABN)** later in this chapter.)

- SNFs, but not hospitals, may bill the beneficiary for holding a bed during a leave of absence.

Charges to Hold a Bed During a SNF Absence

Charges to the beneficiary for admission or readmission are not **allowable**. There is an exception when a resident leaves a SNF temporarily: a resident can choose to make bed-hold payments to the SNF. These are not the same as payments made prior to initial admission, in that the patient is or was already a resident and admitted to the facility. In addition, the resident has a distinguishable living space within the facility.

Bed-hold payments are also different from payments for readmission in that the facility agrees, in advance, to allow a departing resident to reenter the facility upon their return. The bed-hold payments represent remuneration for the privilege of actually maintaining the resident's personal effects in the particular living space that the resident has temporarily vacated. These charges must be calculated on the basis of a per-diem bed-hold rate multiplied by the amount of days the residents is absent, as opposed to a fixed amount at the time the resident left the facility.

Patient Refunds

In the provider agreement between CMS and the provider, the provider agrees to, as promptly as possible, refund any money that they incorrectly collected from the Medicare beneficiary or from someone on their behalf. This includes money incorrectly collected, in any amount, for which the beneficiary is liable because of the deductible and coinsurance requirements. If a provider believed that the patient was not Medicare eligible, but it was determined that the beneficiary was later determined to have been entitled to Medicare benefits, or the beneficiary's entitlement period fell within the time the provider's agreement with CMS was in effect, and such amounts exceed the beneficiary's deductible, coinsurance or noncovered services liability (CMS, 2013a, p. 56).

Provider Treatment of Beneficiaries

In the provider agreement between CMS and the healthcare provider, the provider agrees to accept Medicare beneficiaries for care and treatment. The provider cannot impose any limitations with respect to services provided or treatment to Medicare beneficiaries that it does not impose on all other persons seeking care and treatment. In other words, if the provider does not furnish treatment for certain illnesses and conditions to patients who are not Medicare beneficiaries, it does not need to furnish such treatments to Medicare beneficiaries in order to participate in the Medicare program (CMS, 2013a, p. 56).

Assignment of Payment to Provider

Fiscal Intermediaries (FI) pay benefits due to a provider only to the provider. Carriers are permitted to pay assigned benefits only to the physician, practitioner, or supplier that actually furnished the services. They do not pay the benefits to any other person or organization under assignment or reassignment, power of attorney, or under any other arrangement. The assigned benefits include benefits payable after the death of the enrollee to the physician or other supplier on the basis of an agreement to accept the reasonable charge as payment in full. A power of attorney, for this purpose, means a written authorization by a principal to an agent to receive in the agent's own name amounts due the principal, to negotiate checks payable to the principal, or to receive in any other manner direct payment of amounts due the principal. A payment is considered to be made directly to an ineligible person or organization if that person or organization receiving the payment can convert the payment to its own use and control without the payment first passing through the control of the provider or the party eligible to receive the payment (CMS, 2013a, p. 57).

Payment to Agent

The Fiscal Intermediary can make payments in the name of the provider to an agent who furnishes billing or collection services if the agent receives the payment under an agreement between the provider and the agent. The agent's compensation is not related in any way to the dollar amount billed or collected. The agent's compensation is not dependent upon the actual collection of payment, the agent acts under payment disposition instruction which the provider may modify or revoke at any time, and in receiving the payment, the agent acts only on behalf of the provider (CMS, 2013a, p. 62).

Payment to Bank

Medicare payments due to a provider or supplier may be sent directly to a bank for deposit in the provider/supplier's account so the bank may provide financing to the provider/supplier, as long as the bank states in writing in the loan agreement that it waives its right to offset. Therefore, the bank may have a lending relationship with the provider/supplier and may also be the depository for Medicare receivables. In addition, the account is in the provider/supplier's name only, and only the provider/supplier may issue an instruction on that account. The bank must be bound by the provider/supplier's instructions. To clarify, if a bank is under a standing order from the provider/supplier to transfer funds from the provider/supplier's account to the account of a financing entity in the same or another bank, and the provider/supplier cancels or rescinds that order, the bank will honor this cancellation—even though it will be a breach of the provider/supplier's agreement with the financing entity. Moreover, no matter what the language is in any agreement between a provider/supplier and third party that is providing financing, that third party cannot purchase the provider/supplier's Medicare receivables.

Payment to Employer of a Physician

The carrier may pay Part B benefits for covered physician services under an assignment, provided that under the terms of the physician's employment, only the employer and not the physician has the right to charge or collect charges for the physician's services. There must be an employer–employee relationship between the physician and the person or organization hiring the physician to perform services such that the terms of the employment provide that the employer, and not the physician, has the right to receive the payment for all the latter's services within the scope of the employment. The employer must establish that it qualifies to receive payment for the services of its physicians by submitting the Form CMS-855R. In addition, the employer must provide evidence that the employee is a valid employee by providing the carrier with a W-2 or other acceptable Internal Revenue Service (IRS) document such as a pay stub (CMS, 2013a, p. 64).

Payment under Reciprocal Billing Arrangements

At times, a patient's regular physician may arrange to have services provided to a Medicare beneficiary by a substitute physician on an occasional reciprocal basis if (1) the regular physician is unavailable to provide the visit or service; (2) the Medicare patient has arranged or seeks to receive the visit from the regular physician; (3) the substitute physician does not provide the visit or services to the Medicare patients over a continuous period longer than 60 days; and (4) the regular physician identifies the services as substitute physician services meeting the requirements listed and by entering in item 24d of the Form CMS-1500 a HCPCS code of Q5 modifier, which means that the services were furnished by a substitute physician under a reciprocal billing arrangement, after the procedure code (CMS, 2013a, p. 72).

Generally there is a 60-day limit to this type of relationship, but in a case where a physician is called to active duty in the Armed Forces, the time limit may be longer than the 60 days. A physician can have such reciprocal arrangements with more than one physician, but all arrangements must be in writing. For a Physician Medical

Group, these rules do not apply when different members of the group see the same patient at different times. On the claim form, the physician in the group that provided services to the patient must be identified.

Carrier Claims: Mandatory Assignment

When practitioners provide services under the Medicare program, they are required to accept assignment for all Medicare claims involving clinical diagnostic laboratory services and physician lab services, and physician services to individuals dually entitled to Medicare and Medicaid. This means that the provider must accept the payment from Medicare as payment in full for their services rendered. The patient's liability for the services rendered is limited to any applicable deductible and 20 percent coinsurance (CMS, 2013a, p. 87).

Showing Payment on CMS-1500 Claim Forms

A physician that has collected the copayment of 20 percent, or any other payment, must show this amount on the CMS-1500, as this information is essential for correct payment of benefits. Not displaying this amount on the claim may result in an excessive benefit payment to the provider.

A physician should refrain from billing the patient for any balances due to the practice until receiving the Medicare Summary Notice (MSN) to see what amount was approved, what amount was paid, and what amount is the patient's actual responsibility.

Physician Charge for Missed Appointment

A physician may charge the Medicare beneficiary for a missed appointment as long as they do not discriminate against Medicare beneficiaries but also charge all non-Medicare patients for missed appointments (CMS, 2013a, p. 124).

Timely Filing and Postmark Date as Date of Filing

If the last day for timely filing falls on a Saturday, Sunday, legal holiday, or federal non-work day due to a statute or executive order the claim will be considered timely if it is filed electronically on the next day. When a claim is submitted to the carrier by mail it is considered filed on the day the envelope is postmarked in the United States. For a claim to be filed timely it also must be filed within 1 year, or 12 months, of the date of service.

■ Physician Self-Referral Prohibition

Background

Under Section 1877 of the Social Security Act (42 U.S.C. § 1395nn) a physician may not refer a Medicare beneficiary for certain designated health services (DHS) to an entity with which there is ownership by the physician, or an immediate family member of the physician, unless an exception applies to this particular situation. Section 1877 of the Act also prohibits the DHS entity from submitting claims to Medicare, the beneficiary, or any entity for DHS: clinical laboratory services; radiology and certain other imaging services, including MRIs, CT scans, and ultrasound; radiation therapy services and supplies; durable medical equipment and supplies; orthotics; prosthetics and prosthetic devices; parenteral and enteral nutrients; equipment and supplies; physical therapy; occupational therapy; speech-language pathology services; outpatient prescription drugs; home health services and supplies; and inpatient and outpatient hospital services (CMS, 2013a, p. 296).

Financial Relationship

A **financial relationship** includes both ownership and investment interests along with compensation arrangements that include contractual arrangements between a hospital and a physician for physician services.

Regulations

The statute and regulations enumerate various exceptions and violations of the statute are punishable by denial of payment for all DHS claims, refunds of amounts collected for DHS claims, and civil money penalties for knowing violations of the prohibition.

■ Financial Liability Protections for Beneficiaries

Advance Beneficiary Notice

An Advance Beneficiary Notice (ABN) is a form used to inform a Medicare beneficiary, before he or she receives specified items or services that otherwise might be paid for, that Medicare certainly will not or probably will not pay for the item on that particular occasion. A **Financial Counselor** may be the first person in the healthcare organization to address this with the patient. The ABN also allows the beneficiary to make an educated and informed decision on whether or not to receive the items or services that he or she may have to pay for out of pocket or through other insurance. In addition, the use of the ABN allows the patient/beneficiary to better participate in his or her own healthcare treatment decisions by making informed consumer decisions (CMS, 2013b, p. 30).

If the provider, practitioner, or supplier expects payment for the items or services to be denied by Medicare, the provider, practitioner, or supplier must advise the beneficiary before the items or services are furnished that, in the opinion of the provider/practitioner, the beneficiary will be personally and fully responsible for payment. To be personally liable for payment means that the patient or beneficiary will be liable to make the payment for the services rendered by the provider privately or "out-of-pocket" or have another insurance coverage be liable for payment, or Medicaid or other federal or nonfederal payment type (CMS, 2013b, p. 31).

The provider or supplier must issue an ABN to the patient or beneficiary each time and as soon as they determine that the services or products will not be covered. The provider or practitioner or supplier must notify the beneficiary by means of a timely and effective delivery of a proper notice or document to a qualified recipient such as the beneficiary or the beneficiary's **authorized representative**.

Requirements of the ABN

The ABN, or Form CMS-R-131 or Form CMS-R-296, constitutes a proper notice document. If the notice used is not one of these two forms, the notice is not valid. In addition, if a provider or supplier or practitioner modifies a form, it may render the form defective and not valid as a document confirming a patient or beneficiary was properly given notice, in writing, of the responsibility for payment.

The ABN cannot have italics or any font that is difficult to read, must be as least 12-point font size, must be dark ink on a light background, with no use of block-shade or highlighting, and not have any insertions in the forms and any blank areas must be typed, printed, or legibly handwritten (CMS, 2013b, p. 31).

The ABN must be written in lay language, clearly cite the particular items or services that are likely to not be covered, the reasons for believing that the services or items will not be covered, and be delivered to the qualified beneficiary before those items are delivered. The ABN must be delivered by a qualified notifier so that the beneficiary may have confidence in the accuracy and credibility of the notice. Moreover, the ABN must be delivered well in advance of the delivery of the item or service so as to give the beneficiary enough time to make an informed decision. The ABN should be hand-delivered, but if it is not able to be hand-delivered, the ABN can be sent via mail, fax, over the Internet, etc., but must be executed in advance of the delivery. The carrier will not consider a telephone notice to a beneficiary or authorized representative to be sufficient evidence of proper notice for limiting any potential liability unless the content of the telephone contact can be verified and is not in dispute by the beneficiary (CMS, 2013b, p. 33).

Capable Recipient

A **capable recipient** is considered to be a beneficiary who can comprehend the notice. A comatose person, a person who is confused due to senility, dementia, Alzheimer's disease, or a person who is legally incompetent or under great duress is not able to understand and act on his/her rights and will therefore need the presence of an authorized representative for purposes of this notice. In addition, a person who does not read the language that the notice is written in, or a person who is not able to read any or all of the notice, a person who is functionally illiterate to read any notice, a person who is blind or otherwise visually impaired who cannot see the words on the page, or a person who is deaf and cannot hear the oral part of the notice given by phone, is a person for whom receipt of the usual written notice in English cannot be authorized (CMS, 2013b, p. 34).

In light of the above, the provider or practitioner may take additional steps when an authorized representative is not available, the beneficiary is legally blind or vision-impaired or doesn't speak or read English: the provider can make the notice available in Braille extra-large print, or can use an interpreter to translate the notice for the patient.

If the beneficiary declines the supply, product, or service, the beneficiary cannot properly refuse to sign the ABN and still demand the item or service. If the beneficiary refuses to sign the ABN, the supplier or provider should consider not furnishing the item or service unless the consequences are such that the health and safety of the patient is at risk, and not providing the product or service is not an option.

Authorized Representatives

An authorized representative of the beneficiary in regards to receiving notice should be a person who can be reasonably expected to act in the best interest of the beneficiary. Examples of an authorized representative are a spouse, adult child, parent, adult sibling, a close friend, or someone who has exhibited special care and concern for the patient, with whom the patient is familiar, and who understands the patient's personal values. An authorized representative should be someone who does not have a conflicting interest in areas such as shifting financial liability to the beneficiary and who is qualified to be an authorized representative (CMS, 2013b, p. 36).

Generic and Blanket ABNs

Generic ABNs that are considered to be routine and do nothing more than state that the denial of the Medicare payment is possible, or that state that the notifier never knows whether Medicare will deny such payment, are not considered to be acceptable ABNs.

In addition, blanket ABNs, meaning ABNs that a supplier or provider gives to patients for all claims, are not permitted and are not an accepted practice. Notice must be given to a patient or beneficiary on the basis of a genuine judgment about the possibility of Medicare paying for the individual's claim (CMS, 2013b, p. 37).

ABNs Used When a Patient Is Under Duress

ABNs should not be obtained from a patient that is under duress from a medical emergency or circumstances that are compelling and coercive, since individuals cannot be expected to make a reasoned and informed consumer decision in such circumstances. In genuine emergency situations, the patient and his or her family/friends are under great duress to sign anything in order to obtain help. On the other hand, there is a risk that beneficiaries might actually forego care and/or treatment in the emergency situation if they are faced with a financial burden that they believe they cannot bear. ABNs given to a patient or authorized representative who are under great duress cannot be considered to be a proper notice (CMS, 2013b, p. 40).

A. Notifier:

B. Patient Name: **C. Identification Number:**

Advance Beneficiary Notice of Noncoverage (ABN)

NOTE: If Medicare doesn't pay for **D.** _____ below, you may have to pay.
Medicare does not pay for everything, even some care that you or your health care provider have good reason to think you need. We expect Medicare may not pay for the **D.** _____ below.

D.	E. Reason Medicare May Not Pay:	F. Estimated Cost

WHAT YOU NEED TO DO NOW:

- Read this notice, so you can make an informed decision about your care.
- Ask us any questions that you may have after you finish reading.
- Choose an option below about whether to receive the **D.** _____ listed above.
  Note: If you choose Option 1 or 2, we may help you to use any other insurance
        that you might have, but Medicare cannot require us to do this.

G. OPTIONS: Check only one box. We cannot choose a box for you.

- **OPTION 1.** I want the **D.** _____ listed above. You may ask to be paid now, but I also want Medicare billed for an official decision on payment, which is sent to me on a Medicare Summary Notice (MSN). I understand that if Medicare d oesn't pay, I am responsible for payment, but **I can appeal to Medicare** by following the directions on the MSN . If Medicare does pay, you will refund any payments I made to you, less co-pays or deductibles.
- **OPTION 2.** I want the **D.** _____ listed above, but do not bill Medicare. You may ask to be paid now as I am responsible for payment. **I cannot appeal if Medicare is not billed** .
- **OPTION 3.** I don't want the **D.** _____ listed above. I understand with thi s choice I am **not** responsible for payment, and **I cannot appeal to see if Medicare would pay.**

H. Additional Information :

This notice gives our opinion, not an official Medicare decision. If you have other questions on this notice or Medicare bil ling, call **1-800-MEDICARE** (1-800-633-4227/**TTY:** 1-877-486-2048).
Signing below means that you have received and understand this notice. You also receive a copy.

I. Signature:	J. Date:

According to the Paperwork Reduction Act of 1995, no persons are required to respond to a collection of information unless it displays a valid OMB control number. The valid OMB control number for this information collection is 0938-0566. The time required to complete this information collection is estimated to average 7 minutes per response, including the time to review instructions, search existing data resources, gather the data needed, and complete and review the information collection. If you have comments concerning the accuracy of the time estimate or suggestions for improving this form, please write to: CMS, 7500 Security Boulevard, Attn: PRA Reports Clearance Officer, Baltimore, Maryland 21244-1850.

Form CMS-R-131 (03/11)   Form Approved OMB No. 0938-0566

FIGURE 3.3 Advance beneficiary notification.

■ Appeals of Claims

Overview

According to the regulations at 42 CFR 405.940-405.942 provide that a party to a redetermination that is dissatisfied with an initial determination may request that the contractor make a redetermination. A request for determination must be filed within 120 days after the receipt of the notice of the initial determination. It is presumed that the initial determination will be received 5 days after the date of the notice unless there is evidence to the contrary (CMS, 2013c, p. 15).

The appeals process consists of five levels. Each level must be completed for each claim at issue prior to proceeding to the next level. The appeal must begin at the first level after receiving the initial determination. The appellant may exercise the right to appeal any determination or decision to the next higher level until all appeal rights are exhausted (CMS, 2013c, p. 16).

The second level appeal is an appeal with a Qualified Independent Contractor (QIC), and the time limit is 180 days from the date of receipt of the redetermination. The third level involves an Administrative Law Judge (ALJ) and must be filed 60 days from the date of receipt of the reconsideration. The level four is a Departmental Appeals Board (DAB) and needs to be filed 60 days from the receipt of the ALJ hearing decision. Finally, the fifth level is the Federal Court Review and needs to be filed 60 days from the date of receipt of the Appeals Council decision (CMS, 2013c, p. 17).

General Guidelines

The appeal should be prepared so that the appellant can easily understand both the reason why any of the services were not covered or could not be fully reimbursed by Medicare. In addition, the appellant needs to know what actions it can take if the appellant disagrees with that decision. In addition, the language needs to be as simple as possible, does not use abbreviations, choose a positive rather than a negative tone, avoid short or one sentence paragraphs, use consistent formatting, be polite and neutral, use correct spelling and grammar and punctuation, and summarize your request at the end.

The letter should be formatted in a way that you do not use numerical dates and use full dates that are spelled out such as June 10, 2014. Font size should be 12 point or larger and the font type should be consistent throughout the letter. Use bullet points or other formatting techniques, such as headings and subheadings, that will keep the letter and its intention clear and concise. When citing procedure codes, use the actual name of the procedure code. Finally, never write your letter in all caps. This is unnecessary and inappropriate and will possibly offend the reader. Overall, the letter should be inviting to read and easy to understand for the person on the other end who is reading the appeal for the first time (CMS, 2013c, p. 47).

Required Elements of an Appeal Letter

The following are required elements of the appeal letter (CMS, 2013c, p. 48):

- Name of the beneficiary
- Provider name
  - Physician
  - Supplier
- Address the letter "Dear Sir/Madam:"
- Dates of service
- Send letters to the beneficiaries to keep them in the loop of the communication on the claim for services/payment
- The determination that you are appealing
- Your rationale that describes why the items or services meet the Medicare guidelines
- List any statutory citations accurately and in the format that the person reading the letter will understand
- Contact information for any questions
- Medical documentation supporting the appeal
- Identify in the appeal what amount of the claim is being appealed if there was partial payment

■ Completing the Form CMS-1450 Data Set

Form Locators (FL) 1-15

- FL 1 – Billing provider name, address, and telephone number.
- FL 2 – Billing providers designated pay-to name, address, and Secondary Identification Fields.
- FL 3a – Patient Control Number, which is a unique alpha-numeric control number assigned by the provider to facilitate retrieval of individual financial records (CMS, 2013d, p. 14).
- FL 3b – Medical or Health Record Number.
- FL 4 – Type of Bill, which is a four-digit alphanumeric code that gives three specific pieces of information followed by a leading zero. The second digit identifies the type of facility, the third classifies the type of care that the patient

received, and the forth indicates the sequence of the bill in the episode of care (CMS, 2013d, p. 15).

- FL 5 – Federal Tax Number.
- FL 6 – Statement covers periods (from – through).
- FL 7 – Not used.
- FL 8 – Patient's name/ID number.
- FL 9 – Patient's address.
- FL 10 – Patient's date of birth.
- FL11 – Patient's sex.
- FL 12 – Admission or start of care date.
- FL 13 – Admission hour. This data is not needed.
- FL 14 – Priority or type of admission or visit.
- FL 15 – Point of origin for admission or visit.

Form Locators (FL) 16-30

- FL 16 – Discharge hour is not required.
- FL 17 – Patient discharge status that identifies the discharge status as of the "through" date of the billing period in FL 6 (CMS, 2013d, p. 18).
- FL 18 thru 28 – Condition codes.
- FL 29 – Accident state is not needed and the data will be ignored.
- FL 30 – Untitled. No data is needed.

Form Locators (FL) 31-41

- FL 31 to 34 – Occurrence codes and dates. This is required when there is a condition that applies to the claim (CMS, 2013d, p. 19).
- FL 35 and 36 – Occurrence span code and dates. This is required for inpatient stays (CMS, 2013d, p. 19).
- FL 37 – Not used.
- FL 38 – Responsible party name and address. This field is not required for claims that involve payers of a higher priority than Medicare (CMS, 2013d, p. 20).
- FL 39 to 41 – Value codes and amounts that represent related dollar or unit amounts that are necessary for processing a claim (CMS, 2013d, p. 20).
- FL 42 – Revenue code that is required for the form.

Form Locators (FL) 43-81

- FL 43 – Revenue description, investigational device exemption (IDE), and Medicaid drug rebate. This field is not required.

- FL 44 – Health Insurance Prospective Payment System (HIPPS) rate codes that consists of three character resource utilization group (RUG) followed by a two digit assessment indicator (AI) (CMS, 2013d, p. 22).

- FL 45 – Service date. This is required for outpatient.

- FL 46 – Units of service.

- FL 47 – Total charges. This is not applicable for electronic billers. This is required for the provider sums the total charges for the billing period for each revenue code (CMS, 2013d, p. 23).

- FL 48 – Noncovered charges. This is a required field and pertains to the related revenue codes in FL 42 (CMS, 2013d, p. 24).

- FL 49 – Untitled. No data is entered here.

- FL 50A – (Required).

- FL 50B – (Situational).

- FL 50C – (Situational).

- FL 51A – (Required).

- FL 51B – (Situational).

- FL 51C – (Situational).

- FL 52A/B/C – Release of information indicator. "Y" means that the provider has on file a signed statement permitting release of data to other organizations. An "I" indicates that the informed consent to release medical information for conditions or diagnoses regulated by Federal statues. This is when a provider does not have a signature on file and the state or federal law does not supersede the HIPAA Privacy Rule by requiring a signature be collected (CMS, 2013d, p. 25).

- FL53A/B/C – **assignment of benefits** certification indicator

- FL 54A/B/C – Prior payments. This is situational, in that it is required when the provider has received payments towards the bill.

- FL 55A/B/C – Estimated amount due from patient. This is not required.

- FL 56 – Billing Provider National Provider ID (NPI).

- FL 57 – Other provider ID. Not used.

- FL 58A/B/C – Insured's name.

- FL 59A/B/C – Patient's relationship to insured.

- FL 60A – (Required) B (Situational) C (Situational) insured's unique ID (certificate/social security number/HI claim/identification number [HICN]).
- FL 61A/B/C – Insurance group name.
- FL62A/B/C – Insurance group number.
- FL 63 – Treatment authorization code.
- FL 64 – Document control number (DCN).
- FL 65 – Employer name of the insured.
- FL 66 – Diagnosis and procedure code qualifier (ICD Version Indicator).
- FL 67 – Principal diagnosis code.
- FL 67A–67Q – Other diagnosis codes.
- FL 68 – Reserved.
- FL 69 – Admitting diagnosis. Required for inpatient hospital claims subject to QIO review and the admitting diagnosis is required (CMS, 2013d, p. 28).
- FL 70A–70C – Patient's reason for visit.
- FL 71 – prospective payment system (PPS) code.
- FL 72 – External cause of injury (ECI) codes.
- FL 73 – Reserved. Not used.
- FL 74 – Principal procedure code and date. This is situational and is required on inpatient claims when a procedure was performed (CMS, 2013d, p. 28).
- FL 75 – Reserved. Not used.
- FL 76 – Attending provider name and identifiers (including NPI). This is situational and is required when the claim or **encounter** contains any services other than nonscheduled transportation services. There are secondary qualifiers uses that are 0B for State License Number, 1G for Provider UPIN number, and G2 for provider commercial number (CMS, 2013d, p. 28).
- FL 77 – Operating provider name and identifiers (including NPI). There are secondary qualifiers uses that are 0B for state license number, 1G for provider UPIN Number, and G2 for provider commercial number (CMS, 2013d, p. 29).
- FL 78 and 79 – Other provider name and identifiers (including NPI). This is situational, and the name and ID number of the individual corresponding to the qualifier category is indicated in this section of the claim. DN-referring provider, ZZ-operating physician, 82-rendering provider. Secondary identifier qualifiers are 0B for state license number, 1G for provider UPIN number, and G2 for provider commercial number (CMS, 2013d, p. 29).
- FL 80 – Remarks. This is situational and is for DME billings in which the provider shows the rental rate, cost, and anticipated months of usage.

■ Conclusion

Reimbursement in health care has changed over the years. There have been many additions, edits, and complete changes to the way things were done versus where we are at today. We have changed the responsibility from the patient in the 1960s to the payer in the 2000s. As we see prospective-payment and high-deductible insurance plans, the responsibility is swinging back to almost a center position where the patient has become the most responsible they have been in quite some time. Now we have a mix, or hybrid, of the older models and the patient, payer, and provider are realizing risk in the financial side of health care.

Our evolving marketplace is demonstrating a change from the acute care hospital being the center of care to a more dynamic approach with patients receiving care in physician's offices, ambulatory care centers, and medical homes. Our providers have adapted, and now the suppliers have fallen in line as well. Now with the delivery and payment of care evolving, the processing of medical claims has also changed to meet with the other parts of health care that have changed over time. Now we have new billing forms such as the CMS-1500 that is ICD-10 compliant along with the UB-04 as the two main paper billing forms. The new CMS-1500 form can accommodate up to 12 diagnoses and has a pointer that tells the person or system that is processing the claim what version, ICD-9 or ICD-10, the supplier is operating on currently.

There are many rules and regulations that follow the processing of a claim form for payment. The healthcare administrator must be adept in all facets of claims processing to allow themselves to understand all issues surrounding the processing of a claim and to be able to react to quickly to these changes so as to not compromise the cash flow for the facility. In addition, the healthcare administrator must be familiar with the type of provider or facility that they are managing. The variations in payments in a Skilled Nursing Facility are very different from the processes in the Home Health arena. Things that seem simple, such as a provider accepting assignment, can have a great impact on the overall operation, along with the proper use of an Advance Beneficiary Notice (ABN).

Overall, this chapter demonstrates that not only is the claims-processing portion of health care complex, it is aligned closely to the overall profitability of the healthcare facility. Knowing your reimbursement is critical to the future success of the facility, and most importantly, to the overall satisfaction for the patient and their experience of your facility. You may deliver the best care in the area, but if you can't process a claim correctly, the patient will only remember the bad experience that they had with your collections department when they are incorrectly placed there instead of the claim being processed without any edits or issues. Not only is quality the key for patient care, but quality is the key for claims processing. This process will also be addressed in future chapters with regards to compliance and revenue cycle management.

References

Casto, A.B., & Forrestal, E. (2013a). *Principles of healthcare reimbursement* (4th ed.). Chicago: AHIMA.

Centers for Medicare and Medicaid Services. (2013a). Chapter 1-General billing requirements. *Medicare claims processing manual.* Retrieved from http://www.cms.gov/Regulations-and-Guidance/Guidance/Manuals/Downloads/clm104c01.pdf

Centers for Medicare and Medicaid Services. (2013b). Chapter 30-Financial liability protections. *Medicare claims processing manual.* Retrieved from http://www.cms.gov/Regulations-and Guidance/Guidance/Manuals/Downloads/clm104c30.pdf

Centers for Medicare and Medicaid Services. (2013c). Chapter 29-Appeals of Claims Decisions. *Medicare claims processing manual.* Retrieved from http://www.cms.gov/Regulations-and-Guidance/Guidance/Manuals/Downloads/clm104c29.pdf

Centers for Medicare and Medicaid Services. (2013d). Chapter 25-Completing and processing the Form CMS-1450 Data Set. *Medicare claims processing manual.* Retrieved from http://www.cms.gov/Regulations-and-Guidance/Guidance/Manuals/Downloads/clm104c25.pdf

4 Government Payer Types

Learning Outcomes

After reading this chapter, the student will be able to:

- Understand the differences in the Medicare and Medicaid programs.
- Understand the history of the Medicare and Medicaid programs in the United States.
- Understand the government programs offered outside of the Medicare and Medicaid programs.
- Differentiate between TRICARE and CHAMPVA programs provided for the military personnel and their families.
- Differentiate between the various government-sponsored healthcare plans and to understand how these plans interact with and impact the healthcare system in the United States.

■ Introduction

Healthcare leaders manage the care delivered to various populations, with **Medicare** and Medicaid combined being the largest payers in comparison to the commercial payers types. Medicare and Medicaid are recognized programs for specific populations. Medicare covers, for the most part, the elderly, and Medicaid covers a lower-income population. Each of these programs offers a variety of insurance plans for eligible beneficiaries. In addition to Medicare and Medicaid, there are other government programs such as TRICARE and CHAMPVA that provide programs for military personnel and families. Workers Compensation and Indian Health Services are also part of the government payer types and provide coverage to various populations. In this chapter, we will cover the different programs that are offered by the federal government and state programs. In addition, we will cover the basic characteristics of other state and federal payers and the various populations that they cover. Understanding the different programs will assist the healthcare administrator in better managing the populations covered by

Medicare, Medicaid, and other federal and state payers to better manage the revenue stream realized by the healthcare facility.

■ The History of Medicare

Medicare came out of Title XVIII of the Social Security Act. This was designated as being "Health Insurance for the Aged and Disabled," which is commonly known as Medicare. The Medicare legislation started a program that provided health insurance for persons over the age of 65 to complement other insurances a person may have, such as retirement benefits, survivor's benefits, and disability insurance benefits (Klees, 2009). According to Centers for Medicare and Medicaid Services (CMS), the Health Insurance for the Aged and Disabled Act (title XVIII of the Social Security Act), or as we know it, Medicare, has made this coverage available to almost every American over the age of 65 years old. In addition, this broad program is designed to assist the nation's elderly to meet hospital, medical, and other covered healthcare costs. The program includes two related health insurance programs, which are Hospital Insurance (HI) and a Supplementary Medical Insurance (SMI), which is under Part B (CMS, 2012b).

In the beginning, Medicare just covered beneficiaries, or persons, who were age 65 and older. In years since, Medicare changed their coverage guidelines and became available to a broader population. This change enabled Medicare to cover persons who were entitled to Social Security or Railroad Retirement disability, most persons with end-stage renal disease (ESRD), and other people who were 65 or older and elected to pay a premium for coverage. Another group that was given eligibility for Medicare, without having to wait for the customary 24-month waiting period, was people with Amyotrophic Lateral Sclerosis (ALS) or otherwise known as Lou Gehrig's disease. In addition to Medicare Part A and Part B, there are two other programs that are a part of Medicare known as Medicare Part C, which is sometimes called the Medicare Advantage program. This was established under the Medicare + Choice program by the Balanced Budget Act (BBA) of 1997 and then renamed and modified by the Medicare Prescription Drug, Improvement, and Modernization Act (MMA) of 2003. This program expanded the beneficiaries' options for participation in the private sector healthcare plans (Klees, 2009). Then there is Medicare Part D, which is a prescription drug benefit to assist with coverage of prescription medications that were not covered by Medicare Part A, Part B, or Part C.

Medicare Part A

Health Insurance (HI) is a premium-free program. An individual can be covered based on his or her earnings or those of a parent, spouse, or child. According to the Centers for Medicare and Medicaid Services, the worker must have a specific number of quarters of coverage (QCs); the exact number required is dependent on the basis of age, disability, or presence of end-stage renal disease for the person filing for health insurance. QCs are earned through payment of payroll taxes under the Federal Insurance Contributions Act (FICA) during the years that the person works. Federal employees were exempt from the FICA tax for the HI portion of Medicare until 1983, when they were required to participate by paying the HI portion of the HI FICA tax. The payment of the tax for the HI portion of Medicare did not entitle them to receive monthly social security benefits. State and local government employees, after 1986, must also pay the HI portion of the HI tax (CMS, 2012b).

The age requirement for the HI portion of **Medicare Part A** is 65 years of age or older. The person can apply for the HI benefit when they are at least 6 months away from their 65th birthday. Keep in mind that if the person misses the time frame listed above, they only will be able to get retroactive benefits for 6 months. An example given by CMS is if an individual is born on August 1, the attainment date is July 31, and HI begins with July 1. Entitlement does not end until death (CMS, 2012b).

Hospital insurance for disabled persons who are entitled to Social Security or Railroad Retirement Benefits mandates that persons who are looking to get Medicare Part A need to be on Social Security or Railroad Retirement Benefits for at least 24 months. The last variable for this scenario is that there is a 5-month waiting period for a person who is eligible for HI. This will make the total time frame or pathway to coverage end up being a total of 29 months. The one area that is different from other coverage guidelines is that the qualifying period does not need to be consecutive months. If a person happens to recover from their disability, the HI coverage will end the month after being notified of termination of Disability Determination. According to CMS, if notification is November 15, entitlement ends December 31, but if the individual is working, the Disability Benefit may continue for up to 78 months (CMS, 2012b). An additional coverage that is offered under Medicare Part A is for persons with end-stage renal disease (ESRD) and to the spouses and children of those with ESRD.

Coverage under Medicare Part A

According to CMS, Medicare Part A provided protection against costs of specific medical care for around 45 million people and paid out in benefits over $232 billion in 2008 (Klees, 2009). There are several types of care that Medicare Part A covers: inpatient hospital coverage, care in a skilled nursing facility (SNF), home health care, and hospice care for the terminally ill.

EXHIBIT 4-1   MEDICARE PART A SERVICES

Medicare Part A covers the following:

- Inpatient Hospital Care
- Skilled Nursing Facility
- Long-term Care Hospitals
- Hospice
- Home Health

Data From Centers for Medicare & Medicaid Services. Available at: http://www.Medicare.gov, Accessed on August 18, 2014

EXHIBIT 4-2   MEDICARE PART A COSTS

Medicare Part A Costs

- A deductible for each benefit period of $1,216
- For Days 1–60 is $0 coinsurance for each benefit period
- For Days 61–90 is $304 coinsurance per day of each benefit period
- Days 91 and beyond is $608 coinsurance per each "Lifetime Reserve Day" after day 90 of each benefit period (not to exceed 60 days over beneficiaries lifetime)
- Once you go past the lifetime reserve days all costs fall on the beneficiary

Data from Centers for Medicare & Medicaid Services. Available at: http://www.Medicare.gov, accessed on August 18, 2014.

Inpatient Hospital Coverage

An inpatient stay is defined by CMS as a person who has been admitted to a hospital for bed occupancy for purposes of receiving inpatient hospital services. In addition, they will be formally admitted to the facility with the expectation that he or she will remain at least overnight or transferred to another hospital for care (CMS, 2010). Some of the factors to consider when admitting a patient include the severity of the signs and symptoms, the probability of something adverse happening, and the need for and availability of diagnostic procedures at the location.

Inpatient care and other facility type care is managed or governed by what is called a **benefit period**. This benefit period is time frame that is part of a hospital stay and is subsequently discharged. The time after the discharge and the next admission needs to be at least 60 consecutive days since the last stay in a hospital or skilled nursing facility. With regards to a limit to these benefit periods, there are no limits to the number of these that a person can have over a lifetime. An individual, or patient, can have a hospital stay in a benefit period, but they need to keep in mind that the total number of inpatient hospital days in a benefit period is limited to 90 days. If the patient is in need of additional inpatient days during the benefit period, they can elect to use a pool of 60 days that Medicare provides the insured. These days are nonrenewable and considered a reserve that provides 60 additional days of inpatient care during a benefit period.

Covered items in an inpatient hospital are room and board, nursing services, support services such as social work, drugs and biological, blood products that are furnished while inpatient, supplies, appliances and equipment, diagnostic services, surgical services, medical services, and transportation. Some items that are not covered are physician services that are covered under a physician fee schedule.

Some inpatient settings have private rooms, semiprivate rooms (2, 3, or 4 beds), and some have a ward. If a facility has private rooms and it is not medically necessary for the patient to be in a private room, the facility can charge the patient the difference between the private room and semi-private. According to CMS, the private room differential cannot exceed the difference between the customary charge for the accommodations furnished and the most prevalent semiprivate accommodation rate at the time of the patient's admission (CMS, 2010).

If for any reason the patient is charged the difference for the private room as the facility does not feel that a private room is medically necessary, the patient can appeal the charge to the intermediary. This appeal, or dispute, must be reduced to writing and sent to the intermediary. Upon receipt, the intermediary will review the facts and make a determination regarding the medical necessity of the room. This can be done during the stay in the hospital or after discharge from the facility, and it will be treated as a request for reconsideration. If at any time during the hospital stay in which the patient is appealing the charge for the private room, the hospital agrees that a private room is necessary, the intermediary will immediately rule in favor of this finding.

Skilled Nursing Facility

This service is covered by Medicare Part A, and the skilled nursing facility (SNF) provides care similar to that of an inpatient hospital at a lower level and can include rehabilitation services. The patient is limited to 100 days per benefit period and also be responsible for a copayment for days of care 21–100. If a patient does not require a skilled level of care, skilled nursing, or skilled rehabilitation services, Medicare Part A will not cover the admission.

EXHIBIT 4-3   MEDICARE SKILLED NURSING CARE COVERAGE

Covered services for skilled nursing care

- Semi-private room
- Meals
- Skilled nursing care
- Physical therapy
- Occupational therapy
- Speech language therapy
- Medical social services
- Medications and medical supplies
- Ambulance transportation (some exceptions apply)
- Dietary counseling

Data From: Centers for Medicare & Medicaid Services, Medicare Benefit Policy Manual Chapter 8. Revised April 4, 2014. Available at: http://www.Medicare.gov, accessed on August 18, 2014.

Home Health Care

According to CMS, in order for a patient to be eligible for home health services under both Medicare Part A and Part B, the physician needs to attest that the patient in fact needs home care and is confined to his or her home. They do not have to be bedbound, but considered to be confined to their home environment. This classification of home-bound includes, but is not limited to, going to adult day care centers to receive medical care, outpatient kidney dialysis, and to receive outpatient chemotherapy or radiation therapy (CMS, 2011a). Home health care is provided to a patient for a 60-day period and follows a Plan of Care that is set up for the patient. The home health disciplines that are covered are skilled nursing, home health aide services, physical therapy, occupational therapy, speech therapy, and medical social services. The payment for home health services includes nonroutine medical services that could have been unbundled to Medicare Part B prior to Prospective Payment Systems, but Durable Medical Equipment is excluded from this payment. Durable medical equipment is considered items such as hospital beds, wheelchairs, and low-loss mattresses, just to name a few.

To initiate services for home health, there needs to be a physician's order to start care. A registered nurse will generally be the one to open the case and make the initial visit. Then a Plan of Care will be established that outlines the care needed for the patient. For example, the registered nurse will write the plan of care for visiting nurse 1 time per week × 8 weeks, home health aide 3 times a week × 8 weeks, and physical therapy 3 times a week × 8 weeks. The care needs to be under the supervision of a registered nurse, and the plan of care runs for 60-day intervals. For subsequent episodes, the nurse must communicate with the physician and begin the recertification process before the end of the 60-day period.

There are several different types of payment adjustments in the Home Health Prospective Payment System (HHPPS) such as Low Utilization Payment Adjustment, which entails four or fewer visits paid by discipline. The other adjustment is the Partial Episode Payment (PEP) Adjustment where a beneficiary elects a transfer or reaching the treatment goals in the original plan of care and returning to the same home health agency during the 60-day episode. These will be covered in the chapter on Medicare Prospective Payment Systems.

The delivery and billing of medical supplies have changed over the years where in the past all Durable Medical Equipment (DME) was supplied by a separate provider from the home health agency. Now the agency that is providing the care is the only agency that can bill and receive payment for medical supplies for a patient under a plan of care. This requires the home health agency to contract with a DME supplier to provide the medical equipment and supplies during the plan of care. Once the patient is discharged from care the DME supplier will then bill Medicare directly for the equipment and supplies.

Hospice Care

Hospice care is a benefit under the hospital insurance program. According to CMS, to be eligible to elect hospice care under Medicare, an individual must be entitled to Medicare Part A and be certified as being terminally ill. To be considered terminally ill, the patient's medical prognosis is one that the individual's life expectancy is 6 months or less if the illness runs its normal course (CMS, 2012a). An individual must elect hospice to receive the care, and the first service period is for 90 days. There is no limit as to how long or how many benefit periods a beneficiary can receive hospice care. The next period of care consists of 2 more periods of 90 days, and then after these the patient can have an unlimited number of 60-day periods (CMS, 2012a).

During the time the patient is on hospice services, they must waive all rights to Medicare payments for any hospice care or care related to the reason for which the patient is on hospice. If while on hospice the patient requires care or hospitalization for treatment that is not related to the reason that they are on hospice, Medicare will pay for this treatment.

According to CMS, the timing and content for certification is for the first 90 days of hospice coverage. The hospice must obtain, no earlier than 15 days prior to care and no later than 2 calendar days after hospice is initiated, oral or written certification of the terminal illness by the medical director of the hospice or the physician member of the hospice organization (CMS, 2012a). In addition, the certification must be on file with Medicare prior to submitting a claim. Moreover, subsequent periods of care can be completed up to 15 days prior to the next benefit period; starting no more than 2 calendar days after the first day of the new period, a written certification must be on file (CMS, 2012a). Written certification must include (1) a statement that the individual's medical prognosis includes a life expectancy of 6 months or less; (2) specific clinical findings or other documentation supporting the life expectancy of 6 months or less; and (3) signatures of the physician(s) and the date signed, along with benefit period dates.

After January 1, 2011, the regulations require that a hospice physician or hospice nurse practitioner must have a face-to-face encounter with each hospice patient prior to the beginning of the third benefit period, and prior to each subsequent benefit period (CMS, 2012a). This face-to-face can't be done more than 30 days prior to the start or 30 days after the start of a benefit period, and the physician or nurse practitioner must put in writing that the face-to-face encounter took place and the date of this occurrence.

The discharge of a hospice patient is to happen if they are no longer terminally ill, or if the patient moves outside the coverage area of the servicing hospice; the provider cannot routinely discharge the patient at their discretion. In other words, the beneficiary elected the hospice benefit and the hospice agency cannot revoke the beneficiary's election. Moreover, the hospice should not request that the beneficiary revoke his or her election (CMS, 2012a).

If a Medicare beneficiary is residing in a Skilled Nursing Facility (SNF) or Nursing Facility (NF) they may still elect the hospice benefit if the residential care is paid for by the beneficiary or the beneficiary is eligible for Medicaid and being reimbursed by Medicaid for the beneficiary's care, and if the hospice has a written agreement with the facility where the hospice takes full responsibility for the for the professional management of the individual's hospice care and the facility agrees to provide room and board for the individual (CMS, 2012a).

Hospice is generally provided for a beneficiary in their home. In some instances, the beneficiary can be in a SNF or NF. Another area a beneficiary can receive care is in a short-term inpatient unit. There are two levels of care that are provided for a beneficiary while in an inpatient unit. The first level is respite care for relief of a patient's caregivers. The second level is for general inpatient care, which focuses on pain control and symptom management for events such as medication adjustment, observation, and stabilizing treatment for psychosocial monitoring (CMS, 2012a). General inpatient is not at a level that is equivalent to inpatient care. If a patient receives general inpatient care for 3 days and then revokes hospice, the 3-day stay would be reimbursed at a SNF level for services.

The core services that a hospice must provide directly by their employees on a regular basis are physician services, nursing services, medical social services, and counseling services.

EXHIBIT 4-4   HOSPICE CARE COVERAGE

Hospice care generally covers:

- Doctor services
- Nursing care
- Medical equipment and supplies
- Drugs related to symptom control and/or pain relief
- Home health aide and homemaker services
- Physical therapy
- Occupational therapy
- Speech language therapy
- Social work services
- Dietary counseling
- Grief and loss counseling
- Short-term inpatient care for symptom and pain management
- Short-term respite care
- Any other Medicare covered service needed to manage the pain of the patient

Data From: Centers for Medicare & Medicaid Services. Medicare Benefit Policy Manual Chapter 9. Revised May 1, 2014. Available at: http://www.Medicare.gov, accessed on August 18, 2014.

EXHIBIT 4-5   HOSPICE CARE ELIGIBILITY

A Medicare beneficiary is eligible for Hospice Care if they:

- Are eligible for Medicare Part A.
- Doctor certifies that the patient is terminally ill and are expected to live 6 months or less.
- The patient accepts palliative care for comfort instead of treating the beneficiary's present illness.
- The patient signs a document stating that they choose hospice instead of other routine Medicare benefits.

Data From: Centers for Medicare & Medicaid Services. Medicare Benefit Policy Manual Chapter 9. Revised May 1, 2014. Available at: http://www.Medicare.gov, accessed on August 18, 2014.

> **EXHIBIT 4-6   HOSPICE CARE COSTS FOR A MEDICARE BENEFICIARY**
>
> Hospice Care costs for a Medicare Beneficiary are:
>
> - $0.00 for hospice care
> - Various copayments for prescription drugs (not to exceed $5.00)
> - Up to 5% for respite care
> - Medicare does not cover room and board when the beneficiary receives care in their home or another facility like a nursing home
>
> Data From: Centers for Medicare & Medicaid Services. Medicare Hospice Benefits. Revised August 2013. Available at: http://www.Medicare.gov, accessed on August 18, 2014.

Renal Dialysis Centers

According to CMS, End Stage Renal Disease (ESRD) occurs from the destruction of normal kidney tissues over a long period of time. Often there are no symptoms until the kidney has lost more than half its function, and it is usually irreversible and permanent (CMS, 2013a). Under Medicare Part A, renal dialysis treatments are generally covered in an outpatient setting. For renal dialysis, there are some instances where it will be covered if the patient was in an inpatient setting depending on the patient's condition. Renal disease is usually treated in an inpatient setting for a patient suffering from an acute illness, or for a person with borderline renal failure, or for someone who develops acute renal failure with every illness and requires episodic dialysis or short-term dialysis (CMS, 2010).

Financing Medicare Part A

Medicare Part A is financed through separate payroll contributions paid for by employees, employers, and self-employed persons. The proceeds are deposited to an account called the Federal Hospital Insurance Trust Fund. This fund is only used to pay hospital insurance benefits and administrative expenses (CMS, 2012a).

For federal, state, and local employees who do not pay the full FICA tax, they must pay the Medicare Part A, or the HI portion (CMS, 2012a).

Medicare Part B

To obtain **Medicare Part B**, Supplemental Medical Insurance (SMI), an individual must enroll during an enrollment period and pay the required premiums. SMI provides for payment to participating providers for furnishing covered services after a yearly cash deductible is met (CMS, 2013b). Medicare Part B is designed to supplement voluntary medical insurance that the beneficiary may have coverage with while on Part B.

Medicare Part B covers services and supplies such as drugs and biologicals that are not usually self-administered by the patient, hospital services incident to physicians' services rendered to outpatients and partial hospitalizations. Diagnostic services are covered under Part B that are furnished as an outpatient and for the purposes of diagnostic study. Outpatient services include outpatient physical therapy services, outpatient speech therapy services, and outpatient occupational services. Federally qualified health center services in rural health clinics are covered by Part B. Dialysis supplies for in-home dialysis are covered along with drug clotting factors for hemophilia patients and prescription drugs for immunosuppressive therapy for individuals who receive an organ transplant. Also covered under Part B are physician services, nurse practitioner, and physician assistant services under the supervision of a physician. And other clinician services covered under Part B are certified nurse-midwife, psychologist, and social worker services. Preventative screenings covered are prostate cancer screening, screening for glaucoma, mammography, pap smear and pelvic exam, bone mass measurement, and colorectal cancer screening. Medical nutrition therapy services are covered under Part B along with diagnostic x-ray tests, surgical dressings and splints, ambulance services, prosthetic and orthotic devices (outside of dental) that replace all or part of a body organ, and braces for the body such as the leg and neck (CMS, 2013b).

EXHIBIT 4-7 MEDICARE PART B COVERAGE

Medicare Part B covers

- Medically necessary services
- Preventative services such as flu shots
- Clinical research
- Ambulance Service
- Durable Medical Equipment
- Mental Health (Inpatient/Outpatient/Partial Hospitalization)
- Second opinions
- Limited outpatient prescription drugs

Data From: Centers for Medicare & Medicaid Services. Available at: http://www.Medicare.gov, Accessed on August 18, 2014

Financing Medicare Part B

Medicare Part B is financed by monthly premiums from those beneficiaries that voluntarily enroll in the program. The funds generated by the collection of premiums are deposited in a separate account known as the Federal Supplementary Medical Trust

Fund. The money from this fund is only used to pay for Part B benefits and administrative expenses (CMS, 2012b).

Medicare Part C

Medicare Part C is also known as Medicare Advantage. It is an alternative to the traditional Medicare plan for beneficiaries to choose from instead of Medicare Part A or Part B. The Medicare Part C plans are offered by private insurance companies, which must offer beneficiaries at least what is offered by Part A and Part B, excluding hospice. The plans may, and in certain instances must, provide extra benefits such as dental, vision, or hearing. In addition, they may reduce cost sharing or premiums in lieu of extra benefits (Klees, 2009).

The characteristics of the Medicare Advantage plans are local coordinated plans including health maintenance organizations (HMOs), provider sponsored organizations (PSOs), local preferred provider organizations (PPOs), and other plans. In general, the plans use a network of participating providers and if the beneficiary uses the network providers the out-of-pocket may be lower than if the beneficiary elected to get services outside of the network. In addition to these plans there are Regional PPO (RPPO) plans that have networks similar to the HMOs, PSOs, and PPOs where if the beneficiary gets services inside the network the cost sharing is lower as opposed to if they choose to get services outside the network where they may have to pay larger co-pays and the RPPOs are required to provide the beneficiary with limits to the amount of out-of-pocket the beneficiary will experience (Klees, 2009).

In addition to the plans listed above there are **private fee-for-service plans** that generally do not have provider networks. The members may choose to go to any Medicare provider that will accept the plan's payment for services rendered to the beneficiary. Special Needs Plans (SNPs) are also available only for the beneficiaries that are dual eligible for Medicare and Medicaid, live in long-term care facilities, or have certain severe and disabling medical conditions (Klees, 2009).

Medicare Part D

Medicare Part D started out by providing access to prescription drug discount cards for no more than $30.00 annually. Then the program transitioned into providing subsidized access to prescription drug coverage. This plan is completely voluntary, and the beneficiary has a choice to enroll in a stand-alone prescription drug plan (PDP) or an integrated Medicare Advantage that offers Part D coverage. Part D coverage includes most FDA-approved medications and biologicals. Moreover, there are formularies for the prescriptions covered, and the plan offers different levels of coverage (Klees, 2009).

Medigap Insurance

The term "**Medigap**" is used by a beneficiary to cover healthcare services that are not covered by Part A or Part B. These policies must meet federally imposed standards and are offered by Blue Cross and Blue Shield and various other commercial health insurance companies (Klees, 2009).

■ Medicaid

The History of Medicaid

The federal/state entitlement program that came out of the Title XIX of the Social Security Act that pays for medical assistance for individuals with low income is called **Medicaid**, which became law in 1965. This is a program jointly funded by the federal and state governments. The purpose of this funding is to assist in supplying medical coverage for persons who are in need and eligible for the program. For low-income people in America, the Medicaid program is the largest source of funding for health care (Klees, 2009).

Medicaid at the State Level

The federal government has established guidelines through statutes, regulations, and policy and procedures that requires each state to come up with their own eligibility standards, outline the scope of services provided, duration of services, sets the payment/reimbursement, and acts as its own administrator. In addition, each state structures their Medicaid program differently. With that said, a person of a specific income level may qualify in one state but may not qualify in another state. The programs that each state runs under the name "Medicaid" may have the same content, but each one is run differently in that services offered in one state may not be the same in the other. Moreover, the duration of coverage varies from state to state and the guidelines for eligibility, services, or reimbursement may change at any time.

Scope of Medicaid Services

There is much flexibility for the individual state Medicaid plans to receive funding from the federal government, the individual state needs to provide basic services to the neediest populations. In addition, there are matching funds when there are optional services that states can offer to their Medicaid recipients. The mandatory services include inpatient hospital services, outpatient hospital services, pregnancy-relates services (prenatal and 60-days postpartum), vaccines for children, physician services, nursing facility services (for ages 21 and older), rural health clinic services, home health care, lab and x-ray, pediatric and nurse practitioner services, nurse-midwife services, federally qualified health-center services (FQHC), ambulatory services for

FQHC that are available in other settings, and early and periodic screening, diagnostic and treatment (EPSDT) for children under 21 (Klees, 2009).

Optional services for which states can receive matching funds if they provide them include diagnostic services, clinic services, intermediate care facilities for the mentally retarded, prescription drugs, prosthetic devices, optometrist services and eyeglasses, nursing facility for children under age 21, transportation, rehabilitation and physical therapy services, hospice, home- and community-based care, and targeted case-management services (Klees, 2009).

Duration and Payment for Medicaid Services

Each individual state can determine the duration of services offered under the Medicaid, but must keep in mind that there are restrictions to any limitations that a state can impose on Medicaid beneficiaries. First, any limits imposed must result in a sufficient level of services provided. Second, any limitations in coverage may not discriminate against any beneficiaries based on a medical condition or diagnosis. Overall, states are required to provide a consistent level of benefits, the duration of services, and scope of services to a person receiving Medicaid coverage. There are two exceptions: the state must cover services under EPSDT even if the state does not provide these services, and states can request waivers to pay for otherwise uncovered home and community-based services (Klees, 2009).

Payment can be in a fee-for-service format or in other prepayment arrangements such as a Health Maintenance Organization (HMO). States can determine payment levels to providers; these payments must be at a level to enlist enough providers so that covered services covered by the state Medicaid plan have enough providers enlisted to facilitate these services. Any payments from Medicaid are considered as "Payment in Full." In addition, states can impose coinsurance, deductibles, and copayments on the Medicaid beneficiaries for some services. There are some exclusions to the ability of the state to impose cost-sharing and they are pregnant women, children under 18 years of age, hospital or nursing home patients, emergency services, and family planning services (Klees, 2009).

Medicare–Medicaid Relationship

Medicare beneficiaries who are in the low-income category may be eligible to receive assistance from the Medicaid program. For beneficiaries that are eligible for full Medicaid coverage, the Medicare coverage is supplemented by the services available under the individual state Medicaid program. The additional services may include nursing facility care beyond the 100-day limit that Medicare covers, eyeglasses, and hearing aids. For these persons that have Medicare and Medicaid, any payments made for covered services must come from Medicare first, as Medicaid is always considered the "payer of last resort." In addition to this, if Medicare pays for a service as the primary payer and Medicaid is the secondary payer, the Medicaid program will not make a secondary coverage payment if the amount paid to the provider (at 80% of the allowed charge) is greater than the allowable for the state Medicaid program, no payment is made by Medicaid. The reasoning is that Medicaid will not pay as a secondary payer if the primary payer payment is greater than the allowable amount set forth by Medicaid (Klees, 2009).

■ Other Types of Coverage

Children's Health Insurance Program (CHIP)

State Children's Health Insurance Program (CHIP) is a program that was initiated in 2009 as a result of the Balanced Budget Act (BBA) of 1997. According to CMS, the BBA provided $40 billion dollars in federal funding through the fiscal year (FY) 2007 to be used to provide healthcare coverage to low income children—generally those below 200 percent of the Federal Poverty Level (FPL)—who don't qualify for Medicaid and would otherwise be uninsured. Subsequent legislation, including the Children's Health Insurance Program Reauthorization Act (CHIPRA) of 2009 (Public Law 111-3), extended CHIP funding through FY 2013. Under CHIP, states may elect to provide coverage to qualifying children by expanding their Medicaid programs or through a state program separate from Medicaid (CMS, 2009j).

Eligibility

Medicaid does not provide medical coverage for all persons who are poor. A person's income is only one test for Medicaid eligibility; one is also required to test his or her financial resources against state guidelines. Even under the broadest conditions, if people are very poor they may not be eligible for coverage unless they fit into specific categories. Some of these categories are limited-income families with children, children under the age of 6 whose family is at or below 133 percent of the Federal Poverty Level (FPL), pregnant women whose family income is below 133 percent of the FPL, infants born to Medicaid-eligible women, Supplemental Security Income (SSI) recipients, people who receive assistance for care of adoptive or foster care children, special protected groups, all children under the age of 19 whose family income is at or below the FPL, and certain Medicare beneficiaries (Klees, 2009). There are other groups that are covered under the Medicaid umbrella that are considered related as they have the same characteristics of the groups listed above, but the coverage criteria is more relaxed. These groups are infants up to age 1 and pregnant women covered under the rule that their family income is not above 185 percent of the FPL (amount is set by each state individually), children under the age of 21 who meet certain criteria, institutionalized individuals and individuals in home- and community-based waiver programs, individuals who would be eligible if institutionalized, certain individuals who are blind or disabled, the aged (blind or disabled) who receive state supplementary income payments, certain working individuals with income less than 250 percent of the FPL, TB-infected persons who would qualify financially for Medicaid or SSI, certain insured or low-income women who are screened for breast or cervical cancer, optional targeted low-income children included in CHIP, and medically needy persons (Klees, 2009).

In addition to all of the above, each state may have additional services that are unique to each state. Sometimes these programs are called "state-only" and they put money aside and to provide assistance to those persons that do not qualify for Medicaid. Each state can run a little differently, but there are certain requirements that need to be met with regards to the additional funding. The Medically Needy (MN) option will allow individual states to extend Medicaid eligibility to additional persons that are eligible for Medicaid under the mandatory or optional programs.

The Personal Responsibility and Work Opportunity Reconciliation Act of 1996, known as the "welfare reform" bill, states that a legal resident alien and other qualified aliens who entered the United States on or after August 22, 1996 are ineligible for Medicaid for 5 years and aliens that entered the United States before that date then coverage for those individuals is up to the individual state, but emergency services are mandatory for both alien coverage groups (Klees, 2009).

Coverage for Medicaid can begin as soon as 3 months prior to the application date of the person applying for coverage. When a person stops coverage or no longer meets the criteria or Medicaid eligibility group, at any time during the month, the coverage for this person will end on the last day of the month.

Programs of All-Inclusive Care for the Elderly (PACE)

The **Programs of All-Inclusive Care for the Elderly (PACE)** is a managed-care benefit for the elderly that features a comprehensive medical and social service delivery system using an interdisciplinary team approach. The PACE organization is a not-for-profit, private or public entity, that is primarily engaged in providing PACE services and must have certain characteristics such as a governing board, ability to provide a complete service package, physical site for adult day services, defined service area, safeguards to avoid conflict of interest, fiscal soundness, and a Participant Bill of Rights (CMS, 2011b).

To be eligible for PACE, a person must be 55 years of age or older, meet a Nursing Facility level of care, and live in the network servicing area for the PACE organization. Services provided include social work, prescription, nursing facility care, primary care, restorative therapies, personal care, hospice, nutritional counseling, meals, and mental health services. In addition to these services, PACE provides coverage for over-the-counter medications that are approved by the PACE interdisciplinary team and included in the participants plan of care (CMS, 2011b).

EXHIBIT 4-8   PACE SERVICES

Services offered by PACE:

- Social work
- Prescription drugs
- Nursing facility care
- Primary care
- Restorative therapies
- Personal care
- Hospice
- Nutritional counseling
- Meals
- Mental health services
- Some over-the-counter medications

Temporary Assistance for Needy Families (TANF)

The Personal Responsibility and Work Opportunity Reconciliation Act of 1996 (also known as Welfare Reform) brought about many changes, which included the implementation of **Temporary and Needy Families (TANF)** to replace the Aid to Families with Dependent Children (AFDC). TANF provides states with grant money that is to help low-income families with case assistance. Due to the many changes in Medicaid eligibility, some individuals may not know that they are eligible for this benefit (CMS, 2011).

TRICARE

TRICARE offers comprehensive and affordable healthcare coverage to active duty service members and retirees of the seven uniformed services, their family members, survivors and others who are registered in the Defense Enrollment Eligibility Reporting System (DEERS). The sponsor must enroll their family members and make sure that all information is kept up to date. TRICARE is also available to the members of the National Guard and Reserves and their families (DOD, 2013).

TRICARE Prime

TRICARE Prime is the managed care option offered by the Department of Defense and offers the most affordable and comprehensive coverage for its beneficiaries. Coverage includes emergency care, outpatient visits, preventative care, hospitalization, maternity care, mental health, behavioral health, and prescription coverage. The member is assigned a primary care manager (PCM) either at a military hospital or clinic in the TRICARE network. There are no out-of-pocket costs for the member or their family (TRICARE, 2013).

TRICARE Standard and Extra

TRICARE Standard and Extra is a fee-for-service plan available to all nonactive duty beneficiaries in the United States and enrollment is not required as coverage is automatic as long as the beneficiary is registered in DEERS. TRICARE Standard and Extra provide coverage for emergency care, outpatient and inpatient care, preventive care, maternity care, mental and behavioral health, and prescription coverage. The beneficiary and their family have both in-network and out-of-network benefits and will experience out-of-pocket costs for care after they meet their annual deductible. The TRICARE Extra option will reduce the out-of-pocket costs for the beneficiary and their family (TRICARE, 2013).

TRICARE For Life

TRICARE For Life offers secondary coverage to all Medicare beneficiaries who have both Medicare Part A and Medicare Part B. In addition, coverage is available worldwide, and TRICARE is the primary payer. Medicare will pay its portion for services provided, and TRICARE For Life will pay the coinsurance for TRICARE-covered services. For services that are not covered by Medicare, TRICARE For Life will pay the claim, and the beneficiary will be responsible for any coinsurance, copay, or deductible. For services covered by Medicare but not covered by TRICARE For Life, Medicare will pay their portion and the beneficiary will be responsible for the balance due based on the provider's status with Medicare.

CHAMPVA

The **Civilian Health and Medical Program of the Department of Veterans Affairs (CHAMPVA)** is a comprehensive healthcare program where the Veterans Affairs (VA) shares the cost of care for covered services and supplies. There is some confusion between CHAMPVA and TRICARE. The difference is that CHAMPVA is a Department of Veterans Affairs program, where TRICARE is a regionally managed healthcare program for active and retired members of the military.

To be eligible for CHAMPVA, the beneficiary cannot be eligible for TRICARE and must be the spouse or child of a veteran who has been rated as permanently or totally disabled, who died from a VA-rated service or connected disability, who was at the time of death rated permanently or totally disabled, or who died in the line of duty (not due to misconduct). Eligible CHAMPVA sponsor, spouse, and family can receive care from the VA Healthcare System. If the beneficiary is under the age of 65 and eligible for Medicare, the beneficiary must enroll in Medicare Part A and Medicare Part B. With regards to payments, CHAMPVA is always the secondary payer to Medicare (Veterans Administration, 2013).

Worker's Compensation

The **workers' compensation** benefit is made available to most employees to help cover healthcare costs that are due to a work-related injury. Federal government employees are covered under the Federal Employees' Compensation Act (FECA). Other employees that are covered have their benefits established at a state level. Benefits may include death, income, and medical benefits. Employers can get coverage through their state's non-profit compensation fund. By working with these nonprofit funds the employers, both small and large, are able to obtain coverage that is affordable.

Indian Health Services

Indian Health Services (IHS) is an agency within the Department of Health and Human Services that is responsible for providing federal healthcare services to American Indians and Alaska natives. The IHS is the principal healthcare provider and health advocate for the Indian people. The goal of the agency is to raise their health status to the highest level possible. IHS provides comprehensive healthcare services to the American Indians and Alaska Natives who are members of 566 federally recognized tribes across the United States. The mission of the agency is to raise the physical, mental, social, and spiritual health of American Indians and Alaska Natives to the highest level. The goal of the agency is to assure that comprehensive, culturally acceptable personal and public healthcare services are available. The foundation's mission is to uphold the federal government's obligation to promote healthy American Indian and Alaska Native people, communities, and cultures and to honor and protect the rights of the tribes (IHS, 2013).

The delivery of healthcare services is provided directly by the IHS through contracted and operated healthcare programs and through services purchased from private providers of health care. The system consists of 28 hospitals, 61 health centers, and 33 health stations. The clinical staff consists of approximately 2,640 nurses, 820 physicians, 670 pharmacists, 340 physician assistants, 310 dentists, and various allied health professionals such as nutritionists and health administrators (IHS, 2013).

■ Conclusion

In this chapter, the student was introduced to many government payer types. Government payers play a large role in the reimbursement system for hospitals and other medical providers that service the Medicare beneficiaries. Medicare and Medicaid are the recognized payers, and combined they represent the largest payer in the country for healthcare services. Each program has a variety of coverage to meet the needs of many consumers. As we can see, Medicaid is offered in every state in the United States, but each individual Medicaid plan is different in what they offer outside of the core services as required by the federal government. In addition, the programs TRICARE and CHAMPVA are government programs for military personnel and their families providing inpatient and outpatient care. In addition, we can see that there are several specialty programs like PACE and TANF that cover individuals for services that they may not be eligible to get in other plans or that they cannot afford. Insurance coverage is a key to the profitability of the healthcare facility in that they need to be paid appropriately for the medical services that they supply to the patient. It is important for the healthcare leader to understand and differentiate between the different government payers with regards to coverage, rules, and regulations regarding care and payment. And as we can see, there are quite a few different options of coverage and payment, so the facility must know the proper billing procedures. More importantly, they need to know what services are offered and under what conditions the beneficiary is eligible to receive these services.

References

Centers for Medicare and Medicaid Services. (2010). Inpatient hospital services covered under part A. *Medicare benefit policy manual.* Retrieved from http://www.cms.gov/Regulations-and-Guidance/Guidance/Manuals/Downloads/bp102c01.pdf

Centers for Medicare and Medicaid Services. (2011a, May 6). Home health services. *Medicare benefit policy manual* (p 20). Retrieved from http://www.cms.gov/Regulations-and-Guidance/Guidance/Manuals/Downloads/bp102c07.pdf

Centers for Medicare and Medicaid Services. (2011b, June 9). Programs of all-inclusive care for the elderly (PACE). Retrieved from http://www.cms.gov/Regulations-and-Guidance/Guidance/Manuals/Downloads/pace111c01.pdf

Centers for Medicare and Medicaid Services. (2012a, June 1). Coverage of hospice services under hospital insurance. *Medicare benefit policy manual.* Retrieved from http://www.cms.gov/Regulations-and-Guidance/Guidance/Manuals/Downloads/bp102c09.pdf

Centers for Medicare and Medicaid Services. (2012b, October 26). Medicare general information, eligibility, and entitlement; General program benefits. Retrieved from http://www.cms.gov/Regulations-and-Guidance/Guidance/Manuals/Downloads/ge101c01.pdf

Centers for Medicare and Medicaid Services. (2013a, June 7). End stage renal disease (ESRD) *Medicare benefit policy manual* (p 3). http://www.cms.gov/Regulations-and-Guidance/Guidance/Manuals/Downloads/bp102c11.pdf

Centers for Medicare and Medicaid Services. (2013b, March 1). Hospital services covered under part B. *Medicare benefit policy manual.* Retrieved from http://www.cms.gov/Regulations-and-Guidance/Guidance/Manuals/Downloads/bp102c06.pdf

Indian Health Services. (2013). *IHS fact sheet quick look.* Retrieved from http://www.ihs.gov/newsroom/factsheets/quicklook/

Klees, B. S. (2009). Brief summaries of Medicare & Medicaid; Title XVIII and Title XIX of The Social Security Act. Retrieved from http://www.cms.gov/Research-Statistics-Data-and-Systems/Statistics-Trends-and-Reports/MedicareProgramRatesStats/downloads/MedicareMedicaidSummaries2009.pdf

TRICARE. (2013). TRICARE Overview. Retrieved from http://www.tricare.mil/Welcome/Plans/Prime.aspx

Veterans Administration. (2013). CHAMPVA Overview. Retrieved from http://www.va.gov/hac/forbeneficiaries/champva/champva.asp

5 | Affordable Care Act

Learning Outcomes

After reading this chapter, the student will:

- Describe the 10 titles that address a critical component of the Patient Protection and Affordable Care Act (PPACA) reform.
- Explain the timeline of the PPACA and the influence that it has on the quality of care that is delivered to the beneficiary.
- Identify the role of the Center for Consumer Information and Insurance Oversight (CCIIO) for assisting in implementing various parts of the PPACA.
- Describe the healthcare insurance marketplace and the process that individuals can follow to purchase healthcare benefits in the PPACA era.
- Describe the process for filing an appeal for healthcare-related services that are delayed and/or denied by the insurance company.
- Understand and explain the components of the Summary of Benefit and Coverage documents that are provided to individuals who are looking to purchase healthcare benefits through the PPACA.

■ Introduction

The Patient Protection and Affordable Care Act (PPACA, also referred to as ACA) was designed to ensure that all Americans have access to quality health care that is affordable and that will ultimately reduce healthcare costs, which have been on the rise over the years. "The Congressional Budget Office (CBO) has determined that the Patient Protection and Affordable Care Act is fully paid for, will provide coverage to more than 94% of Americans while staying under the $900 billion limit that President Obama established" (DPC, 2014, p. 1), with the thought behind the program of impacting the curve of the healthcare cost in a positive way and reducing the country's deficit over the time period of 10 years and beyond.

◼ The Patient Protection and Affordable Care Act

The Patient Protection and Affordable Care Act (PPACA) contains 10 titles that address a critical component of the ACA reform. They are as follows:

Title 1: Quality, Affordable Health Care for All Americans

Title II: The Role of Public Programs

Title III: Improving the Quality and Efficiency of Health Care

Title IV: Prevention of Chronic Disease and Improving Public Health

Title V: Health Care Workforce

Title VI: Transparency and Program Integrity

Title VII: Improving Access to Innovative Medical Therapies

Title VIII: Community Living Assistance Services and Supports

Title IX: Revenue Provisions

Title X: Reauthorization of the Indian Health Care Improvement Act

The PPACA was enacted on March 23, 2010; shortly after the name of the act was changed to the **Health Care Reconciliation Act of 2010**. The goal of the act was to expand the coverage of health insurance, and at the same time, reduce the medical expenditures that Medicare has been facing over the years. In addition, the PPACA will increase the Hospital Insurance (HI) payroll tax that employers pay by 0.9 percent for those high-income individuals and families. "The PPACA also established a 3.8 percent unearned-income Medicare contribution on income from interest, dividends, annuities, and other nonearning sources for high-income taxpayers" (DHHS, 2010, p. 1).

It is estimated that the average net savings to the Medicare Part A Trust Fund will be that the estimated exhaustion of the fund assets will be extended by 12 years from 2017 to 2029 under the PPACA. However, with that said, the projected savings through efficiencies and productivity gains are not fully realized or sustainable through the projected extension, the overall savings, and projected date that the Medicare Part A Trust Fund will be shortened. The impact on the Medicare Part B will be where the premiums will be reduced as a result of the manufacturers and importers of brand-name drugs having fees imposed upon them for importing prescription drugs into the United States. The savings in Medicare Part B can be used to offset other federal costs that can include any costs associated with the PPACA coverage expansions.

This chapter will address the 10 components of the PPACA to bring a better understanding of the changes that will be impacting all aspects of the healthcare delivery model for individuals and **providers**.

Title I: Quality, Affordable Health Care for All Americans

The PPACA is designed to put business owners, families, and individuals in complete control of their health care. The goal of the act is to reduce premiums by providing tax relief for millions of small businesses and working families, which will end up being the largest tax cut for the middle class in the history of the United States. The PPACA also addresses the amount that the families will have to pay by reducing this amount through limiting the amount of out-of-pocket costs that the families have to pay. In addition, there will be preventative services offered to the families that may have not been offered in the past, which will be completely covered by the insurance coverage that they have; the goal is to eliminate the out-of-pocket expenses they have experienced in the past. One thing to keep in mind is that if a person or family is satisfied with their current healthcare coverage, they do not have to change their coverage to a plan that is offered through the PPACA (DHHS, 2014a, p. I).

The PPACA provides individuals and families without coverage the ability to select an insurance plan that is best for their needs. For the current uninsured or underinsured, this is a comforting option, as they can get a healthcare plan that fits their needs and they don't have to worry about whether the plan is reputable and good enough. This pool of insurance companies will be the very same pool of providers from which all members of Congress will be required to select for their insurance needs. To achieve affordable plans, the insurance exchange will combine their buying power to reduce premiums such that the insurance companies have to compete for their members—an approach that is completely different from past practices. Moreover, the insurance companies will have to abide by the rules of not denying coverage for a person due to a pre-existing condition. Along with this, an individual will have new-found power to appeal insurance company decisions to deny a service or procedure that a doctor has ordered and found to be medically necessary. Assistance made available to small businesses and families to help them better navigate the healthcare marketplace and understand their rights will support better management of the healthcare dollars that are spent in the United States.

Title II: The Role of Public Programs

The PPACA reaches the Medicaid level for each state in the country and promotes treating each one equally across the board. The PPACA will ensure the viability of the Children's Health Insurance Program (CHIP) that services children in each state and will simplify the enrollment process for the families that are in need of this coverage. The PPACA also will work towards strengthening the community-based services that the people with disabilities rely on and look towards expanding homecare services to those people who are requiring long-term care or services in the home. This focus on home care is extremely helpful, in that the shift of care is moving more and more towards the delivery of services in the home as this will also help to reduce costs in the long run (DHHS, 2014b, p. II).

The PPACA also affords flexibility at the state level for improvements to care given to beneficiaries and the overall coordination of care for Medicare and Medicaid patients. Moreover, with more people gaining insurance the states' payments for the uninsured who receive care will diminish and the focus on prescription medications will reduce costs that are shouldered by the individual taxpayers.

Title III: Improving the Quality and Efficiency of Health Care

The PPACA will address the status of Medicare and ensure that it protects the Medicare Trust Fund and the overall commitment to the American seniors who rely on the coverage. Not only do they rely on the coverage of services, they also rely on saving money on out-of-pocket expenses for such necessities as prescription medications and reducing the "donut hole" that the Medicare beneficiary may experience throughout the year. In addition to managing the pharmacy expenses for the Medicare beneficiary, the primary care physicians, nurses, and hospitals will be incentivized to improve the care given to the beneficiary and reduce any unnecessary tests and errors that can cause harm to the patient. In addition to reducing costs and improving access to the Medicare beneficiaries in urban areas, the PPACA focuses on improving access to areas outside of the city that are in rural areas. These areas will experience improved access to healthcare services and this will help to improve outcomes and reduce costs to the beneficiary.

In addition to reducing costs and improving access and quality care for the Medicare beneficiary, the PPACA will help to tighten up and reduce the overpayments to the insurance companies. The cost savings of tens of billions of dollars from avoiding overpayments to insurance companies will help to validate the commitment to preserving Medicare for the next generation of beneficiaries so they can get the care that they have come to expect through the years that they were contributing to the program. As the PPACA evolves and the number of Americans without health insurance decreases, these changes will ensure that people have credible healthcare coverage prior to entering the Medicare program; they will ultimately be healthier as they enroll in the program. In addition, the need for caring for the uninsured will decrease and so will the need for Medicare to pay hospitals for the care of the uninsured. To support these initiatives of reducing costs and improving access, there will need to be an oversight committee to oversee the decisions surrounding quality care for our seniors and this will be accomplished by having a group of doctors and various healthcare experts and they will be charged with coming up with the best possible ideas to improve all areas of the healthcare delivery model relating to access, cost, and quality (DHHS, 2014a, p. III).

Title IV: Prevention of Chronic Disease and Improving Public Health

The PPACA provides for unprecedented funding and commitment to the areas of prevention, wellness, and public health. The PPACA will develop a national model for health promotion and disease prevention that will look to incorporate the most effective and obtainable methods to improve the overall health of the American citizen. Moreover, the PPACA will look to reduce the likelihood of preventable illness and disabilities that are present in the United States. Areas that the PPACA will focus on are areas like nutrition that will give families the proper tools to better manage the nutrition of their family members and make available prevention and screenings and making these available to Medicare beneficiaries without having to pay a copayment to receive the services (DHHA 2014a, IV).

Title V: Health Care Workforce

There are areas of the country that are in need of primary care physicians, nurses, physician assistants, mental health providers, and dentists. The PPACA will address these issues by making available to the clinicians in these areas scholarships and loan repayment programs that will help these clinicians in areas of the country that they are needed the most. In addition, the PPACA also addresses the shortage of nurses in the country and will take a comprehensive approach of offering enhanced educational opportunities. The PPACA will also focus its efforts on the overall supply of professionals in the public health sector. This focus will help to increase the supply of public health professionals in the United States and better prepare everyone for the possibilities health emergencies that may arise from time to time. The PPACA also provides the individual states the flexibility and resources to create recruitment strategies to enhance the healthcare workforce. In addition, the PPACA offers individual states the necessary funding to expand, construct, and operate community healthcare centers to improve access to care across the United States (DHHS, 2014a, p. V).

Title VI: Transparency and Program Integrity

The PPACA allows individual patients to take more control of the decisions that they make surrounding their health care and make these decisions with additional information being made available to them so their decisions work better for them. The PPACA also provides to the physicians cutting edge medical research information to enhance the decision process and have the decisions that are being made ones that are made with all the facts and possibilities so as the decision is a comprehensive one and most beneficial to the patient and caregiver.

The PPACA improves the access to information surrounding nursing home care and helping the patient and their family select the right place for the beneficiary. In addition, the PPACA provides for enhanced training for the staff members of the nursing home that will ultimately improve quality and help to reduce costs. Some of the areas of focus for the PPACA and nursing homes are (1) promoting safety by empowering the facility to self-correct their errors; (2) requiring background checks for the employees that provide direct patient care; and (3) implementing programs to prevent and eliminate the issue of elder abuse that is present today in the nursing home environment (DHHS, 2014a, p. VI).

Finally, the PPACA seeks to reduce waste in the nursing home environment. It strives to reduce fraud and abuse by implementing new disclosure requirements that will help to identify any provider that is a high risk to the American taxpayer. In addition, it will allow states to prohibit providers from operating in that state if they have had issues in other states or have been penalized in the past, which will help to avoid duplication of these improper business practices in multiple states. In addition, the states will have increased flexibility to look at tort reforms that address several areas such as reducing healthcare errors, improving patient safety, boosting the efficient resolution of disputes, and improving the access to liability insurance (DHHS, 2014a, p. VI).

Title VII: Improving Access to Innovative Medical Therapies

The PPACA looks to save consumers money by promoting innovation, extending drug discounts to those providers who take care of the low-income patients or may be a disproportionate-share hospital. Moreover, the PPACA looks to create a pathway for the current brand name biological drugs to be manufactured in in a generic version that will give all the providers the ability to utilize the most efficient and cost effective alternative to the more expensive brand-name medications (DHHS, 2014a, p. VII).

Title VIII: Community Living Assistance Services and Supports Act (CLASS Act)

The purpose of this section of the PPACA is to provide American citizens with a new option to finance long-term care services. This is designed so that when someone encounters a disability, there will be insurance coverage to help with the expenses. This is a self-funded program, a voluntary long-term care option, and workers will pay into the program through premiums. If the worker develops a disability, then a daily cash benefit is available to offset the loss of income. The need is based on the ability of the patient to perform basic Activities of Daily Living (ADLs) and the benefit can be used for a wide variety of community services from respite care to home care. The program will seek to reduce Medicaid spending as the goal is to allow the patient to continue to work while they still reside in their home. This will reduce the amount of spending on nursing home care that Medicaid would usually provide. There will be measures in place to make sure that the premiums collected will be sufficient to cover the costs of the plan option (DHHS, 2014a, p. VIII).

Title IX: Revenue Provisions

The PPACA will offset the premiums for healthcare insurance by providing the middle class tax cuts that will allow the families and small businesses to benefit from more affordable healthcare coverage. These credits will allow tens of millions of families to benefit from reduced premium costs and the enhanced ability to purchase health insurance. Families that make less than $250,000 per year will realize the tax credits that are provided through this plan. The goal of the PPACA is to have this reform funded by the savings that the Act will provide and reduce our country's deficit by more than $100 billion over the next 10 years (DHHS, 2014a, p. IX).

Title X: Reauthorization of the Indian Health Care Improvement Act

This part of the PPACA reauthorized the Indian Health Care Improvement Act (IHCIA) that provides care for the American Indians and Alaskan Natives. This program will ultimately modernize the healthcare system and improve the care delivered to the over 1.9 million beneficiaries that are currently being served under the program (DHHS, 2014a, p. XI).

■ Timeline of the PPACA

2010 New Consumer Protections

In 2010 the PPACA put insurance coverage online for the consumer to allow them to compare coverage between plans and to pick the best one for their needs. The rules were changed to prohibit insurance companies from denying coverage to children under the age of 19 due to a pre-existing condition. The Act also stops the insurance companies from looking for a technical mistake or oversight to deny coverage or payment for services if the beneficiary ended up becoming ill, and made this type of practice illegal. In addition, the PPACA eliminated lifetime limits on insurance coverage and regulating the limits that insurance companies generally put on the annual amounts of coverage a person could receive. The Act also set up a consumer assistance program to help the consumer to navigate the private health insurance networks and to make the way that a person could appeal coverage determinations through an external review process.

In 2010, there was a push to improve quality and at the same time lower costs. The PPACA provided small businesses tax credits to help them to provide health insurance benefits to their employees. The Act also looked at offering relief to Medicare beneficiaries who hit the "donut hole" in their prescription drug coverage and gave them a one-time rebate check in the amount of $250 that was not taxable. Part of the program was a focus on preventative care to combat diseases and illnesses that were avoidable. These initiatives included smoking cessation to combating obesity along with providing preventative services such as mammograms and colonoscopies without charging the beneficiary any copays or deductibles. Another initiative was addressing healthcare fraud; in doing so, lawmakers returned more than $2.5 billion dollars to the Medicare Trust Fund in 2009 (DHHS, 2014b).

The PPACA looked to increase access to health care to individuals who have been uninsured because of a pre-existing condition for at least 6 months. The Act also extended coverage for young adults so that they could stay on their parents' plan until they reached

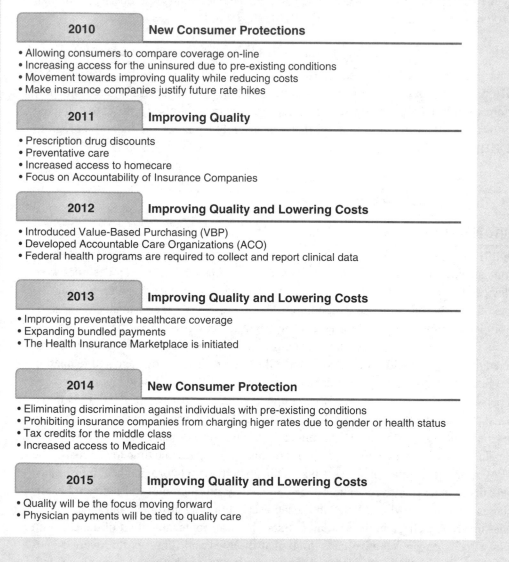

| 2010 | New Consumer Protections |

• Allowing consumers to compare coverage on-line
• Increasing access for the uninsured due to pre-existing conditions
• Movement towards improving quality while reducing costs
• Make insurance companies justify future rate hikes

| 2011 | Improving Quality |

• Prescription drug discounts
• Preventative care
• Increased access to homecare
• Focus on Accountability of Insurance Companies

| 2012 | Improving Quality and Lowering Costs |

• Introduced Value-Based Purchasing (VBP)
• Developed Accountable Care Organizations (ACO)
• Federal health programs are required to collect and report clinical data

| 2013 | Improving Quality and Lowering Costs |

• Improving preventative healthcare coverage
• Expanding bundled payments
• The Health Insurance Marketplace is initiated

| 2014 | New Consumer Protection |

• Eliminating discrimination against individuals with pre-existing conditions
• Prohibiting insurance companies from charging higer rates due to gender or health status
• Tax credits for the middle class
• Increased access to Medicaid

| 2015 | Improving Quality and Lowering Costs |

• Quality will be the focus moving forward
• Physician payments will be tied to quality care

FIGURE 5.1   Timeline for the PPACA.

the age of 26. The new exchanges would provide expanded care for early retirees that would retire without an employer-sponsored insurance plan before they would be eligible for Medicare benefits. The plan also looked to improve or increase the number of primary care physicians, nurses, and physician assistants. Finally, in 2010, the PPACA would hold insurance companies responsible for unreasonable rate hikes and make them justify the rate increases. The Act also looked to allow more people to be covered under Medicaid and increased the payments for rural healthcare providers and provided new funding to support the construction of community health centers (DHHS, 2014b).

2011 Improving Quality

In 2011 the PPACA offered prescription drug discounts and free preventative care for seniors. In addition, CMS would start looking at different ways to deliver care to patients and look to improve care for seniors that are at a high risk for hospitalizations or unnecessary readmissions. To further bring the cost of health care down, the act would entertain proposals that would focus on extending the life of the Medicare trust fund by targeting waste in the system, and at the same time, look at improving quality and outcomes for patients.

The PPACA focused in 2011 on increasing access to home care in the community that would help to shift the care from the nursing home to the patient's home. Accountability was also a focus, and the insurance companies were required to bring the cost of care down by spending more of the premium dollars that they collected directly on patient care. The goal was that at least 85 percent of all premium dollars collected from large employers were spent on healthcare services and supported quality improvement. In addition, overpayments to insurance companies to cover the Medicare Advantage enrollees were looked at and it was found that insurance companies were paid $1,000 more per person than the average person receiving traditional Medicare (DHHS, 2014b).

2012 Improving Quality and Lowering Costs

The PPACA had the focus of improving quality and at the same time, lowering costs. **Value-Based Purchasing (VBP)** was established and it offered financial incentives to hospitals to improve the quality of care delivered to the patient. This was done through publicly reporting data on heart attacks, heart failure, and patient's perception of care that was delivered to them while in the hospital. The Act also looked at providing incentives for physicians to join together and to develop **Accountable Care Organizations** that would ultimately allow the physician to better coordinate patient care and improve quality through decreased infections and reducing unnecessary admissions to the hospital. The Act looked at reducing paperwork and administrative costs by standardizing billing and look at electronic exchanges to transfer healthcare information through the use of electronic health records. Finally, to reduce constant healthcare disparities the law required that federal health programs collect and report racial, ethnic, and language data. The Act in 2012 also targeted increasing access to affordable care through voluntary long-term care insurance programs (DHHS, 2014b).

2013 Improving Quality and Lowering Costs

In 2013 the PPACA focused on improving preventative healthcare coverage for the Americans receiving preventative care. It also looked at expanding the use of bundled payments to providers. This shifted the risk to the provider to deliver quality care and lower costs; this was done through the bundle payment, in that the provider was entirely responsible for their profit and loss on a patient, but had to balance out quality care and access at the same time. In addition, in 2013 the Act looked at increasing the reimbursement to primary care physicians who treated Medicaid patients. The last element to the act in 2013 was the initialization of the **Health Insurance Marketplace**, which allowed individuals and small businesses to purchase affordable health insurance in a competitive environment (DHHS, 2014b).

2014 New Consumer Protection

The PPACA prohibits insurance companies from discriminating against or refusing to sell coverage to an individual because of their pre-existing conditions. Moreover, the insurance companies are prohibited from charging higher rates to individual or small groups due to their gender or health status. The PPACA eliminated the annual limits on healthcare coverage and looked to ensure that insurance companies could not drop an individual if they choose to be part of a clinical trial.

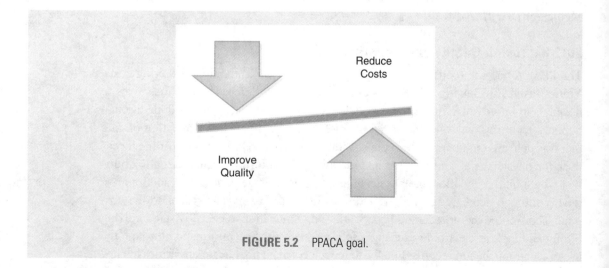

FIGURE 5.2   PPACA goal.

The PPACA will look to make care more affordable through providing tax credits for the middle class to afford coverage. This benefit will be given to the individual in advance towards monthly premiums instead of waiting for tax season to get reimbursed. The Health Insurance Marketplace will be able to provide access to insurance if the individual's employer does not offer coverage. The marketplace will offer the individual a choice of health plans that meet certain cost standards and benefits. The small business tax credit will enter its second phase in 2014 where the credit will be up to 50 percent of the employer's contribution to provide health coverage for its employees.

Finally, through 2014 the PPACA will provide for increased access to Medicaid for Americans who earn less than 133 percent of the federal poverty level. The states will receive funding to support this expanded coverage. And the act will look to promote individual responsibility to get health coverage by charging those who can afford coverage and who do not obtain it a fee for not complying. This fee will go towards helping those who cannot afford coverage to offset their expense through an exemption.

2015 Improving Quality and Lowering Costs

Quality has been the focus, and in 2015, the idea of providing quality care to individuals will fall on the shoulders of the physician. Physician payments will be tied to the quality care that they provide. The payments to physicians will be modified in that those who provide higher quality care will receive higher payments and those who provide lower quality care will receive lower payments.

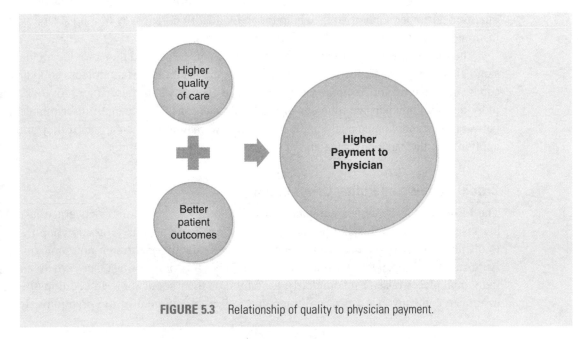

FIGURE 5.3 Relationship of quality to physician payment.

■ The Center for Consumer Information and Insurance Oversight

The Center for Consumer Information and Insurance Oversight (CCIIO) is responsible for assisting in implementing various parts of the PPACA. CCIIO oversees the portion of the Act relating to the implementation of private health insurance and working with states to initiate the Health Insurance Marketplace. The overall mission of the CCIIO is to work closely with the stakeholders to make sure that the PPACA serves the American public in the most effective and efficient manner. The CCIIO handles areas such as the Health Insurance Marketplace and Summary of Benefits and Coverage.

Health Insurance Marketplace

The Marketplace is a new way to shop for healthcare coverage if you currently have coverage or are looking for coverage and you need options. The Marketplace will help you learn if you can find coverage at a lower rate and compare different plans side-by-side. The individual will need to provide some basic information about themselves such as household size and income. The Marketplace will show you plans in the individual's area that best fit their needs. In addition, the Marketplace will let the individual know if they qualify for lower cost coverage through Medicaid or CHIP (HealthCare.gov, 2014).

The individual can apply online by phone or in person. There is support available to the individual 24 hours a day 7 days a week. There is also a Navigator or other qualified customer support staff to help the individual find their way around selecting insurance coverage for themselves or family members.

The Marketplace is a service offered by private companies and they provide all the same elements of insurance for the individual or family. In the Marketplace, nobody can be turned down for coverage and no insurance company can charge more for those individuals with expensive illnesses or medical conditions. They cannot discriminate between men and women such that they charge a woman more than a man if they are applying for the same coverage and have the same medical conditions.

Cracking Down on Policy Cancellations

The PPACA stops insurance companies from canceling an individual's coverage just because they made a mistake on their insurance application. This protection applies to all health plans for those who get coverage individually or through an employer. An insurance company can still cancel coverage, but it is only for instances where an individual places false or incomplete information on their application. In addition, the insurance company can cancel coverage due to lack of payment of the premiums. If the policy is to be cancelled, the insurance company will need to give at least 30 days' notice of a proposed cancellation. This way the individual can have enough time to obtain new coverage.

Doctor Choice and Out-of-Network Services

In the PPACA an individual has the right to choose the doctor that they want to care for them from the insurance companies list of network providers. The individual can also use an out-of-network emergency room provider without penalty. The selection of providers can be from any provider in the network and for services involving OB-GYN there is no need for a referral to visit this type of specialist. In the event of a need to visit an emergency room the individual will not need a prior approval to visit and they will not be required to pay a higher copayment or coinsurance if the individual goes to an emergency room that is not in network. It is always a safe option to check your plan restriction to make sure you understand all covered services and limitations.

Policy Lifetime and Yearly Limitations

The PPACA stops insurance companies from placing limits on coverage for both yearly benefits and lifetime benefits. For yearly benefits after January 1, 2014, insurance companies cannot put limitations on the individual for essential health benefits. For policies that are before January 1, 2014, plans can still set yearly limits such as $2 million dollars for coverage during a calendar year. For lifetime benefits, insurance companies can no longer place limits on what an individual can spend on essential health benefits during the time that they are enrolled in the plan.

Rate Review and the 80/20 Rule

The use of **Rate Review** and the 80/20 Rule are two ways that the PPACA can keep healthcare costs down. The rate review is where it protects individuals from excessive or unreasonable rate increases. If a rate increase is greater than 10 percent, the insurance company must publicly justify the rate increase before raising the premium.

The 80/20 Rule is where insurance companies are to spend at least 80 percent of the money that they take in through premiums and spend this on health care and quality improvement as opposed to overhead and administrative or marketing costs. This 80/20 Rule is also known as the **Medical Loss Ratio (MLR)**. In the instance where an insurance company is selling insurance to a group of greater than 50 individuals, then the amount that the insurance company needs to spend on healthcare costs and quality is 85 percent. If for any reason, the insurance plan does not meet the 80/20

Rule, then the insurance company may be required to issue a rebate to individuals or a reduction in future premiums.

Filing an Appeal

When an individual has payment for services denied, the individual patient can now appeal the decision of the insurance company by putting in writing an appeal questioning the decision of the insurance company. Once the insurance carrier receives the written appeal, they must then review their own decision to deny coverage and determine if this was done according to policy or not.

When an insurance company denies a claim they must notify the patient in writing the reason why the claim was denied, that the individual has a right to file an appeal, that the individual has the right to request an external review, and (if applicable) the availability of a Consumer Assistance Program to help the patient.

Summary of Benefits and Coverage

The Summary of Benefits and Coverage (SBC) will outline the following for the individual looking to purchase coverage (CMS, 2014):

- The insurance company will be listed at the top.
- The plan option will be listed at the top.
- The coverage period that this plan will cover.
- Who will be covered on the plan (individual, individual and spouse, family).
- The annual deductible per person and total for family.
- It will identify other deductibles for prescription drugs.
- It will identify any out-of-pocket expenses and the limits for these expenses (per person/family and if the individual uses a nonparticipating provider).
- What is not included in the out-of-pocket limits.
- It will identify what the annual plan limits are.
- Whether the plan uses a network of providers.
- Whether you need a referral for a specialist.
- Identify any services that the plan does not cover.
- Define copayments, coinsurance, allowed, deductible, and identify if the individual uses a participating provider it can lower deductibles, copayments, and coinsurance.
- Scenarios for costs if you visit a provider for care in the office or clinic.
- Scenarios for costs if you have a diagnostic test.

Insurance Company 1: Plan Option 1

Coverage Period: 01/01/2014 –12/31/2014

Summary of Benefits and Coverage: What this Plan Covers & What it Costs

Coverage for: Individual + Spouse | Plan Type: PPO

⚠️ **This is only a summary.** If you want more detail about your coverage and costs, you can get the complete terms in the policy or plan document at www.[insert] or by calling 1-800-[insert].

Important Questions	Answers	Why this Matters:
What is the overall deductible?	**$500** person / **$1,000** family Doesn't apply to preventive care	You must pay all the costs up to the **deductible** amount before this plan begins to pay for covered services you use. Check your policy or plan document to see when the **deductible** starts over (usually, but not always, January 1st). See the chart starting on page 2 for how much you pay for covered services after you meet the **deductible**.
Are there other deductibles for specific services?	Yes. **$300** for prescription drug coverage. There are no other specific **deductibles**.	You must pay all of the costs for these services up to the specific **deductible** amount before this plan begins to pay for these services.
Is there an out-of-pocket limit on my expenses?	Yes. For participating providers **$2,500** person / **$5,000** family For non-participating providers **$4,000** person / **$8,000** family	The **out-of-pocket limit** is the most you could pay during a coverage period (usually one year) for your share of the cost of covered services. This limit helps you plan for health care expenses.
What is not included in the out-of-pocket limit?	Premiums, balance-billed charges, and health care this plan doesn't cover.	Even though you pay these expenses, they don't count toward the **out-of-pocket limit**.
Is there an overall annual limit on what the plan pays?	No.	The chart starting on page 2 describes any limits on what the plan will pay for *specific* covered services, such as office visits.
Does this plan use a network of providers?	Yes. See www.[insert].com or call 1-800-[insert] for a list of participating providers.	If you use an in-network doctor or other health care **provider**, this plan will pay some or all of the costs of covered services. Be aware, your in-network doctor or hospital may use an out-of-network **provider** for some services. Plans use the term in-network, **preferred**, or participating for **providers** in their **network**. See the chart starting on page 2 for how this plan pays different kinds of **providers**.
Do I need a referral to see a specialist?	No. You don't need a referral to see a specialist.	You can see the **specialist** you choose without permission from this plan.
Are there services this plan doesn't cover?	Yes.	Some of the services this plan doesn't cover are listed on page 4. See your policy or plan document for additional information about **excluded services**.

Questions: Call 1-800-[insert] or visit us at www.[insert].
If you aren't clear about any of the underlined terms used in this form, see the Glossary. You can view the Glossary at www.[insert] or call 1-800-[insert] to request a copy.

OMB Control Numbers 1545-2229, 1210-0147, and 0938-1146

Released on April 23, 2013 (corrected)

1 of 8

August 18, 2014

FIGURE 5.4 Sample summary of benefits and coverage. *(continued)*

Insurance Company 1: Plan Option 1

Coverage Period: 01/01/2014 –12/31/2014

Summary of Benefits and Coverage: What this Plan Covers & What it Costs

Coverage for: Individual + Spouse | Plan Type: PPO

- **Copayments** are fixed dollar amounts (for example, $15) you pay for covered health care, usually when you receive the service.
- **Coinsurance** is *your* share of the costs of a covered service, calculated as a percent of the **allowed amount** for the service. For example, if the plan's **allowed amount** for an overnight hospital stay is $1,000, your **coinsurance** payment of 20% would be $200. This may change if you haven't met your **deductible**.
- The amount the plan pays for covered services is based on the **allowed amount**. If an out-of-network **provider** charges more than the **allowed amount**, you may have to pay the difference. For example, if an out-of-network hospital charges $1,500 for an overnight stay and the **allowed amount** is $1,000, you may have to pay the $500 difference. (This is called **balance billing**.)
- This plan may encourage you to use participating **providers** by charging you lower **deductibles**, **copayments** and **coinsurance** amounts.

Common Medical Event	Services You May Need	Your Cost If You Use a Participating Provider	Your Cost If You Use a Non-Participating Provider	Limitations & Exceptions
If you visit a health care provider's office or clinic	Primary care visit to treat an injury or illness	$35 copay/visit	40% coinsurance	——none——
	Specialist visit	$50 copay/visit	40% coinsurance	——none——
	Other practitioner office visit	20% coinsurance for chiropractor and acupuncture	40% coinsurance for chiropractor and acupuncture	——none——
	Preventive care/screening/immunization	No charge	40% coinsurance	
If you have a test	Diagnostic test (x-ray, blood work)	$10 copay/test	40% coinsurance	——none——
	Imaging (CT/PET scans, MRIs)	$50 copay/test	40% coinsurance	——none——

Questions: Call 1-800-[insert] or visit us at www.[insert].
If you aren't clear about any of the underlined terms used in this form, see the Glossary. You can view the Glossary at www.[insert] or call 1-800-[insert] to request a copy.

2 of 8

FIGURE 5.4 Sample summary of benefits and coverage. (*continued*)

Insurance Company 1: Plan Option 1

Coverage Period: 01/01/2014 –12/31/2014

Summary of Benefits and Coverage: What this Plan Covers & What it Costs

Coverage for: Individual + Spouse | **Plan Type:** PPO

Common Medical Event	Services You May Need	Your Cost If You Use a Participating Provider	Your Cost If You Use a Non-Participating Provider	Limitations & Exceptions
If you need drugs to treat your illness or condition More information about **prescription drug coverage** is available at www.[insert].	Generic drugs	$10 copay/ prescription (retail and mail order)	40% coinsurance	Covers up to a 30-day supply (retail prescription); 31-90 day supply (mail order prescription)
	Preferred brand drugs	20% coinsurance (retail and mail order)	40% coinsurance	——none——
	Non-preferred brand drugs	40% coinsurance (retail and mail order)	60% coinsurance	——none——
	Specialty drugs	50% coinsurance	70% coinsurance	——none——
If you have outpatient surgery	Facility fee(e.g., ambulatory surgery center)	20% coinsurance	40% coinsurance	——none——
	Physician/surgeon fees	20% coinsurance	40% coinsurance	——none——
If you need immediate medical attention	Emergency room services	20% coinsurance	20% coinsurance	——none——
	Emergency medical transportation	20% coinsurance	20% coinsurance	——none——
	Urgent care	20% coinsurance	40% coinsurance	——none——
If you have a hospital stay	Facility fee (e.g., hospital room)	20% coinsurance	40% coinsurance	——none——
	Physician/surgeon fee	20% coinsurance	40% coinsurance	——none——

Questions: Call 1-800-[insert] or visit us at www.[insert].
If you aren't clear about any of the underlined terms used in this form, see the Glossary. You can view the Glossary at www.[insert] or call 1-800-[insert] to request a copy.

FIGURE 5.4   Sample summary of benefits and coverage. *(continued)*

Insurance Company 1: Plan Option 1

Summary of Benefits and Coverage: What this Plan Covers & What it Costs

Coverage Period: 01/01/2014–12/31/2014

Coverage for: Individual + Spouse | Plan Type: PPO

Common Medical Event	Services You May Need	Your Cost If You Use a Participating Provider	Your Cost If You Use a Non-Participating Provider	Limitations & Exceptions
If you have mental health, behavioral health, or substance abuse needs	Mental/Behavioral health outpatient services	$35 copay/office visit and 20% coinsurance other outpatient services	40% coinsurance	—none—
	Mental/Behavioral health in patient services	20% coinsurance	40% coinsurance	—none—
	Substance use disorder outpatient services	$35 copay/office visit and 20% coinsurance other outpatient services	40% coinsurance	—none—
	Substance use disorder inpatient services	20% coinsurance	40% coinsurance	—none—
If you are pregnant	Prenatal and postnatal care	20% coinsurance	40% coinsurance	—none—
	Delivery and all inpatient services	20% coinsurance	40% coinsurance	—none—
If you need help recovering or have other special health needs	Home health care	20% coinsurance	40% coinsurance	—none—
	Rehabilitation services	20% coinsurance	40% coinsurance	—none—
	Habilitation services	20% coinsurance	40% coinsurance	—none—
	Skilled nursing care	20% coinsurance	40% coinsurance	—none—
	Durable medical equipment	20% coinsurance	40% coinsurance	—none—
	Hospice service	20% coinsurance	40% coinsurance	—none—
If your child needs dental or eye care	Eye exam	$35 copay/ visit	Not Covered	Limited to one exam per year
	Glasses	20% coinsurance	Not Covered	Limited to one pair of glasses per year
	Dental check-up	No Charge	Not Covered	Covers up to $50 per year

Questions: Call 1-800-[insert] or visit us at www.[insert].
If you aren't clear about any of the underlined terms used in this form, see the Glossary. You can view the Glossary at www.[insert] or call 1-800-[insert] to request a copy.

4 of 8

FIGURE 5.4 Sample summary of benefits and coverage. *(continued)*

Insurance Company 1: Plan Option 1

Coverage Period: 01/01/2014 –12/31/2014

Summary of Benefits and Coverage: What this Plan Covers &What it Costs   **Coverage for:** Individual + Spouse | **Plan Type:** PPO

Excluded Services & Other Covered Services:

Services Your Plan Does NOT Cover (This isn't a complete list. Check your policy or plan document for other **excluded services**.)

- Cosmetic surgery
- Dental care (Adult)
- Infertility treatment

- Long-term care
- Non-emergency care when traveling outside the U.S.
- Private-duty nursing

- Routine eye care (Adult)
- Routine foot care

Other Covered Services (This isn't a complete list. Check your policy or plan document for other covered services and your costs for these services.)

- Acupuncture (if prescribed for rehabilitation purposes)
- Bariatric surgery

- Chiropractic care
- Hearing aids

- Most coverage provided outside the United States. See www.[insert]
- Weight loss programs

Questions: Call1-800-[insert] or visit us at www.[insert].
If you aren't clear about any of the underlined terms used in this form, see the Glossary. You can view the Glossary at www.[insert] or call1-800-[insert] to request a copy.

5 of 8

FIGURE 5.4 Sample summary of benefits and coverage. (*continued*)

Insurance Company 1: Plan Option 1

Coverage Period: 01/01/2014 –12/31/2014

Summary of Benefits and Coverage: What this Plan Covers & What it Costs

Coverage for: Individual + Spouse | **Plan Type:** PPO

Your Rights to Continue Coverage:

** Individual health insurance sample –

Federal and State laws may provide protections that allow you to keep this health insurance coverage as long as you pay your **premium.** There are exceptions, how ever, such as if:

- You commit fraud
- The insurer stops offering services in the State
- You move outside the coverage area

For more information on your rights to continue coverage, contact the insurer at [contact number]. You may also contact your state insurance department at [insert applicable State Department of Insurance contact information].

OR

**Group health coverage sample –

If you lose coverage under the plan, then, depending upon the circumstances, Federal and State laws may provide protections that allow you to keep health coverage. Any such rights may be limited in duration and will require you to pay a **premium,** which may be significantly higher than the premium you pay while covered under the plan. Other limitations on your rights to continue coverage may also apply.

For more information on your rights to continue coverage, contact the plan at [contact number]. You may also contact your state insurance department, the U.S. Department of Labor, Employee Benefits Security Administration at 1-866-444-3272 or www.dol.gov/ebsa, or the U.S. Department of Health and Human Services at 1-877-267-2323 x61565 or www.cciio.cms.gov.

Your Grievance and Appeals Rights:

If you have a complaint or are dissatisfied with a denial of coverage for claims under your plan, you may be able to **appeal** or file a **grievance.** For questions about your rights, this notice, or assistance, you can contact: [insert applicable contact information from instructions].

Does this Coverage Provide Minimum Essential Coverage?

The Affordable Care Act requires most people to have health care coverage that qualifies as "minimum essential coverage." **This plan or policy [does/ does not] provide minimum essential coverage.**

Does this Coverage Meet the Minimum Value Standard?

The Affordable Care Act establishes a minimum value standard of benefits of a health plan. The minimum value standard is 60% (actuarial value). **This health coverage [does/does not] meet the minimum value standard for the benefits it provides.**

———————*To see examples of how this plan might cover costs for a sample medical situation, see the next page.*———————

Questions: Call 1-800-[insert] or visit us at www.[insert].
If you aren't clear about any of the underlined terms used in this form, see the Glossary. You can view the Glossary at www.[insert] or call 1-800-[insert] to request a copy.

6 of 8

FIGURE 5.4   Sample summary of benefits and coverage. *(continued)*

Insurance Company 1: Plan Option 1
Coverage Examples

Coverage Period: 1/1/2014 – 12/31/2014
Coverage for: Individual + Spouse | Plan Type: PPO

About these Coverage Examples:

These examples show how this plan might cover medical care in given situations. Use these examples to see, in general, how much financial protection a sample patient might get if they are covered under different plans.

This is not a cost estimator.

Don't use these examples to estimate your actual costs under this plan. The actual care you receive will be different from these examples, and the cost of that care will also be different.

See the next page for important information about these examples.

Having a baby
(normal delivery)

■ Amount owed to providers: $7,540
■ Plan pays $5,490
■ Patient pays $2,050

Sample care costs:

Hospital charges (mother)	$2,700
Routine obstetric care	$2,100
Hospital charges (baby)	$900
Anesthesia	$900
Laboratory tests	$500
Prescriptions	$200
Radiology	$200
Vaccines, other preventive	$40
Total	$7,540

Patient pays:

Deductibles	$700
Copays	$30
Coinsurance	$1320
Limits or exclusions	$0
Total	$2,050

Managing type 2 diabetes
(routine maintenance of a well-controlled condition)

■ Amount owed to providers: $5,400
■ Plan pays $3,520
■ Patient pays $1,880

Sample care costs:

Prescriptions	$2,900
Medical Equipment and Supplies	$1,300
Office Visits and Procedures	$700
Education	$300
Laboratory tests	$100
Vaccines, other preventive	$100
Total	$5,400

Patient pays:

Deductibles	$800
Copays	$500
Coinsurance	$500
Limits or exclusions	$80
Total	$1,880

Note: These numbers assume the patient is participating in our diabetes wellness program. If you have diabetes and do not participate in the wellness program, your costs may be higher. For more information about the diabetes wellness program, please contact: [insert].

Questions: Call 1-800-[insert] or visit us at www.[insert].
If you aren't clear about any of the underlined terms used in this form, see the Glossary. You can view the Glossary at www.[insert] or call 1-800-[insert] to request a copy.

FIGURE 5.4 Sample summary of benefits and coverage. (continued)

Reproduced from: Office of Management and Budget. Published April 23, 2013. Available at: https://www.cms.gov/...and.../sample-completed-sbc-accessible.pdf, accessed August 18, 2014

Insurance Company 1: Plan Option 1

Coverage Examples

Coverage Period: 1/1/2014–12/31/2014

Coverage for: Individual + Spouse | Plan Type: PPO

Questions and answers about the Coverage Examples:

What are some of the assumptions behind the Coverage Examples?

- Costs don't include **premiums.**
- Sample care costs are based on national averages supplied by the U.S. Department of Health and Human Services, and aren't specific to a particular geographic area or health plan.
- The patient's condition was not an excluded or preexisting condition.
- All services and treatments started and ended in the same coverage period.
- There are no other medical expenses for any member covered under this plan.
- Out-of-pocket expenses are based only on treating the condition in the example.
- The patient received all care from in-network **providers.** If the patient had received care from out-of-network **providers,** costs would have been higher.

What does a Coverage Example show?

For each treatment situation, the Coverage Example helps you see how **deductibles, copayments,** and **coinsurance** can add up. It also helps you see what expenses might be left up to you to pay because the service or treatment isn't covered or payment is limited.

Does the Coverage Example predict my own care needs?

✗ **No.** Treatments shown are just examples. The care you would receive for this condition could be different based on your doctor's advice, your age, how serious your condition is, and many other factors.

Does the Coverage Example predict my future expenses?

✗ **No.** Coverage Examples are **not** cost estimators. You can't use the examples to estimate costs for an actual condition. They are for comparative purposes only. Your own costs will be different depending on the care you receive, the prices your **providers** charge, and the reimbursement your health plan allows.

Can I use Coverage Examples to compare plans?

✓ **Yes.** When you look at the Summary of Benefits and Coverage for other plans, you'll find the same Coverage Examples. When you compare plans, check the "Patient Pays" box in each example. The smaller that number, the more coverage the plan provides.

Are there other costs I should consider when comparing plans?

✓ **Yes.** An important cost is the **premium** you pay. Generally, the lower your **premium,** the more you'll pay in out-of-pocket costs, such as **copayments, deductibles,** and **coinsurance.** You should also consider contributions to accounts such as health savings accounts (HSAs), flexible spending arrangements (FSAs) or health reimbursement accounts (HRAs) that help you pay your out-of-pocket expenses.

8 of 8

Questions: Call 1-800-[insert] or visit us at www.[insert].
If you aren't clear about any of the underlined terms used in this form, see the Glossary. You can view the Glossary at www.[insert] or call 1-800-[insert] to request a copy.

FIGURE 5.4 Sample summary of benefits and coverage. *(continued)*

- Scenarios for costs if you have a prescription filled.
- Scenarios for costs if you have outpatient surgery.
- Scenarios for costs if you have the need for immediate medical attention.
- Scenarios for cost if you have an inpatient hospital stay.
- Scenarios for cost if you utilize mental health benefits.
- Scenarios for cost if you are pregnant.
- Scenarios for cost for other special health needs.
- Coverage for eye exams and dental care.
- Services that are not covered.
- Your rights as a consumer.
- Appeal or grievance process.
- Provide coverage examples.
- Provide plan contact information.

■ Conclusion

PPACA is designed to ensure that all Americans have access to quality health care that is affordable and will ultimately reduce the costs that have been on the rise over the years. This is an important process as we learn the titles and implementation timeline. Changes will impact consumers of health care as well as insurers and it is of the utmost importance for the healthcare administrator to know the process and potential impacts to the healthcare facility or organization that he or she manages.

References

Centers for Medicare and Medicaid Services. (2014). Center for Consumer Information and Insurance Oversight. Retrieved from http://www.cms.gov/CCIIO/Resources/Forms-Reports-and-Other-Resources/Downloads/sample-completed-sbc-accessible.pdf

Democratic Policy and Communications Center. (2014). The Patient Protection and Affordable Care Act: detailed summary. Retrieved from http://www.dpc.senate.gov/healthreformbill/healthbill04.pdf

Department of Health and Human Services. (2010). Estimated effects of the "Patient Protection and Affordable Care Act," as amended, on the year of exhaustion for the part A trust fund, part B premiums, and part A and part B coinsurance amounts. Retrieved from https://www.cms.gov/Research-Statistics-Data-and-Systems/Research/ActuarialStudies/downloads/PPACA_Medicare_2010-04-22.pdf

Department of Health and Human Services. (2014a). HHS.gov/HealthCare: Read the law. Retrieved from http://www.hhs.gov/healthcare/rights/law/index.html

Department of Health and Human Services. (2014b). HHS.gov/HealthCare: Key features of the Affordable Care Act by year. Retrieved from http://www.hhs.gov/healthcare/facts/timeline/timeline-text.html

HealthCare.gov. (2014). What is the health insurance marketplace? Retrieved from https://www.healthcare.gov/what-is-the-health-insurance-marketplace/

6 Managed Care Organizations

Learning Outcomes

After reading this chapter, the student will be able to:

- Define the different types of managed care plans.
- Explain the differences between the various types of managed care plans.
- Identify and explain the cost controls utilized by managed care health plans.
- Explain the Contract Management and Financial Incentives tools used by managed care plans.
- Explain the functions of the National Committee for Quality Assurance (NCQA) and the impact that it has on driving the quality of care delivered by managed care organizations.
- Identify the purpose and goals of the Healthcare Effectiveness Data and Information Set (HEDIS) in measuring performance on important measures of care and services.
- Describe the components of Medicare Managed Care and how they impact the Medicare beneficiary.

■ Introduction

The purpose of **managed care** is to provide quality and affordable health care to the plan beneficiaries. Managed care looks at delivering health care to its members and takes into account the financial, administrative costs, and services, and combines this with a clinical approach focused on quality. In addition, managed care looks at managing the three critical parts of health care that are access, cost, and quality (Casto & Forrestal, 2013, p. 105).

Managed care is a generic term for prepaid health plans and ultimately the goal of the managed care organizations (MCOs) is to control the cost of health care that is delivered to the member and, at the same time, offer the services their members need and to manage the delivery of these services in a cost effective manner. The MCO will also manage the care that is provided to their members to ensure that the appropriate level of care is provided to the member and that the access to the most expensive levels of care are controlled and delivered as medically appropriate.

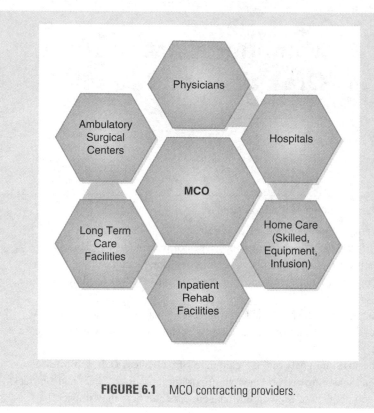

FIGURE 6.1 MCO contracting providers.

An MCO will contract with providers such as physicians, hospitals, homecare companies, durable medical equipment companies, inpatient rehabilitation facilities, long-term care, and ambulatory surgical centers just to name a few. In addition to contracting with these providers and facilities, the MCO will negotiate discounted rates that they will pay the providers for caring for their members.

There are several types of managed care plans such as Health Maintenance Organizations (HMOs), Preferred Provider Organizations (PPOs), Point of Service (POS), **Exclusive Provider Organizations (EPOs)**, and Integrated Delivery Systems (IDSs). Medicare and Medicaid both offer several managed care options to its enrollees such as the HMO, PPO, and POS. Moreover there are agencies that provide oversight to the managed care organizations which are the National Committee for Quality Assurance (NCQA) and the Healthcare Effectiveness Data and Information Set (HEDIS).

Health Maintenance Organization (HMO)

Preferred Provider Organization (PPO)

Point of Service (POS)

Exclusive Provider Organization (EPO)

Integrated Delivery System (IDS)

■ Health Maintenance Organizations

An HMO is a voluntary health plan that will provide healthcare services to its members in return for a monthly premium for their membership in the HMO. According to LaTour, "HMO Premiums are based on a projection of the costs that are likely to be involved in treating the plan's average enrollee over a specified period of time" (LaTour & Eichenwald Maki, 2013, p. 427).

HMOs usually only pay for care that takes place within their network. The patient will choose a primary care physician (PCP) who will act as a gatekeeper and coordinate all of the care provided to the patient. The PCP will ensure that the patient stays within the network of providers or the patient can potentially be responsible for payment. There are different types of HMOs and all have different characteristics, but the same goal of providing quality care along with managing cost and access.

Today, with much of the focus on health care surrounding access, cost, and quality, most employers offer some version of an HMO to their employees. This type of plan will benefit the employer in that they will realize cost savings as the employer, and the employee will realize cost savings in the form of out-of-pocket expenses as long as they stay within the plan's network. The premiums are generally lower than that of the traditional fee-for-service or point of service (POS) plans.

Group Model HMOs

Group Model HMOs are considered a closed panel where the physicians are not permitted to treat other managed care patients outside the managed care plan that they are contracted with. The group model HMO is where the HMO enters into an agreement with the physician group that is a multispecialty group that can provide medical services to the plan members. The group may provide services to other plan types that are not an HMO and they may agree to devote a specific percentage of the practice to serving the members of the managed care. In addition, there may be instances where the plan will own part of the practice.

Independent Practice Associations

An **Independent Practice Association (IPA)** operates as an HMO, but not like the group model, where they are limited in who they can treat. The IPA can treat patients from any managed care organization or other payer. The IPA is comprised of an organized group of physicians that get together to form the IPA, but they do not give up ownership of their individual practices. The group of practices that form the IPA will allow the IPA to serve as the intermediary during any contract or pricing negotiations with a payer (LaTour & Eichenwald Maki, 2013, p. 427).

The IPA will manage the payments from the payer and distribute the funds appropriately to each individual physician or practice. The IPA will negotiate the fees that the payer will reimburse for the services rendered to the patients of the insurance company. The practices still keep their physical locations and staff along with the day-to-day responsibility to run their practice and service the patients of the payers that they are contracted to serve.

Network Model HMOs

The **Network Model HMO** is similar to the group model HMO, but the network model HMO will contract with multiple multispecialty groups to provide care for their members. The members will be given a list of providers that they can see when they need care and the member must select a physician from the group to act as their primary care physician.

Staff Model HMOs

In a **Staff Model**, the HMO will directly employ the physicians and various other healthcare professionals to provide healthcare services to their members. The staff model HMO is a closed panel which means that the practice does not see any patients outside those of the HMO. Moreover, the patient pays their premiums to the HMO and the staff model HMO will provide all services for the members; any services that the staff model HMO does not provide, the patient will be provided by other facilities in the corporate network.

Preferred Provider Organizations

The **Preferred Provider Organization (PPO)** is considered to be a large group of hospitals and physicians that are under contract to service members of a managed care plan. Healthcare providers in the PPO provide services to the members for a prenegotiated fee. There are copayments that will apply to the patient for the services rendered by the PPO. Plan members who use providers not in the PPO will face higher

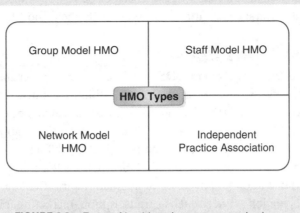

FIGURE 6.2   Types of health maintenance organizations.

out-of-pocket costs than if they were serviced by a provider in the PPO (Patient Advocate Foundation, 2014).

Point-of-Service Plan

The **Point-of-Service Plan** is similar to the HMO plans in that the subscriber must select a physician to be what is referred to as the primary care physician (PCP) for the patient. This type of plan is the fastest growing plan in the managed care marketplace and is the plan that gives the patient the most flexibility in choices for care. The patient, or consumer, can choose a provider in the network and have a reduced out-of-pocket or they can choose to go outside the plan and receive care and have a larger out-of-pocket expense (Patient Advocate Foundation, 2014).

The PCP is a physician that can be a family physician, pediatrician, internist, or obstetrician/gynecologist. The PCP will control access for the patient and guide them through the services that they may need to ensure that they are managing costs based on the plan guideline and network providers, and they ensure that appropriate, quality care is delivered to the patient (Patient Advocate Foundation, 2014).

Exclusive Provider Organizations

An **Exclusive Provider Organization (EPO)** is similar to the PPO, except that the patients enrolled in the plan are to receive healthcare services only from the EPO network providers. This is a closed plan and the patient cannot be reimbursed for care outside the network. The EPO requires that the member choose a PCP and the care must be coordinated by the PCP. In terms of being regulated, the EPOs are regulated by the state insurance department (LaTour & Eichenwald Maki, 2013, p. 428).

Integrated Delivery Systems

Integrated Delivery System (IDS) is a healthcare provider that furnishes coordinated healthcare services through a number of affiliated medical facilities. Most IDSs are comprised of multiple facilities that can provide care along the continuum of care for the patient and their family. They consist of physician's offices, ambulatory surgical centers, outpatient clinics, and acute care facilities. (LaTour & Eichenwald Maki, 2013, p. 428).

There are several models of IDS, such as Group Practices without Walls (GPWWs) that allows a physician to maintain their office individually but to share in business operation services such as transcription, marketing, billing, and other administrative functions and services. This process enables the practice to better function as a stronger group when it comes to negotiating managed care contracts.

The next IDS is Integrated Provider Organizations (IPOs). These groups manage the care delivered by multiple providers and multiple facilities. The IPO will generally provide the full spectrum of care from physician services, acute care, ambulatory care services, and services of a skilled nursing facility. These organizations are sometimes considered or referred to as health delivery networks and integrated service networks.

The next type is the Physician-Hospital Organization (PHO), and this type of organization is one that provides healthcare services through a contractual arrangement between a hospital or hospitals and a physician or multiple physicians. This type of entity gives them a unified front when negotiating with a managed care or other type of insurance company in that all of the parties involved are viewed as one entity.

Lastly, there are Management Service Organizations (MSOs) that are there to support multiple practices in the administrative and support functions that they need to operate. The difference here is that there is one entity that handles medical records, release of information, billing, general office staff, registration, and other administrative functions.

■ Managed Care Cost Controls

There are several ways that managed care plans will look to contain costs, all while maintaining quality. These include service management tools, reimbursement tools, and financial incentives to the providers. The reimbursement mechanism that focuses on cost reduction for the MCO is episode-of-care reimbursement. The financial incentives are found both on the provider side and the patient side of the care delivered.

Medical Necessity

The American College of Medical Quality has defined medical necessity as "accepted healthcare services and supplies provided by healthcare entities, appropriate to the evaluation and treatment of a disease, condition, illness or injury and consistent with applicable standard of care" (ACMQ, 2010, p. 1). These cost controls are designed to control costs along with monitoring the use of healthcare services by balancing the level of need with the level of treatment.

Utilization Review

Utilization Management is defined as "the evaluation of the medical necessity, appropriateness, and efficiency of the use of healthcare services, procedures, and facilitates these under the provisions of the applicable health benefits plan" (URAC, 2014).

Utilization Management, sometimes called **Utilization Review** (UR), is responsible "for the day-to-day provisions of the hospital's utilization plan as required by the Medicare Conditions of Participation (LaTour & Eichenwald Maki, 2013, p. 464).

The UR personnel are required to perform a review of the medical record and use this information to make a decision based on UR. They must apply all criteria objectively for admission, during the stay, and discharge readiness; provide around the clock all services needed in the UR field; review all patients medical records within 24 hours of being placed in an inpatient bed; screen and coordinate elective and emergency admissions, transfers, outpatient observation beds, and any conversions; and provide UR services to all admissions regardless of the payer that the patient has. They are also required to review on a scheduled basis all continued stays/admissions; screen for the timeliness and appropriateness of all hospital services; meet weekly on all complex or high-dollar cases; and complete all retrospective or focused reviews as directed (LaTour & Eichenwald Maki, 2013, p. 464).

Primary Care Physician as a Gatekeeper

A Primary Care Physician (PCP) in a **gatekeeper** role is defined as "a primary care physician who controls a patient's access to certain tests, treatments, and specialty physicians in a managed care plan (Patient Advocate Foundation, 2014).

This access will revolve around a PCP determining if a referral is warranted for medical specialists, diagnostic or therapeutic sites, or referrals to hospitals. This will also include determining if the level of healthcare personnel or the healthcare setting is appropriate for the patient in the continuum of care.

Prior Authorization

A Prior Authorization (PA) is also considered a cost control measure for the MCOs. This process is where a healthcare provider will have to follow an administrative process to obtain a PA for a procedure, test, or hospital stay prior to the services being rendered to the patient. The need for a PA can include a visit to a specialist, an elective procedure, an expensive procedure, a sophisticated procedure, expensive diagnostic test, or for services such as mental health. The MCO will assign a PA number to the case and the provider must submit their claim referencing the PA given by the payer. Even if a PA is obtained by a healthcare provider, this is not a guarantee of payment. Each healthcare policy may be different, and the provider must research the patient's policy requirements or limitations to determine what procedures need a PA and which ones do not need a PA.

Case Management

Case Management is defined by the Case Management Society of America as "a collaborative process of assessment, planning, facilitation, care coordination, evaluation, and advocacy for options and services to meet an individual's and family's comprehensive health needs through communication and available resources to promote quality, cost-effective outcomes" (CMSA, 2014).

The Case Manager helps the patient to identify appropriate providers that fit the patient's needs and to make sure that the provider fits the patient's insurance company provider listing to ensure the continuum of care for the patient is uninterrupted by having to change providers as one may not be in network or accept the payer that the patient is a member with currently. Generally, the highest-cost beneficiaries tend to have an inpatient hospital admission during the year that results from a lack of early diagnosis, noncompliance to treatment recommendations, or postacute hospital care not meeting the patient's needs. This type of intervention has been proven to have successfully reduced costs in patients with conditions such as congestive heart failure (CHF) (Schore et al, 1999, p. 87).

The overall goal of the case manager is to improve quality, provide access to care and services, all the while balancing the needs of the patient and the payer to find the optimum situation for all. Today's case manager role has evolved to include partnering with physicians during rounds and participating in treatment plan progress reporting, questioning duplicate services that are not in line with evidence-based protocols, collaborating with other nurses to identify any obstacles to keep the treatment plan moving forward, initiating communication between primary care physicians and consultative physicians, advocating for the patient and family, and initiating the planning discussion for transitioning the patient from one level of care to the next (LaTour & Eichenwald Maki, 2013, p. 464).

The case manager is charged with coordinating care between the current place of care to the next place of care, keeping in mind the needs of the patient and family, all the while balancing those needs with the clinical team involved and the payer guidelines. The case manager looks to expedite all parts of the care process to make sure that there are no delays in care, delays in discharge, delays in admission to the next provider or facility, and no delays to the patient receiving the necessary treatment to continue progressing in their healing or management of symptoms.

Prescription Management

A prescription **formulary**, as part of **prescription management**, can be used as a cost control measure to manage a patient's prescriptions. This formulary is a means for the patient to share in the costs of medications, but it is not only a means of cost control; it is a comprehensive approach that includes patient education, electronic screening, alerts for drug interactions, and decision support tools along with criteria for drug utilization. Some systems include electronic transmission of the patient's medication order to their pharmacy that eliminates the need for paper prescriptions, faxes, or calling in prescriptions to the patient's pharmacy in most instances. Moreover, the prescription formulary is a way to manage the dispensing of medications from generic to name-brand medications that can be a way to enhance quality, reduce costs for both the plan and the patient, all the while focusing on safety and quality outcomes for the patient (Casto & Forrestal, 2013, p. 110).

Prescription Benefit Managers

There are specialty management organizations, or **Prescription Benefit Managers (PBMs)**, and they administer the prescription portion of health benefit plans. These PBMs administer developing and managing formularies, negotiating contracts with drug manufacturers that includes discounts and rebates, managing prior authorization and drug utilization, processing claims for payment, analyzing claims data, and mail-order pharmacy operations (Casto & Forrestal, 2013, p. 110).

◾ Contract Management and Financial Incentives

Episode-of-Care Payment Method

This payment mechanism referred to as Episode-of-Care (EOC) payment, or sometimes called a bundled payment, is a method that involves making a lump sum payment to healthcare providers to cover all services that were delivered to a patient for a specific illness that was treated during a specific period of time. These payments will cover all services that were provided by one or multiple providers during the care for the patient for the specified period. EOC includes payment methods such as **capitation** and global payment.

Capitation

This type of payment is not based on a specific procedure or hospital stay, as it is based on a per-member-per-month (PMPM) methodology. In the managed care environment, the plan will negotiate with a large group, employer, or a government agency and contracts to cover the agreed upon population and provide all contracted services listed in the agreement for a set monthly fee per member. This fee will be payable by the group that the managed care organization contracts with and this contract will generally last for a specified period of time. The details of the contract will specifically outline what services and products that the MCO will have to provide to the member and the price that the group will have to pay on a PMPM basis. The group will pay the monthly premium, no matter the amount of contracted services that were utilized during the month and then the MCO will pay the providers that actually provide the services to the patients. In some instances, the MCO assumes all the risk, and in other instances the risk is shared with the PCPs who are acting as gatekeepers for the plan (LaTour & Eichenwald Maki, 2013, p. 430).

Global Payment

The global payment methodology can be applied to procedures that are associated with technical components. This global payment is a lump-sum payment that can be distributed among all the physicians who either performed the procedure or interpreted the results of the procedure. There is a professional component and a technical component in the procedure. The professional component is provided by the physician and the technical component is the portion of the procedure that involves supplies or equipment (LaTour & Eichenwald Maki, 2013, p. 430).

Financial Incentives

Financial incentives are designed to work for both providers and members. In addition, they can be a positive incentive or a negative incentive. Positive incentives are for when physicians meet targets that surround cost efficiency such as managing the referrals to specialists, the use of laboratory and other ancillary services, inpatient admissions, setting of care, physician productivity, and the use of pharmaceuticals. In these instances a provider may receive an incentive for meeting cost targets, and on the other hand, a negative incentive or penalty. For a negative incentive, it may include a reduction in the PCP's salary for not meeting the cost targets. In addition, the PCP may realize a loss in the contingency reserves called a "withhold," or a part of a provider's salary or capitation payment that is held in reserve and if they meet the productivity, or costs management associated with referrals to specialists, they will be paid the withhold amount that was taken from the provider's capitated payment (LaTour & Eichenwald Maki, 2013, p. 111).

The financial incentives for members of the plan can include different rates of cost sharing. In a positive example, the member will experience a lower amount of out-of-pocket expenses if they stay in the network and follow the prescription formulary and go with generics versus brand prescriptions. Where the incentive can go to the negative is when a patient decides to go out of network for care or insists on using a brand prescription when a suitable generic is available. In this example, the patient's out-of-pocket expense will be far greater than if they stayed in network or selected to use a generic drug (LaTour & Eichenwald Maki, 2013, p. 111).

Contract Management

Contract management is a very important part of the episode-of-care payment method and it requires that the providers of care, along with the plans, have to be as precise as possible in projecting expenditures in order to negotiate a contract that will cover the costs involved in treating the members of the plan. In this scenario, if a plan or provider underestimates the utilization for the population they are serving, the outcome will be a negative one, in that the utilization will be higher than the projected and the plan or provider loses money. Once a contract is established, there needs to be constant monitoring of costs and evaluation of the utilization of its members, and if there are variances to the projections there needs to be adjustments or corrective measures in a timely manner (LaTour & Eichenwald Maki, 2013, p. 111).

■ National Committee for Quality Assurance

The **National Committee for Quality Assurance (NCQA)** is an accrediting entity as identified by the Department of Health and Human Services (HHS) for Qualified Health Plan. NCQA is a private, not-for-profit organization that focuses on accreditation, certification, and recognition of health plans and reports on the overall quality of managed care plans in the United States.

The NCQA provides accreditation programs for health plans that cover various disciplines such as health plan accreditation for interim, first, and renewal accreditation and provide flexible programs for the health plans to follow working towards accreditation. They also offer disease management that covers patients with asthma, diabetes, chronic obstructive disease (COPD), heart failure, and ischemic vascular disease (IVD). For **case management**, NCQA offers a program that addresses how case management is delivered while looking at the coordination and quality of care delivered. A new program at NCQA is wellness and health promotion and this accreditation uses evidence-based standards to assess how wellness programs are implemented in the workplace and the coaching provided to the members along with protection of private health information (PHI). There is an accreditation process for new health plans that entails on-site and off-site evaluations and the program has demonstrated that accredited plans deliver greater value through improved quality care for the patient. Another new program offered by the NCQA is Managed Behavioral Healthcare Organization Accreditation. This program focuses on care coordination to reduce fragmented care, complex case management, and data exchange between health plans and behavioral healthcare organizations. Finally, the NCQA offers programs for provider organizations such as Accountable Care Organizations.

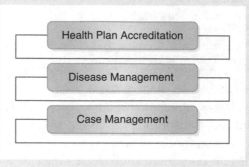

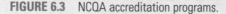

FIGURE 6.3   NCQA accreditation programs.

Secondly, the NCQA offers certification programs that are a subset of the accreditation product that they offer and these programs focus on the organizations that provide a specialty or a more specific line of care and not the comprehensive programs that other organizations provide. They consist of on-site and off-site evaluations conducted by people that are considered experts in the field that they are surveying. In addition, they use physicians when appropriate in this process. These certifications include such programs as Credentials Verifications Organizations, Disease Management, Health Information Products, Multicultural Health Care, Physician and Hospital Quality, PCMH Content Expert Certification, Utilization Management and Credentialing, Wellness and Health Promotion, and Accreditation Users Group.

EXHIBIT 6-2   NCQA CERTIFICATION PROGRAMS

Credentials Verifications Organizations

Disease Management

Health Information Products

Multicultural Health Care

Physician and Hospital Quality

PCMH Content Expert Certification

Utilization Management and Credentialing

Wellness and Health Promotion

Accreditation Users Group

Finally, the NCQA offers Recognition Programs that focus on the employers, health plans, patients, and consumers to allow them to make informed healthcare decisions based on quality (NCQA 2014a). The first program is Research and Industry Resources which provides research articles and other support for NCQA Recognition Programs. The second program is Patient-Centered Specialty Practice Recognition that recognizes specialty practices that have coordinated care with other primary care practices and that provide timely access to care along with continuous quality improvement. The third program is **Patient-Centered Medical Home**, which recognizes clinical practices that are functioning in the patient-centered mode. The fourth program is the Government Recognition Initiative that works with government agencies that utilize a Patient-Centered Medical Home model in their delivery model. The fifth program is the Diabetes Recognition Program that recognizes clinicians that provide high-quality care to the patients they serve that have diabetes. The sixth program is the Heart/Stroke Recognition Program that recognizes those that give high-quality care to patients that have suffered a stroke or who have heart conditions. The seventh program is Physician Practice Connections that recognizes physician practices that use up-to-date information systems with the goal of providing quality patient care. The last program is the Back Pain Recognition Program that looks at those practices with a patient-centered approach and that delivers care through utilizing evidence-based guidelines (NCQA, 2014).

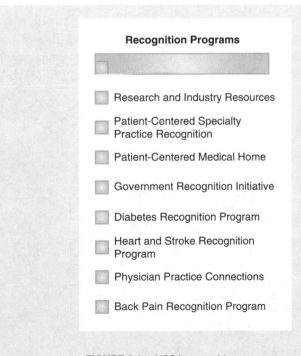

FIGURE 6.4 NCQA recognition programs.

■ Healthcare Effectiveness Data and Information Set

The **Healthcare Effectiveness Data and Information Set (HEDIS)** was originally developed by National Committee for Quality Assurance (NCQA) along with a group of various health plans and employers. One of the main ideas with the development of HEDIS was to allow employers to see what they are getting for their healthcare dollars. The Health Care Financing Administration (HCFA) "contracted with the NCQA to develop a database of HEDIS measures that would be used to measure the performance of the Medicare Program" (Lied & Sheingold, 2001, p. 150).

With regards to measures the Centers for Medicare and Medicaid Services "arguably has the most comprehensive health-related performance measurement database in the world to support its Managed Care Program. This system can support policy development, monitor and enforce contract standards, inform beneficiaries about their choices, and guide targeted quality improvement efforts" (Lied & Sheingold, 2001, p. 149).

It is felt that performance measures alone will contribute to improved outcomes for patients. The NCQA found in 1999 that managed care plans that consistently monitored quality demonstrated significant improvements in quality. Moreover, NCQA "also found that plans that have the most satisfied members continually score high on clinical quality" (Lied & Sheingold, 2001, p. 149).

Overall, HEDIS will have targeted goals of helping beneficiaries make informed choices with regards to choosing a managed care plan, improving managed care's quality of care, allowing not only the consumer, but government and other payers to make informed purchasing decisions (LaTour & Eichenwald Maki, 2013, p. 427).

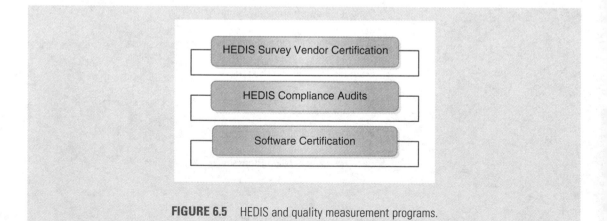

FIGURE 6.5   HEDIS and quality measurement programs.

■ Medicare Managed Care

The Balanced Budget Act of 1997 created the Medicare Part C or **Medicare Managed Care**. Then the plan changed its name to Medicare+Choice (M+C) in 1999. CMS is able to contract with private or public organizations to offer various health plans to their beneficiaries that include traditional insurance and managed care plans. There were four types of M+C plans that were authorized under Medicare Part C. The first plan was called the Coordinated Care Plans. The second plan was the Medicare Medical Savings Account (MSA) plan. The third plan was the Private Fee-For-Service (PFFS) plan. And finally, the fourth plan was the Religious Fraternal Benefit (RFB) plan.

In 2003, the M+C program was added to the Medicare Advantage (MA) Program which was part of the Medicare Prescription Drug, Improvement, and Modernization Act of 2003 (MMA). The MMA updated and improved the types of plans that beneficiaries could choose from and how the benefits and payments were made under the program. This change made it possible for the beneficiaries to choose from other plan options. These options included such plans as the Regional PPO (RPPO) plans and Special Needs Plans (SNPs). In addition to all of this with MA, the Medicare Part D plan was established to cover prescription drugs for Medicare beneficiaries.

The MA plan is established by using the competitive process of bidding by various MA organizations that offer the plan. The MA organizations submit an annual aggregate bid for each MA plan; this bid is based on the estimate of the costs for the upcoming year to provide healthcare benefits in the area that they cover. The bid includes all services that are considered to be nondrug-related benefits. The goal is to make sure that the MA organizations offer benefit packages that meet the needs of the beneficiaries and, that this information regarding the plan and its benefits are made available to the public so as they can make an informed decision on the plan that will best fit their coverage needs (CMS, 2011, p. 3).

Through this process, the MA organizations are encouraged to provide a variety of high quality benefits at a reduced cost to Medicare beneficiaries along with constantly striving to improve the benefits offered, reduce the premiums to the beneficiary, and to improve their provider networks that will allow the plan to achieve the goal of gaining or retaining market share of the plan. Another area of focus is to make sure that the MA organization offers an integrated delivery model that includes disease prevention, disease management, and other coordinated services (CMS, 2011, p. 4).

■ Coordinated Care Plan

A **Coordinated Care Plan (CCP)** includes a network of providers that are under a contractual arrangement to deliver the benefit package that is approved by CMS. CMS must approve the network, and this is done to ensure that all applicable requirements are met for access, cost, and quality. CCPs can use various mechanisms to help control utilization that are similar to the ones that MCOs use such as requiring referrals, the use of gatekeepers to manage the flow of services for the patient, and the use of financial arrangements that offer incentives and penalties to ensure that cost-effective and high-quality care is ultimately provided to the beneficiary. CCPs include plans similar to the ones that are offered by many preferred provider organizations, health maintenance organizations, and various senior housing facilities (CMS, 2011, p. 5).

Health Maintenance Organization

A **Health Maintenance Organization (HMO)** is generally a more restrictive model than the others offered as it controls utilization through the use of referrals from the primary care practitioner (PCP) and restricts the patient's access to a network of providers to receive routine, nonurgent, or emergency services. The HMO may offer a **Point of Service Plan (POS)** to its beneficiaries that will allow them to utilize services from providers that are outside the network. In the POS plan, the beneficiary must get a referral or prior authorization before receiving services from the provider and they may experience a larger out-of-pocket expense than if they were utilizing services from a network provider.

Preferred Provider Organization

A **Preferred Provider Organization (PPO)** is a plan that is not licensed as an HMO under state law and has providers under contract to provide services for the covered benefits offered by the plan. In addition, the PPO must provide for reimbursement for all covered benefits both in-network and out-of-network.

There are local PPOs that will cover county, partial county, and multiple county service areas and regional PPOs that cover expanded areas to provide access to beneficiaries in rural areas. The RPPOs are risk-bearing entities that can offer both health insurance and health benefits coverage within their region. A RPPO can operate in multiple states, and each health plan must hold a state license in the state in which it is doing business and meet all applicable Medicare requirements (CMS, 2011, p. 12).

■ Special Needs Plans

Special Needs Plans (SNPs) are a Medicare Advantage coordinated care plan that meets all the requirements for CMS and offers a Part D plan for prescriptions. In addition, has an approval to operate as an SNP. The SNPs will target a specific population, or special needs individuals, that include institutionalized individuals and other high-risk groups of individuals who have one or more disabling chronic conditions that are specified by CMS and their enrollment in this plan will be beneficial to them for their care.

According to CMS, there are three categories that are related to targeted populations and they are Chronic Conditions SNPs (S-SNPs) that are designed for beneficiaries with severe or disabling chronic conditions that would benefit from enrollment in a coordinated plan of care. Second, there is a dual-eligible SNPs (D-SNPs) that are for beneficiaries entitled to Medical Assistance under both Medicare and a state's Medicaid program. And finally, an institutionalized SNP (I-SNP) is one that serves beneficiaries who reside, or are scheduled to reside, in a long-term care facility for 90 days or longer (CMS, 2011, p. 13).

An institutionalized individual is defined at 42 DFR 422.2 "as an individual residing or expected to reside for 90 days or longer in a **skilled nursing facility** (SNF), nursing facility (NF), SNF/NF, intermediate care facility for the mentally retarded (ICF/MR), or inpatient psychiatric facility (IPF)" (CMS, 2011, p. 13).

■ Senior Housing Facility Plans

The Affordable Care Act established **Senior Housing Facility Plans** that limit enrollment to residents of Continuing Care Retirement Communities and are receiving health-related services under an agreement that is in place for a specified period or the life of the enrollee. In addition, the facility will need to provide primary care services on-site and supply transportation services for the beneficiaries to receive services outside of the facility.

■ Medical Savings Account Plans

Medicare Medical Savings Account (MSA) Plans combine a high-deductible MA plan and a medical savings account that is used to pay for qualified medical expenses for the account holder. The MSA plan pays for services that an enrollee has incurred that are countable expenses that are equal to the annual deductible of the plan. The MSA account is a custodial account that is established for the purposes of paying for qualified expenses of the account holder. The funds come from contributions from CMS under the MA program or from a rollover from another MA MSA of the same account holder. The money that CMS will pay into the account can be used for their health care before the high deductible is reached. At the time the deductible is met, the MA is responsible for payment of expenses related to covered services. The maximum annual deductible is set by law and updated annually (CMS, 2011, p. 14).

■ Private Fee-for-Service Plans

A **Private Fee-for-Service (PFFS)** plan is a MA plan that provides on a fee-for-service basis without placing the provider at risk, and the rates are not subject to vary based on utilization, and does not restrict enrollees' choices of providers that are authorized to provide services and accept the plan's payment terms and conditions. Although a PFFS plan is not permitted to vary the payment rates based on utilization, the PFFS can vary the reimbursement rates based on the type of provider, specialty, or location. The freedom of the PFFS plan allows the beneficiary to see any provider, in a physician setting or hospital setting, anywhere in the country and if the provider agrees to accept the plan's reimbursement then the provider is an eligible provider. This process can take place each time the provider sees a PFFS member (CMS, 2011, p. 15).

Employer Group Health Plan

An **Employer Group Health Plan (EGHP)** is a group plan that is sponsored by an employer or labor organization. The employers and unions can sponsor a group plan by enrolling their members in one of three plan (EGHP) options. First, they may enroll their members in a Medicare plan that is open to general enrollment, or an employer or union-only group waiver plan (EGWP) where the enrollment is restricted to individuals that are beneficiaries or participants in the employer or union-sponsored group plan (CMS, 2011, p. 5).

■ Religious Fraternal Benefit Plans

The **Religious Fraternal Benefit (RFB)** plans are MA plans that are offered to a society that is a religious fraternal society. The enrollment is limited to only the members of the RFB society. An RFB is a society that is described in the Internal Revenue Code of 1986 and is exempt from taxation under that act and is affiliated with and carries out the tenets of and shares a religious bond with the church, convention, association, or affiliated group of churches and may have a MA plan that is a PFFS, MSA, or CCP.

■ Conclusion

This chapter defines what managed care organizations are and the types of managed care programs that are used in our healthcare delivery system. The healthcare administrator needs to understand, at the highest level possible, the different type of payment models that managed care uses. If the administrator does not understand these models, the facility can experience negative financial outcomes. Moreover, the healthcare professional needs to better understand the entities that oversee the managed care organizations such as NCQA and HEDIS. Understanding these components will supply the healthcare professional with the necessary tools to fully understand one of the major payer systems that impact their facility. To go along with this, being able to navigate through the cost controls will also help in facilitating, not only better financial outcomes, but a better delivery model that can increase quality for the patient. Moreover, as a consumer, and as well as an administrator, it is helpful to understand the different health plans and how they cover the different populations that are served. Summarizing the relationship between the MCO and the facility, the administrator must remember that managed care is complex and is an important model for healthcare administrators to understand and the more knowledge they have of this type of coverage, the better they can run their healthcare organization from the patient care side, the cost management side, the contract management side, and the quality outcomes side, all of which impacts the profitability side of the healthcare organization.

References

American College of Medical Quality. (2010). Policy 8: Definition and application of medical necessity. Retrieved from http://www.acmq.org/policies/policy8.pdf

Case Management Society of America. (2014). What is a case manager? Retrieved from http://www.cmsa.org/Home/CMSA/WhatisaCaseManager/tabid/224/Default.aspx

Casto, A.B., & Forrestal, E. (2013). *Principles of healthcare reimbursement* (4th ed.). Chicago: AHIMA.

Centers for Medicare and Medicaid Services. (2011a). *Medicare managed care manual.* Retrieved from http://www.cms.gov/Regulations-and-Guidance/Guidance/Manuals/downloads/mc86c01.pdf

LaTour, K.M., & Eichenwald Maki, S. (2013). *Health information management; Concepts, principles, and practice* (4th ed.). Chicago: AHIMA.

Lied, T. R., & Sheingold, S. (2001). HEDIS performance trends in Medicare managed care. *Health Care Financing Review* 23(1). Retrieved from http://www.cms.gov/Research-Statistics-Data-and-Systems/Research/HealthCareFinancingReview/downloads/01fallpg149.pdf

Medicare Learning Network. (2012). *Medicare fraud & abuse: Prevention, detection, and reporting.* Retrieved from http://www.cms.gov/Outreach-and-Education/Medicare-Learning-Network-MLN/MLNProducts/downloads/Fraud_and_Abuse.pdf

NCQA. (2014). Recognition. Retrieved from http://www.ncqa.org/Programs/Recognition.aspx

Patient Advocate Foundation. (2014). Managed care glossary. Retrieved from http://www.patientadvocate.org/index.php?p=384

Schore, J.L., Brown, R.S., & Cheh, V.A. (1999). Case management for high-cost Medicare beneficiaries. *Health Care Financing Review* 20(4). Retrieved from https://www.cms.gov/Research-Statistics-Data-and-Systems/Research/HealthCareFinancingReview/downloads/99summerpg87.pdf

URAC. (2014). About URAC. Retrieved from https://www.urac.org/about-urac/about-urac/

7 | Medicare Prospective Payment Systems

Learning Outcomes

After reading this chapter, the student will be able to:

- Explain the history of Medicare and the prospective payment systems that are in use today.
- Define the key elements of prospective payment and the impact on the health care at a facility.
- Differentiate the Medicare coverage for acute care, rehabilitation, and psychiatric care.
- Define the components, process, and impact of the MS-DRG on healthcare systems related to the coding and billing process in a healthcare facility.
- Define HIPPS and the impact on healthcare facilities today and going forward.

■ Introduction

Medicare prospective payment has a huge impact on the delivery and reimbursement for health care. The plan covers specific populations. The development of Medicare Severity DRGs (MS-DRG) has further defined the reimbursement process for acute care facilities. This chapter will cover the acute care arena, where there are a variety of factors to consider with regard to reimbursement and prospective payment. This includes high cost outliers to help capture additional revenues that are over and above the established threshold amount. It also includes indirect medical education for the facilities that are an educational facility. We will cover transfer cases for patients that start off in an acute care setting and then move to another acute care setting or nonacute setting. Also included in this chapter are billing of transplant services; rehabilitation and psychiatric settings are also further defined in this chapter. Finally we will cover the Health Insurance Prospective Payment System (HIPPS). Medicare is a complex yet vital program for not only the population that they cover but the facilities that service this covered population.

Overall, prospective payment shifts the responsibility of profit or loss from the insurance carrier to the healthcare provider. With the prospective payment system developing payment for cases based on averages and grouping patients in like resource groups, the healthcare facility is now more than ever responsible for making a profit based on averages and managing the care to deliver the highest quality possible to the patient.

History of Prospective Payment Systems

Over the years, Medicare expenditures have been on the rise. The reason for this is that in the past, Medicare and other payers have reimbursed providers in a retrospective cost-based reimbursement environment. In this payment structure, the provider was paid interim payments throughout the fiscal year. At the end of the year, the hospital would file a cost report, and the payments made during the year were reconciled with the allowable costs. This was done by using the cost-to-charge ratio to bring the number down to an allowable figure. Under this payment system the costs for the Medicare program increased from $3 billion in 1967 to $37 billion annually in 1983 (CMS, 2001, p. 3).

In 1982 the United States Congress required the creation of a **prospective payment system (PPS)** to be developed with the focus on controlling costs. There were several states that were implementing the PPS model and they decided to go with the New Jersey PPS mode (CMS, 2001, p. 3). This DRG system was created at Yale University in the late 1960s through the early 1970s and the system was designed to monitor the quality, care, and use of services in a hospital setting (Casto & Forrestal, 2013, p. 126). The Prospective Payment System (PPS) was implemented in 1983 as part of the Public Law 98-21. The PPS model is designed to reimburse a hospital an amount based on Diagnosis Related Groups (DRG) that would be assigned to each patient based on their diagnosis at the time of discharge (LaTour & Eichenwald Maki, 2013, p. 16). This system is a per-case reimbursement mechanism and Medicare pays hospitals a flat rate per case for inpatient hospital care. In addition, the DRG was based on relating the type of patients a hospital treats or by the Case Mix Index (Averill et al., 2001, p. 83). The result of using the DRG system was that it puts the responsibility for profit or loss entirely on the hospital where the efficient hospitals are rewarded and the inefficient hospitals are incentivized to become more efficient (CMS, 2001, p. 3).

Congress had four chief objectives in creating the PPS, according to CMS, which were ensure fair compensation for services rendered and not compromise access, update payment rates that would account for new medical technology and inflation, monitor the quality of hospital services, and provide a mechanism to handle complaints (CMS, 2001, p. 5).

The overall concept of PPS was to make sure that payment rates were established in advance and they would be fixed for the FY in which they apply, payment rates were not automatically determined by the hospital's past or current cost, payment rates are considered to be payment in full, and the hospital retains the profit or suffers the loss as a result from the difference between the payment and the cost for the admission (Casto & Forrestal, 2013, p. 126).

All information pertaining to inpatient and outpatient payment systems is posted in the *Federal Register*. Published every federal working day, the *Federal Register* is the official journal of the U.S. government. According to Casto & Forrestal (2013), it contains rules, regulations, and legal notices of federal administrative agencies, of departments of the executive branch, and of the president. The contents are organized alphabetically by agency and all notices regarding federal payment systems are listed under Centers for Medicare and Medicaid Services (CMS) (Casto & Forrestal, 2013, p. 125). All proposed changes are publicized in advance through a process called Notice of Proposed Rulemaking (NPRM). Once these proposed changes are posted there is a comment period and at the close of this the final rule will be published. All comments will be analyzed and posted along with the final rule.

■ Acute Care Prospective Payment System

This Inpatient Prospective Payment System (IPPS) is designed for an acute care inpatient setting and the single payment does not include payment for any professional services that are provided during the patient's hospital stay. From 1966 until 1983, all hospital inpatient claims that were submitted to Medicare were paid based on the cost of services. Then the first large-scale application of the DRGs was done by the New Jersey State Department of Health to reimburse hospitals a fixed rate based on a specific DRG for each patient treated. Then in 1982, the Tax Equity and Fiscal Responsibility Act (TEFRA) modified the section 223 Medicare hospital reimbursement limits to include a case-mix adjustment based on DRGs, and in 1983 Congress amended the Social Security Act to include a national DRG-based hospital PPS for all Medicare patients (Averill et al., 2001, p. 83).

Under the IPPS, each patient admission is assigned a DRG upon discharge. The weight assigned to it that is based on the average amount of resources used in treating the patient during their stay. The payment is then divided up into a labor-related and nonlabor-related share. The labor share is adjusted by a variable called the wage index (CMS, 2013d). The wage index is the ratio that reflects the average salary level that is applicable to the area where the healthcare organization is located versus the national average for that particular healthcare setting. There are several other types of adjustments in calculating payment in the prospective payment model. The first one is for the states of Alaska and Hawaii, where there is a Cost of Living Adjustment (COLA) and this will be an additional calculation added to the totals (CMS, 2013a, p. 25). The next type of adjustment is if the hospital is an approved teaching hospital. If so, the hospital will receive an additional payment called an Indirect Medical Education

(IME) payment for each case under the PPS (CMS, 2013b). Then there is an adjustment for cases that involve the use of new technology that has been approved by CMS for a special add-on payment. Finally, there is an outlier calculation (CMS, 2013c) that covers additional costs that are incurred by the hospital that exceed a certain amount and then the hospital will receive an additional payment for the patient's hospital stay.

Medicare Severity Diagnosis-Related Group Classification System (MS-DRG)

The Medicare Severity DRGs (MS-DRGs) is a classification system that provides a means of grouping together similar types of patients a hospital treats. For example, their case mix is a tool that takes all the DRGs and calculates the average case mix and then compare this number to the costs incurred by the hospital. The payment for the hospital services is made based on a rate per discharge that varies in accordance to the MS-DRG that was assigned that represents the patient's stay in the facility. All inpatient and transfers, from both PPS and non-PPS facilities, are classified by the Grouper software program into one of 745 diagnosis-related groups (DRGs) (CMS, 2013e, p. 24).

Inpatient Hospital Payments Under PPS

Payments for hospital inpatient stays under PPS are based on predetermined prospectively set rates. These predetermined rates are set for each hospital discharge. The hospital discharge is classified according to the listing of the 745 DRGs.

The payment consists of a base payment rate. This rate is made up of a labor-related share or portion and a nonlabor-related share or portion. The labor related share is directly influenced by the wage index that is representative of the area that the facility is located. The balance of the calculation is the non-labor related portion. There is an adjustment here if the facility is located in Alaska or Hawaii. In this instance, the nonlabor related portion is adjusted by a cost-of-living factor. The final outcome is then the base rate that will be multiplied by the DRG relative weight.

Disproportionate Share Adjustment

If a hospital treats a high percentage of low-income patients, it will receive a percentage add-on payment that will be applied to the DRG-adjusted base payment rate, which is known as a **disproportionate share hospital** (DSH) adjustment (CMS, 2013a, p. 25). The resulting adjustment will be an increase to the payment based on statutory formulas that are designed to appropriately identify hospitals that fit the DSH category. The statutory formula takes into account Medicare inpatient days for patients eligible for Medicare Part A, Medicare Advantage, Supplemental Security Income (SSI), and total inpatient days for patients eligible for Medicaid but not Medicare Part A (Casto & Forrestal, 2013, p. 133). This additional payment will help to offset the unbalanced share of low-income patients that the facility services in the community.

There are two methods of qualification for a hospital to become a DSH facility. First, a hospital may qualify for the qualification if they exceed 15 percent on the statutory formula. The second method for DSH qualification applies to large urban hospitals. In this scenario if a large urban hospital can demonstrate that more than 30 percent of their net inpatient care revenues come from state and local governments for indigent care, excluding Medicare and Medicaid, then they can be granted DSH status (CMS, 2013a).

Changes to the DSH status will take place in FY 2014 as a result of the Affordable Care Act. Effective in FY 2014, hospitals will receive 25 percent of the amount that they previously would have received under the current formula. The additional payment, equal to 75 percent of what was to be paid in the previous DSH calculation will become available for an uncompensated care payment after being reduced for changes in the percentage of patients that are uninsured at the time of delivering care.

Each hospital's uncompensated care payment is the product of three factors. The three factors are as follows (CMS, 2013a):

1. 75 percent of the estimated DSH payments that would otherwise be made under the old DSH methodology [Section 1886 (d)(5)(F) of the Social Security Act];

2. 1 minus the percent change in the percent of individuals under the age of 65 who are uninsured (minus 0.1 percentage points for FY 2014, and minus 0.2 percentage points for FY 2015 through FY 2017); and

3. A hospital's amount of uncompensated care relative to the amount of uncompensated care for all DSH hospitals expressed as a percentage.

Indirect Medical Education

Section 1886(d)(5)(B) of the Social Security Act "provides that PPS hospitals that have residents in an approved Graduate Medical Education (GME) program will receive an additional payment for a Medicare discharge" (CMS, 2013b). This higher payment will reflect the additional costs that are incurred by teaching hospital as opposed to a facility that is not a teaching facility.

The regulations surrounding the calculation of this additional payment to hospitals is to offset the costs of medical education that is known as the **Indirect Medical Education** (IME) adjustment are located at 42 CFR § 412.105. The additional payment is calculated by using the hospital's ratio of residents to beds. In the following equation the ratio of resident to beds is "r" and the multiplier "c" is set by Congress.

$$C \times [(1 + r).405 - 1]$$

Overall, "the amount of the IME payment that a hospital receives is based on the number of residents the hospital trains and the current level of the IME multiplier set by Congress" (CMS, 2013b).

Hospital Wage Index

Section 1886(d)(3)(E) of the Social Security Act requires that, as part of the methodology for determining prospective payments to hospitals, the Secretary must adjust the standardized amounts "for area differences in hospital wage levels by a factor (established by the Secretary) reflecting the relative hospital wage level the geographic area of the hospital compared to the national average hospital wage level" (CMS, 2013d).

The **Hospital Wage Index** is an adjustment based on the geographical location of a hospital and their area wage level as compared to the national average and this is adjusted annually. The data that supports the calculation is based on wage-related information from acute care hospitals and short-term hospitals and includes information obtained from Medicare Cost Reports, hospital's payroll records, and other wage-related documentation. The wage index is computed for each labor area by taking the total wage costs divided by the total hours for all hospitals in a geographic area. Then compare the results to the national average hourly wage and the value will be the ratio of the wages in the local area to the national average hourly wage. If the labor market area's average hourly wage is greater than the national average, the area's wage index value will be greater than 1.0000, or if the area's average hourly wage is less than the national average the index value will be less than 1.0000 (CMS, 2013d, p. 26). The wage index adjustment factor is only applied to the labor portion of the DRG payment calculation.

High Cost Outliers

Section 1886(d)(5)(A) of the Social Security Act provides for Medicare payments to Medicare-participating hospitals in addition to the basic prospective payments for cases incurring extraordinarily high costs (CMS, 2013c). For a facility to have a Medicare discharge qualify for a High Cost Outlier payment the case must have costs that exceed the fixed-loss threshold plus the DRG payment for the discharge.

Cost to Charge Ratios

The **Cost to Charge Ratio** (CCR) is applied to the covered charges for a case to determine whether the costs of a case exceeds the fixed-loss outlier threshold. This ratio reduces the Medicare charge down to a net number to calculate if the charges exceed the threshold that would make the stay eligible for an additional payment.

Calculation of Charges

The following is an example of a Medicare beneficiary who was admitted to Hospital Anywhere, U.S.A. with congestive heart failure in a situation where no Operating Room procedures were performed. Hospital Anywhere, U.S.A. is in a large urban area, and their Wage Index will be 1.45; it is not a teaching facility, and it is not a Disproportionate Share Hospital.

The following is a step-by-step outline for calculating payment for a Medicare Beneficiary discharge:

Step 1: Determine the Federal Operating Payment with IME and DSH

Step 2: Determine the Federal Capital Payment with IME and DSH

Step 3: Determine the Operating and Capital Costs

Step 4: Determine the Operating and Capital Outlier Threshold

Step 5: Determine the Operating and Capital Outlier Payment Amount

---

EXHIBIT 7-1   (CALCULATION THAT DOES NOT QUALIFY FOR OUTLIER PAYMENT)

OUTLIER EXAMPLE

The following example simulates the outlier payment for a case at a generic hospital in the Mid-Atlantic Area, which is a large urban area. The patient was discharged on or after October 1, 2006 and the hospital incurred Medicare approved charges of $150,000. The DRG assigned to the case was 428. The hospital is 100% federal for capital payment purposes.

Table of Operating Values Used in Calculation		Table of Capital Values Used in Calculation	
DRG 428 Relative Weight:	0.6723	DRG 498 Relative Weight:	0.6723
Labor-Related	$4,225.14	Federal Capital Rate	$425.00
Nonlabor-Related	$1,845.47	Large Urban Add On	1.03
Mid-Atlantic CBSA Wage Index	1.45	Mid-Atlantic CBSA GAF	1.2897
Cost-of-Living Adjustment (COLA)	1	Cost-of-Living Adjustment	1
IME Operating Adjustment Factor	1	IME Operating Adjustment Factor	1
DSH Operating Adjustment Factor	1	DSH Operating Adjustment Factor	1
Labor-Related Portion	0.696	Capital Cost-to-Charge Ratio	0.019
Nonlabor-Related Portion	0.304		
Operating Cost-to-Charge Ratio	0.236		

Other Factors	
Billed Covered Charges	$150,000
Fixed Loss Outlier Threshold	$25,000
Marginal Cost Factor	0.8

(continued)

EXHIBIT 7-1   (CALCULATION THAT DOES NOT QUALIFY FOR OUTLIER PAYMENT) (CONTINUED)

Step 1: Determine Federal Operating Payment with IME and DSH:

Federal Rate for Operating Costs = {DRG Relative Weight × [(Labor Related Large Urban Standardized Amount × Mid-Atlantic CBSA Wage Index) + (Nonlabor Related National Large Urban Standardized Amount × Cost of Living Adjustment)] × (1 + IME + DSH)}

Federal Operating Payment With IME and DSH = $16,078.57

Step 2: Determine Federal Capital Payment with IME and DSH:

Federal Rate for Capital Costs = [(DRG Relative Weight × Federal Capital Rate × Large Urban Add-On × Geographic Cost Adjustment Factor × COLA) × (1 + IME + DSH)]

Federal Capital Payment With IME and DSH = $1,138.67

Step 3: Determine Operating and Capital Costs:

Operating Costs = Billed Charges × Operating Cost-to-Charge Ratio

Operating Costs = $35,400

Capital Costs = Billed Charges × Capital Cost-to-Charge Ratio

Capital Costs = $2,850

Step 4: Determine Operating and Capital Outlier Threshold

A. Operating CCR to Total CCR = Operating CCR / (Operating CCR + Capital CCR)

Operating CCR to Total CCR =   0.9255

B. Capital CCR to Total CCR = Capital CCR / (Operating CCR + Capital CCR)

Capital CCR to Total CCR =   0.0745

C. Operating Outlier Threshold = {[(Fixed Loss Threshold × (Labor related portion × Mid-Atlantic CBSA Wage Index) + Nonlabor related portion) × (Operating CCR to Total)] + Federal Payment with IME and DSH}

Operating Outlier Threshold = $46,462.74

D. Capital Outlier Threshold = (Fixed Loss Threshold × Geographic Adj. Factor × Large Urban Add-On × Capital CCR to Total CCR) + Federal Payment with IME and DSH

Capital Outlier Threshold = $3,612.80

EXHIBIT 7-1   (CALCULATION THAT DOES NOT QUALIFY FOR OUTLIER PAYMENT) (CONTINUED)

Step 5: Determine Operating and Capital Outlier Payment Amount

A. Determine if Total Costs are Greater than Combined Threshold = [if (operating costs+ capital costs) > (operating threshold + capital threshold)]

Determine if Total Costs are Greater than Combined Threshold	**FALSE, No Outlier Payment Will be Made**

B. Operating Outlier Payment = (Operating Costs − Operating Outlier Threshold) × Marginal Cost Factor

Operating Outlier Payment =	FALSE, No Operating Outlier Payment Will be Made

C. Capital Outlier Payment = (Capital Costs − Capital Outlier Threshold) × Marginal Cost Factor
    Note: If Capital Outlier Payment Amount is Negative, we default this amount to 0

Capital Outlier Payment =	FALSE, No Capital Outlier Payment Will be Made

---

EXHIBIT 7-2   (CALCULATION THAT DOES QUALIFY FOR OUTLIER PAYMENT)

OUTLIER EXAMPLE

The following example simulates the outlier payment for a case at a generic hospital in the Mid-Atlantic Area, which is a large urban area. The patient was discharged on or after October 1, 2006 and the hospital incurred Medicare approved charges of $250,000. The DRG assigned to the case was 428. The hospital is 100% federal for capital payment purposes.

Table of Operating Values Used in Calculation		Table of Capital Values Used in Calculation	
DRG 428 Relative Weight:	0.6723	DRG 498 Relative Weight:	0.6723
Labor-Related	$4,225.14	Federal Capital Rate	$425.00
Nonlabor-Related	$1,845.47	Large Urban Add On	1.03
Mid-Atlantic CBSA Wage Index	1.45	Mid-Atlantic CBSA GAF	1.2897
Cost-of-Living Adjustment (COLA)	1	Cost-of-Living Adjustment	1
IME Operating Adjustment Factor	1	IME Operating Adjustment Factor	1
DSH Operating Adjustment Factor	1	DSH Operating Adjustment Factor	1
Labor-Related Portion	0.696	Capital Cost-to-Charge Ratio	0.019
Nonlabor-Related Portion	0.304		
Operating Cost-to-Charge Ratio	0.236		

Other Factors	
Billed Covered Charges	$2,50,000
Fixed Loss Outlier Threshold	$25,000
Marginal Cost Factor	0.8

(continued)

EXHIBIT 7-2   (CALCULATION THAT DOES QUALIFY FOR OUTLIER PAYMENT) (CONTINUED)

Step 1: Determine Federal Operating Payment with IME and DSH:

Federal Rate for Operating Costs = {DRG Relative Weight × [(Labor Related Large Urban Standardized Amount × Mid-Atlantic CBSA Wage Index) + (Nonlabor Related National Large Urban Standardized Amount × Cost of Living Adjustment)] × (1 + IME + DSH)}

Federal Operating Payment With IME and DSH = $16,078.57

Step 2: Determine Federal Capital Payment with IME and DSH:

Federal Rate for Capital Costs = [(DRG Relative Weight × Federal Capital Rate × Large Urban Add-On × Geographic Cost Adjustment Factor × COLA) × (1 + IME + DSH)]

Federal Capital Payment With IME and DSH = $1,138.67

Step 3: Determine Operating and Capital Costs:

Operating Costs = Billed Charges × Operating Cost-to-Charge Ratio

Operating Costs = $59,000

Capital Costs = Billed Charges × Capital Cost-to-Charge Ratio

Capital Costs = $4,750

Step 4: Determine Operating and Capital Outlier Threshold

A. Operating CCR to Total CCR = Operating CCR / (Operating CCR + Capital CCR)

Operating CCR to Total CCR =   0.9255

B. Capital CCR to Total CCR = Capital CCR / (Operating CCR + Capital CCR)

Capital CCR to Total CCR =   0.0745

C. Operating Outlier Threshold = {[Fixed Loss Threshold × (Labor related portion × Mid-Atlantic CBSA Wage Index) + Nonlabor related portion)] × (Operating CCR to Total) + Federal Payment with IME and DSH}

Operating Outlier Threshold = $46,462.74

D. Capital Outlier Threshold = (Fixed Loss Threshold × Geographic Adj. Factor × Large Urban Add-On × Capital CCR to Total CCR) + Federal Payment with IME and DSH

Capital Outlier Threshold = $3,612.80

EXHIBIT 7-2   (CALCULATION THAT DOES QUALIFY FOR OUTLIER PAYMENT) (CONTINUED)

Step 5: Determine Operating and Capital Outlier Payment Amount

A. Determine if Total Costs are Greater than Combined Threshold = [if (operating costs + capital costs) > (operating threshold + capital threshold)]

Determine if Total Costs are Greater than Combined Threshold	TRUE, Continue With The Next Step

B. Operating Outlier Payment = (Operating Costs − Operating Outlier Threshold) × Marginal Cost Factor

Operating Outlier Payment =	$10,029.81

C. Capital Outlier Payment = (Capital Costs − Capital Outlier Threshold) × Marginal Cost Factor
      Note: If Capital Outlier Payment Amount is Negative, we default this amount to 0

Capital Outlier Payment =	$909.76

Transfer Cases

There are three types of transfer cases under the Inpatient Prospective Payment System which are a transfer between IPPS hospitals (Transfer Type 1), transfers from IPPS hospital to hospitals/facility excluded from IPPS (Transfer Type 2), and transfers from IPPS hospital to hospitals or units excluded from IPPS that fall within a DRG that is subject to the Post-Acute Care Transfer Policy (Special Payment Transfer). The incentive for Medicare is to avoid paying the full amount to two facilities for the same patient stay. By calculating the payment based on a per-diem rate and following the payment calculations for each type of transfer, Medicare can save a considerable amount of money and hospitals will not be artificially incentivized to transfer patients early.

In Transfer Type 1, a transfer between IPPS hospitals, the transferring hospital will be paid a per-diem rate for the days that the patient spends at the facility. Outlier calculations will apply to this admission proportionately based on the number of days spent at the transferring facility. The process will be to take the total cost divide it by the **Geometric Mean Length of Stay** (GMLOS) and multiply by the total days spent at the transferring facility and then add one. The receiving hospital will be paid the full prospective payment rate. Outlier calculations will also be applicable to the receiving facility and calculated for the full stay.

Transfer Type 2 is a transfer that takes place between a hospital and a facility that is excluded from IPPS. In this type of transfer, the transferring facility is paid for the full admission, and any outlier calculations will apply for the full admission. The receiving facility will receive payment based on the type of payment system that the facility falls under in the Medicare payment system. There are exceptions to this rule known as post-acute-care transfer (PACT) policy for Type 2 transfers. In this situation, if the DRG is one of the 275 MS-DRGs that qualify for the PACT policy, the transfer is treated like a Transfer Type 1 rather than a discharge (Casto & Forrestal, 2013, p. 135).

For the remaining 30 MS-DRGs, there is a Special Payment Transfer where the transfer is taking place from an IPPS hospital to a hospital or facility that is excluded from IPPS that fall within a DRG that is subject to the Post-acute Care Transfer Special Payment Policy. The transferring hospital will be paid 50 percent of the full MS-DRG payment plus the per-diem rate for the first day and then 50 percent of the per-diem rate for each day thereafter. The 30 MS-DRGs in this category have a significantly higher cost per admission (Casto & Forrestal, 2013, p. 145).

Calculation of Transfer Cases

EXHIBIT 7-3   (TRANSFER TYPE 1)

Post-Acute Transfer Policy Type 1 Example:

MS-DRG 064 Intracranial hemorrhage or cerebral infarction with MCC

Relative Weight	1.8555
GMLOS	4.9
Hospital Base Rate	$8,500

Full MS-DRG payment (based on if the patient is discharged home)

Relative weight * Hospital base rate

$15,771.75

Post-acute transfer payment for 2 days stay

Patient Length of Stay is 2 days
Transfer to Skilled Nursing Facility

Full MS-DRG payment divided by GMLOS

$3,218.72

Payment calculations

Day 1	Per-diem rate plus 1 day	$3,218.72
Day 2	Per-diem rate	$3,218.72
Plus 1 day		$3,218.72
Total		$9,656.16
	Total MS-DRG Payment	$15,771.75
	Total Transfer Type 1 Payment	$9,656.16
	Difference	$6,115.59

EXHIBIT 7-4   (TRANSFER TYPE 2)

Post-Acute Transfer Policy Type 2 Special Payment Example:

MS-DRG 477 Biopsies of musculoskeletal system & connective tissue with MCC

Relative Weight	3.4596
GMLOS	9
Hospital Base Rate	$8,500

Full MS-DRG payment (based on if the patient is discharged home)

Relative weight * Hospital base rate

$29,406.60

Post-acute transfer special payment for 2 days stay

Patient Length of Stay is 2 days

Transfer to Inpatient Rehab Facility

Full MS-DRG payment divided by GMLOS

$29,406.60	divided by 9.0
$3,267.40	per day

Payment Calculations

Day 1	50% full payment + per-diem rate
	$14,703.30 plus $3,267.40
	$17,970.70
Day 2	50% per-diem rate
	$3,267.40*50%
	$1,633.70
Total	$19,604.40

Full MS-DRG Payment	$29,406.60
Special Payment	$19,604.40
Difference	$9,802.20

■ Billing of Transplant Services

Kidney Transplant

A major treatment for patients with end-stage renal disease (ESRD) is kidney transplantation. This process involves removing a kidney, usually from a living relative of the patient or from an unrelated person who has died, and according to CMS, "surgically placing the kidney into the patient. After the beneficiary receives a kidney transplant, Medicare pays the transplant hospital for the transplant and appropriate standard acquisition charges" (CMS, 2013e, p. 149).

A hospital that performs transplant surgery may acquire cadaver kidneys by excising them from cadavers that are located in its own hospital. In addition, they can accomplish this acquisition through arrangements with a freestanding organ-procurement organization (OPO) that provides cadaver kidneys to any transplant hospital. A hospital that is also certified as an OPO may acquire kidneys by having its own team/staff excise kidneys from cadavers in other hospitals, through arrangements with participating hospitals, and arrangements with an OPO that services the transplant hospital as a member of the networks (CMS, 2013e, p. 150).

The cost for excising the cadaver kidney differs from a transplant hospital and nontransplant hospital. The transplant hospital will include cost of the procedure in the kidney acquisition costs when they also excise the cadaver kidney. When the transplant hospital excises the kidney and provides it to another hospital it can charge the standard cadaver kidney acquisition charge or its standard detailed charges to that hospital.

If the transplanting hospital's organ transplant team excises a kidney at another hospital, then the cost of the operating team is included in the transplanting hospital's kidney acquisition costs, in addition to reasonable charges for its services.

The two basic standard charges that must be developed by transplant hospitals are the standard charge for acquiring a live donor kidney and the standard charge for acquiring a cadaver kidney. The standard charge is not based on the cost of a specific kidney, but the charge that reflects the average cost associated with each type of acquisition of a kidney. When the transplant hospital bills for the transplant the revenue code used is 081X. These charges are not considered for the IPPS outlier calculation when a procedure code of 556 is reported (CMS, 2013e, p. 151).

These services are billed from the excising hospital to the transplant hospital and no billing form is submitted to the Fiscal Intermediary. In addition, the charges reflected in the transplant hospital's acquisition cost for the kidney are used in determining the standard charge for acquiring a live donor's kidney. These charges are all inclusive, or bundled, and include everything from tissue typing to post-operative evaluation.

In billing for cadaveric donor services, the various tests performed to assess the suitability of the cadaver kidney by the excising hospital can include the related charges on its bill to the transplant hospital or to the OPO. Billing for physician services differ from pre to post transplant services. The costs involved in excisions involving live donors and recipients as well as all physicians' services are considered Part A hospital services. After transplantation, all physician services rendered to the transplant recipient are billed to the Medicare program with all other Medicare B services during the stay. All donor physician services must be billed to the recipient using modifier Q3 so that (Live Kidney Donor and Related Services) appears on the claim.

Heart Transplant

Heart transplants are covered under Medicare, but only when performed by a facility that is approved by Medicare as meeting the coverage criteria and are considered medically reasonable and necessary when performed in facilities that meet the criteria published in "Criteria for Medicare Coverage of Heart Transplants" that was published in the *Federal Register* on April 6, 1987 (Ruling 87-1) (CMS 2013e, p. 155).

According to CMS, "Medicare Part B covers all immunosuppressive drugs following a covered transplant in an approved facility based on the Criteria for Medicare Coverage of Heart Transplants" (CMS, 2013e, p. 156). Moreover, Medicare will not cover any transplant, or retransplants in facilities, that have not been approved as meeting the facility criteria. If a patient did end up receiving a heart transplant from a hospital that was not approved as a transplant facility, and later requires services as a result of the noncovered transplant, the patient's treatment or services they received will be covered by Medicare as long as they are reasonable and necessary in all other respects (CMS, 2013e, p. 156).

The charges incurred by the excising hospital are billed to the OPO. Then the OPO will bill the transplant (implant) hospital for the applicable services/charges. The transplant hospital must keep an itemized statement of account that reflects services rendered, applicable charges, the person receiving the service (donor/recipient) and if this person is a potential transplant donor or recipient. All charges that for services in the acquisition of a heart transplant including, but not limited to, tissue typing and post-operative evaluation (CMS, 2013e, p. 156).

Medicare does not cover artificial hearts, for temporary or permanent replacement for a human heart. Medicare does cover Ventricular Assist Device (VAD) as a bridge to a heart transplant and to assist in pumping blood for a damaged or weakened heart.

Liver Transplant

Under Medicare liver transplants are considered medically reasonable and necessary for specified conditions when performed in facilities that meet specific coverage guidelines. Effective for claims after June 21, 2012, contractors may, at their discretion, cover adult liver transplantation for patients with extrahepatic unresectable cholangiocarcinoma (CCA), liver metastases due to neuroendocrine tumor (NET), or hemangioendothelima (HAE) when an approved Liver Transplant Center furnishes the services (CMS, 2013e, p. 163).

Each facility must develop a standard charge for acquiring a cadaver liver. The transplant hospital keeps an itemized statement that tracks all services rendered, charges, and person receiving the treatment (donor/recipient), and the potential transplant donor. All charges for services required in the acquisition of a liver such as tissue typing, transportation, and surgeon's retrieval fees are all included.

The contractor deducts liver acquisition charges for IPPS hospitals prior to processing through the prices. The costs of the liver acquisition incurred by an approved liver transplant facility are not included in the liver transplant prospective payment. They are paid on a reasonable cost basis and are processed through as a "pass-through" cost for which interim payments are made. Moreover, all claims for liver transplant must be accompanied by an operative report (CMS, 2013e, p. 164).

Pancreas Transplants with Kidney Transplants

Effective July 1, 1999, Medicare covered pancreas transplantation when performed simultaneously with or following a kidney transplant. A pancreas transplantation is performed to induce an insulin independent, euglycemic state in diabetic patients. The procedure is generally limited to those patients with severe secondary complications of diabetes including kidney failure. With that said, pancreas transplantation is sometimes performed on patients with labile diabetes and hypoglycemic unawareness (CMS, 2013e, p. 166).

In the past Medicare had a policy of not covering pancreas transplantation, but after 1994 they found reasonable graft survival outcomes for patients receiving either simultaneous pancreas-kidney (SPK) transplantation or pancreas after kidney (PAK) transplantation.

Unlike other types of transplants, Managed Care Plans are required to provide all Medicare covered services. Moreover, Medicare does not restrict which hospitals or physicians that can perform a pancreas transplantation.

If a kidney and pancreas transplants are performed simultaneously, the claim should contain a diabetes diagnosis code and a renal failure diagnosis code or one of the hypertensive renal failure diagnosis codes. In addition, this claim should contain two transplant codes. If the claim is for a pancreas transplant only, the claim should only contain a diabetes diagnosis code and a V-code to indicate a previous kidney transplant. If the V-code is not on the claim for the pancreas transplant, the contractor will perform a search on the beneficiary's claim history for a V-code (CMS, 2013e, p. 168).

All immunosuppressive drugs will be covered for a pancreas transplant that occurs after the kidney transplant from that date of discharge from the inpatient stay for the pancreas transplant.

Pancreas Transplants Alone (PA)

Pancreas transplants are performed to induce an insulin-independent, euglycemic state in diabetic patients. The procedure is generally limited to those patients with severe secondary complications of diabetes, including kidney failure. But as previously stated, pancreas transplantation is sometimes performed on patients with labile diabetes and hypoglycemic unawareness. Medicare has a long-standing policy of not covering pancreas transplantation as the safety and effectiveness of the procedure has not been demonstrated (CMS, 2013e, p. 169). Medicare contractors shall pay for Pancreas Transplantation Alone (PA) effective for services on or after April 26, 2006 when performed in facilities that are Medicare-approved for kidney transplantation. In addition to being done in an approved facility, the beneficiary must have a diagnosis of type 1 diabetes.

■ Inpatient Rehabilitation Facility Prospective Payment System (IRF PPS)

Section 1886(j) of the Social Security Act authorized implementation of a Prospective Payment System for **Inpatient Rehabilitation Facilities**. The system was referred to as IRF PPS and was effective after January 1, 2002. IRF PPS payments cover all services rendered to a patient in the facility that includes routine, ancillary, **bad debts**, capital-related costs, and other costs that are not covered under the PPS (CMS, 2013e, p. 215).

The IRF PPS pays for inpatient hospital services in an inpatient rehabilitation hospital or a rehabilitation unit of a hospital. It is required that the IRF PPS maintains the criteria necessary to remain an excluded entity from an IPPS. In addition, any changes to the IRF must be put in writing to the Fiscal Intermediary (FI) and Medicare Administrative Contractor (MAC) that pertain to their operations such as increasing their bed size, square footage, moving to a new location, change of ownership, merging, or other similar changes to the ownership or operations of the facility.

The criteria that is necessary for an IRF to be excluded from the IPPS are the facility must serve an inpatient population that at least 60 percent of the patients require intensive rehabilitative services for medical conditions such as a stroke, spinal cord injury, congenital deformity, amputation, major multiple trauma, fracture of femur (hip fracture), brain injury, neurological disorders (multiple sclerosis, muscular dystrophy, Parkinson's disease, etc.), burns, active polyarticular rheumatoid arthritis, psoriatic arthritis, systemic vasculidities with joint inflammation, severe or advanced osteoarthritis, or knee or hip joint replacement. For knee or hip joint replacement, the patient needs to have undergone bilateral knee or bilateral hip joint replacement surgery while admitted in an inpatient facility, or the patient must be extremely obese with a Body Mass Index (BMI) of at least 50 at the time of admission to the IRF, or the patient was 85 or older at the time of admission (CMS, 2013e, p. 218).

Comorbidities

Comorbidities are a specific patient condition that is secondary to a patient's principle diagnosis. A patient with a comorbidity can be counted towards the required percentage of the population (60 percent) if the patient is admitted to the facility for a medical condition that is not an approved condition for admission, the patient has a comorbidity that falls in one of the medical conditions listed above, or when a comorbidity has caused significant decline in functional ability that even in the absence of the admitting condition the individual would require intensive rehabilitation treatment that is unique to the IRF (CMS, 2013e, p. 219).

IRF Qualifications

From the first cost reporting period through all subsequent reporting periods, the IRF must meet the requirements to be an approved facility. If at any time the facility does not meet the requirements to be an IRF, CMS will adjust the payments to the facility. The preadmission screening procedures include determining if the patient would benefit significantly from an admission for an intensive rehabilitation program. A rehabilitation physician must review and approve the patient's admission to the facility. The IRF must have one physician who serves as the Director of Rehabilitation who is full-time at a facility or at least 20 hours in a rehabilitation unit, holds the degree of doctor of medicine (MD) or doctor of osteopathy (DO), is licensed under the state to practice medicine or surgery, and has completed the 1-year hospital internship and have at least 2 years of training or experience in the management of patients requiring intensive rehabilitation services. A plan of treatment must be in place for each inpatient that is admitted and must be reviewed and revised as needed by a physician in consultation with other clinical personnel who provide services to the patient.

During the stay the patient must receive close medical attention and have at least three face-to-face visits per week by a licensed physician with specialized training in rehabilitative medicine. In addition to the physician services, the IRF must furnish qualified personnel such as rehabilitation nursing, physical therapy, occupational therapy, speech-language therapy, social services, psychological services, and orthotic and prosthetic services (CMS, 2013e, p. 220).

Additional criteria for the inpatient rehabilitation unit are that the unit must be part of an institution that is participating as a hospital and is not excluded from the IPPS, have written admission criteria for all patients, have their own medical record and needs to be kept separate from the inpatient medical records, be licensed in accordance with all applicable requirements (local, state, and federal), separate standards for utilization review for the type of care offered by the unit, all beds for the unit must not be comingled with beds that are not in the unit, be a separate cost center, there may only be one type of each rehab unit (psychiatric/rehabilitation) and not excluded from the IPPS.

Data Collection and Reporting

The IRF PPS features an 85-item rehabilitation-specific tool that is called the IRF PAI. This tool is the driver for calculating payment for the facility. The IRF PAI must be completed upon admission and upon discharge for each patient. The IRF PAI consists of patient information gathered such as identification information, admission, payer, medical, medical needs, function modifiers and independence assessment information, discharge information, and quality measures.

The assignment of codes for the patient will take place on the fourth day of the admission. The codes will reflect the reason for admission/rehabilitation, etiology of the impairment by using ICD-9-CM codes, any comorbidities and complications using ICD-9-CM codes, and the reason for any interruption of the stay (transfer or death) using ICD-9-CM codes. The functional abilities of the patient must be assigned and this is done by using the Functional Independence Assessment Tool.

Patients are grouped into a case mix that represents the resource intensity that would be associated with the admission and the patient's physical condition. The cases are grouped into Rehabilitation Impairment Categories, which is reflective of the primary reason for admission. The cases are further placed into Case Mix Groups (CMG) that have all patients with like diagnosis and resource consumption. Then the patients are grouped into one of four tiers within each CMG according to the patient's comorbidity. A comorbidity is a condition that will require the IRF to use more resources to treat the patient. Each tier, from low to medium to high, can add a higher payment to the case. Tier 1 is the highest cost, Tier 2 is a medium cost, and Tier 3 is the lowest cost. There are excluded comorbidities that will not affect the payment to the facility.

In addition to the other assessments, there is a Functional Independence Assessment that the IRF will use in assessing the patient. A functional status is the patient's ability to function effectively in their Activities of Daily Living (ADL). CMS has organized this assessment tool to be focusing on motor and cognitive functioning. There are 18 items on the measurement tool and each item is scored from a Minimum ability that equals a one or complete dependence to a Maximum of seven, which means complete independence. There is also a score of zero which means that the item was not assessed. At this point the scores are totaled for the motor and cognitive functioning and the total score is then assigned a case-mix group.

Inpatient Rehabilitation Facilities must report quality data to CMS electronically. They use the program called Inpatient Rehabilitation Validation and Entry or IRVEN. There are time frames for submission of the data, and if the facility is not compliant with these time frames, they could see a 25 percent reduction in their payments.

Overall, the process for classification goes from establishing an Impairment Group Category for the patient. Then the patient is assigned a Rehabilitation Impairment Category and then the patient is moved into a Case-mix Group. There are a total of five special CMGs that cover short-stay cases (3 days or less) and four CMGs for expired patients. A special payment will be established for an interrupted stay and a transfer case.

IRF PPS Payment Calculation

Basically the payment is calculated by the **Health Insurance Prospective Payment System** (HIPPS) code assigned to the patient. The HIPPS code is a five character alphanumeric code that encompasses the information about the case-mix group and comorbidity into this one code. The first character designates the comorbidity level and uses the characters A, B, C, and D. The last four characters are the four-digit CMG. For example, if a patient was to have Tier 2 comorbidity they would have the letter "D" assigned in the first position. Then if they had a CMG of 0108 they would have a HIPPS Code of D0108. There is only one HIPPS code permitted per IRF admission.

To calculate a payment for an IRF patient you need to have the HIPPS code that was assigned to the patient and see what Tier (1, 2, or 3) was assigned. Then you take the weight assigned and multiply it by the Standard Payment Conversion Factor to come up with the unadjusted rate or dollar amount. Then you multiply the labor portion by the local wage index and the nonlabor portion by the nonlabor-related ratio. Then you add the labor-related and nonlabor-related numbers together to get the final payment. There are some adjustments that are present in the IRF PPS that are the rural adjustment, disproportionate share or share of low-income patients, and a teaching hospital adjustment.

■ Inpatient Facility Prospective Payment System (IPF PPS)

In Section 124 of the Medicare, Medicaid, and SCHIP (State Children's Health Insurance Program) Balanced Budget Refinement Act for 1999 (BBRA) it mandated that the Secretary develop a per diem PPS for inpatient hospital services furnished in psychiatric hospitals and psychiatric units and include in the PPS an adequate patient classification system that reflects differences in patient resources used, maintain budget neutrality, permit the Secretary to require that psychiatric hospitals and psychiatric units supply information for the development of the PPS, and submit a report to Congress (CMS, 2013e, p. 347).

This newly created prospective payment system for inpatient psychiatric hospitals and units is IPF PPS. The IPF is certified under Medicare as an inpatient psychiatric hospital. This means that the facility is primarily providing psychiatric services under the direction or supervision of a physician for the treatment of mentally ill patients. There are several hospitals that are not reimbursed under the IPF PPS model: Veterans Administration hospitals, hospitals reimbursed under the state cost control system, hospitals reimbursed according to demonstration projects, nonparticipating hospitals, and foreign hospitals (CMS, 2013e, p. 348).

IPF PPS Payment Structure

The payment for an IPF PPS facility is determined by a federal per-diem base rate. This rate is based on inpatient operating costs and capital-related costs, but not certain pass-through costs such as bad debt, direct graduate medical education, and nursing and allied health education. The federal per-diem base rate is comprised of a labor and nonlabor portion and has the availability of patient and facility adjustments.

Budget Neutrality

The budget neutrality portion of IPF PPS requires that the total expenditures of the program in a prospective payment model not exceed what would have been spent in a fee-for-service model had the IPF PPS model not have been created. There are several Budget Neutrality components under the IPF PPS model. First there is an outlier adjustment which will adjust the payment if the costs for care were above the prospective payment plus the fixed threshold amount. Second, there is a Stop-Loss Adjustment that insures that the IPF's total PPS payments are no less than a minimum percentage of their former payment model if the IPF PPS had not been developed. Third, there is a Behavioral Offset, which may result in certain changes in IPF practices with respect to coding comorbid medical conditions. Medicare implemented an adjustment, which is known as the Behavioral Offset, that reduces the IPF PPS payment 2.66 percent to accommodate for behavioral changes with regards to coding comorbid conditions (CMS, 2013e, p. 350).

Comorbidity Adjustment

Comorbidity adjustments are specific patient conditions that are secondary to the patient's principle diagnosis that require treatment during the stay. The IPF PPS has 17 comorbidity categories that will each receive a grouping-specific adjustment. There can only be one comorbidity adjustment per comorbidity category. The comorbidity categories are as follows:

TABLE 7.1   IPF PPS comorbidity categories.

Description of Comorbidity	Adjustment Factor
Developmental Disabilities	1.04
Coagulation Factor Deficits	1.13
Tracheostomy	1.06
Renal Failure, Acute	1.11
Renal Failure, Chronic	1.11
Oncology Treatment	1.07
Uncontrolled Diabetes-Mellitus with or without complications	1.05
Severe Protein/Calorie Malnutrition	1.13
Eating and Conduct Disorders	1.12
Infectious Disease	1.07
Drug and/or Alcohol Induced Mental Disorders	1.03
Cardiac Conditions	1.11
Gangrene	1.10
Chronic Obstructive Pulmonary Disease	1.12
Artificial Openings – Digestive and Urinary	1.08
Severe Musculoskeletal and Connective Tissue Diseases	1.09
Poisoning	1.11

Data From Centers for Medicare and Medicaid Services. 2013. Medicare Claims Processing Manual; Chapter 3-Inpatient Hospital Billing. Retrieved from CMS: http://www.cms.gov/Regulations-and-Guidance/Guidance/Manuals/Downloads/clm104c03.pdf

Age Adjustment

In addition to the Budget Neutrality and Comorbidity adjustments there is an age adjustment for IPF PPS. There are 9 categories and range from under 45 to 80 and over. The IPF facility will receive an adjustment for each day the patient stays in the facility.

Calculation of IPF PPS Payment

To calculate a payment for an IPF PPS facility you would do the following:

1. Multiply the federal per-diem base rate by the labor share
2. Multiply the resulting amount by the appropriate wage index factor
3. Multiply the federal per-diem base rate by the nonlabor share
4. Multiply the resulting amount by any applicable Cost of Living Adjustment (COLA)

TABLE 7.2 IPF PPS age adjustments.

Age	Adjustment Factor
Under 45	1.00
45 and under 50	1.01
50 and under 55	1.02
55 and under 60	1.04
60 and under 65	1.07
65 and under 70	1.10
70 and under 75	1.13
75 and under 80	1.15
80 and over	1.17

5. Add the adjusted labor portion of the rate to the adjusted nonlabor portion of the rate

6. Multiply Step 5 by any applicable facility and patient level adjustments (comorbidity, age adjustment, and variable per-diem adjustment)

■ Health Insurance Prospective Payment System (HIPPS)

According to CMS, **Health Insurance Prospective Payment System (HIPPS)** rate codes represent specific sets of patient characteristics or case-mix groups on which payment determinations are made under several prospective payment systems. For the payment systems that use HIPPS codes, clinical data is the basic input used to determine which case-mix group applies to a particular patient (CMS, 2010, p. 1).

HIPPS codes are alphanumeric and are five digits in length. Each code contains intelligence, with certain positions of the code indicating the case mix group itself and other positions providing additional information. The structure of the code may vary from payer to payer.

HIPPS codes are used for Inpatient Rehabilitation Facilities (IRF) and Home Health Agencies (HH) along with Skilled Nursing Facilities (SNF). In addition to Medicare, HIPPS codes are used in TRICARE (Department of Defense) for SNF and many of the state Medicaid programs also use HIPPS codes and Minimum Data Set (MDS) patient assessment instruments (CMS, 2010, p. 2).

SNF PPS uses a case-mix adjusted payment for varying numbers of days of SNF care and is made using 66 Resource Utilization Groups Version IV or RUG-IV. The first three places in a code for a SNF represent the case-mix group. The fourth and fifth positions of the code represent an Assessment Indicator (AI) that identifies the reason and time frame for the completion of the MDS.

For Home Health Prospective Payment system, HH PPS, a case-mixed adjusted payment is for a period of 60 days. This 60-day period is also part of the Plan of Care that lasts 60 days. There are 80 Home Health Resource Groups (HHRG), and they are represented as HIPPS codes. The codes are determined by using the assessments made using the Outcome and Assessment Information Set (OASIS) system. The first position used to be a fixed letter "H" to designate home health. The first character is a numeric value and the second, third, and fourth positions reflect the three domains of the HHRG coding system. The fifth position indicates a severity group for nonroutine supplies. The fifth position will have values from S through X.

Examples for coding are as follows:

- First episode, 15 therapy visits with low scores in the clinical, functional, and service domains and low supply severity level and nonroutine supplies were not given = HIPPS code is 2BGL2

- Third episode, 19 visits, moderate scores in the clinical, functional, and service domains and supply severity level 4 = HIPPS code 4CHMV

- Third episode 26 therapy visits, clinical domain is moderate, function domain is low, service domain score is high, and supply severity level 5 = HIPPS code 5CGNW

Overall, in the HH PPS, there are 153 case-mix groups identified in the 2007 HH PPS final rule that fit in the first four positions of the code. All of the case-mix groups can be combined with any nonroutine supplies (NRS) level that results in 918 HIPPS codes in all (i.e., 153 case-mix groups times 6 NRS severity levels). The end result is that each HIPPS code will represent a distinct payment amount without any duplication of payment weights across codes (CMS 2010, p. 7).

For IRF PPS the first position of the code represents a comorbidity tier. The first position of the IRF PPS HIPPS codes will only allow alphabetical characters. The valid positions are as follows:

A = without comorbidities

B = comorbidity in tier 1 (high)

C = comorbidity in tier 2 (medium)

D = comorbidity in tier 3 (low)

The second, third, and fourth position represent the CMG itself. The fifth position will only allow numeric characters. The first 87 CMGs can be used in association with any of the four comorbidity tier indicators (CMS, 2010, p. 8).

EXHIBIT 7-5 (HIPPS HH PPS GRID)

Position #1	Position #2	Position #3	Position #4	Position #5		
Grouping Step	Clinical Domain	Functional Domain	Service Domain	Supply Group – supplies provided	Supply Group – supplies not provided	Domain Levels
Early Episodes (1st & 2nd) 1 (0–13 Visits)	A (HHRG: C1)	F (HHRG: F1)	K (HHRG: S1)	S (Severity Level: 1)	1 (Severity Level: 1)	= min
2 (14–19 Visits)	B (HHRG: C2)	G (HHRG: F2)	L (HHRG: S2)	T (Severity Level: 2)	2 (Severity Level: 2)	= low
Late Episodes (3rd & later) 3 (0–13 visits)	C (HHRG: C3)	H (HHRG: F3)	M (HHRG: S3)	U (Severity Level: 3)	3 (Severity Level: 3)	= mod
4 (14–19 Visits)			N (HHRG: S4)	V (Severity Level: 4)	4 (Severity Level: 4)	= high
Early or Late Episodes 5 (20 + Visits)			P (HHRG: S5)	W (Severity Level: 5)	5 (Severity Level: 5)	= max
				X (Severity Level: 6)	6 (Severity Level: 6)	
6 thru 0	D thru E	I thru J	Q thru R	Y thru Z	7 thru 0	Expansion values for future use

■ Conclusion

Medicare prospective payment for inpatients is a complex system basing reimbursements on averages and grouping patients into like resource categories. The patients in the acute care environment including rehabilitation and psychiatry continue to have access to coverage and care at their normal facilities, but the system has changed with regards to the way the facility is paid. With this new system, Medicare will save money, but they are also looking at making sure that the cost savings do not impact the level of quality delivered to the patient.

The acute care payment system is also impacted by variables that are local such as hospital wage index and high cost outliers. The healthcare administrator needs to understand the complexity and requirements of the program to maintain a healthy financial environment. If the healthcare administrator does not understand the transfer policy or high cost outliers, the facility can suffer financially. Moreover, the balancing of the prospective payment system and delivering the highest quality of care to the patient is a must.

References

Averill, R. F., Goldfield, N. I. Eisenhandler, J., Hughes, J. S., & Muldoon, J. (2001). Clinical risk groups and the future of healthcare reimbursement. In L.M. Jones (Ed.), *Reimbursement methodologies for healthcare services*. Chicago: American Health Information Management Association (AHIMA). Retrieved from http://www.montgomerycollege.edu/faculty/~csmith/public_html/AHIMA.pdf#page=114&zoom=auto,0,444

Casto, A.B., & Forrestal, E. (2013). *Principles of healthcare reimbursement* (4th ed.). Chicago: AHIMA.

Centers for Medicare and Medicaid Services. (2001). Medicare hospital prospective payment System: How DRG rates are calculated and updated. Retrieved from http://oig.hhs.gov/oei/reports/oei-09-00-00200.pdf

Centers for Medicare and Medicaid Services. (2013a). Disproportionate share hospital (DSH). Retrieved from http://www.cms.gov/Medicare/Medicare-Fee-for-Service-Payment/AcuteInpatientPPS/dsh.html

Centers for Medicare and Medicaid Services. (2013b). Indirect medical education (IME). Retrieved from http://www.cms.gov/Medicare/Medicare-Fee-for-Service-Payment/AcuteInpatientPPS/Indirect-Medical-Education-IME.html

Centers for Medicare and Medicaid Services. (2013c). Outlier payments. Retrieved from http://www.cms.gov/Medicare/Medicare-Fee-for-Service-Payment/AcuteInpatientPPS/outlier.html

Centers for Medicare and Medicaid Services. (2013d). Wage index (WI). Retrieved from http://www.cms.gov/Medicare/Medicare-Fee-for-Service-Payment/AcuteInpatientPPS/wageindex.html

Centers for Medicare and Medicaid Services. (2013e). Chapter 3: Inpatient hospital billing. In *Medicare claims processing manual*. Retrieved from http://www.cms.gov/Regulations-and-Guidance/Guidance/Manuals/Downloads/clm104c03.pdf

Centers for Medicare and Medicaid Services, Division of Institutional Claims Processing. (2010). *Definition and uses of health insurance prospective payment system codes*. Retrieved from http://www.cms.gov/Medicare/Medicare-Fee-for-Service-Payment/Prosp-MedicareFeeSvcPmtGen/downloads/hippsusesv4.pdf

LaTour, K.M., & Eichenwald Maki, S. (2010). *Health information management: Concepts, principles, and practice* (3rd ed.). Chicago: AHIMA.

8

Hospital Outpatient Prospective Payment System (OPPS)

Learning Outcomes

After reading this chapter, the student will:

- Describe the role of HCPCS codes, indicators, and APC payment groups.
- Differentiate between the prospective payment systems for outpatient, home health, physician and nonphysician practitioners, and ambulatory surgical settings.
- Describe the responsibilities of the practitioners in each clinical setting.
- Define the basic language of the Medicare Prospective Payment Systems surrounding the Hospital Outpatient Prospective Payment System.

■ Introduction

The **Hospital Outpatient Prospective Payment System (OPPS)** has a set of rules and regulations separate from the delivery of care in the acute setting. Outpatient, home health, physician and nonphysician practitioners, and ambulatory surgery have rules and regulations related to billing. From the actual procedure to the coding to the billing, each site has unique and comprehensive requirements. It is important for the healthcare leaders to differentiate the settings and meet the site-specific regulations. In this chapter we will discuss all components of OPPS, the home health prospective payment system (HH PPS), and Resource Based Relative Value Scale (RBRVS) for physician payments. This will help the student to understand the many variables to payment in the outpatient setting.

■ Hospital Outpatient Prospective Payment System

History

The Social Security Act as amended by the Balanced Budget Act (BBA) of 1997 authorized the Centers for Medicaid and Medicare Services (CMS) to implement a Prospective Payment System for hospital outpatient services. These services included partial hospitalizations, services to beneficiaries that do not have Medicare Part A,

Hepatitis B vaccines and certain services provided by Home Health Agencies (HHA), and various supplies provided to patients on **hospice care** for treatment of nonrelated illness to their terminal diagnosis (CMS, 2012, p. 12).

The Balanced Budget Refinement Act of 1999 (BBRA) contains provisions that impact the development of the OPPS. The first item was to create a system under OPPS that would be budget neutral based on 1999 allowable amounts, maintain the agreed upon reduction in operating costs of 5.8 percent, and a reduction in capital costs of 10 percent. The OPPS payment rates, weights, and adjustments are required to be updated annually. In addition to these steps it is required that an annual consultation with an expert provider panel to review payment groups, establish budget neutral outlier adjustments adjusted to costs, allow transitional pass-through for additional costs for medical devices along with drugs and biologicals, payment for implantable devices, limit provider losses under OPPS by providing additional payments for Community Mental Health Centers (CMHC) and cancer hospitals, and place a ceiling on the beneficiary coinsurance for services under OPPS not to exceed the inpatient hospital deductible (CMS, 2012, p. 13).

In addition to the revisions mentioned above, the Medicare, Medicaid, and SCHIP Benefits Improvement Act of 2000 (BIPA) introduced the accelerated reduction in a beneficiary's co-payment, increase in the market basket update in 2001, transitional corridor provision for transitional outpatient payments (TOPs), and a special transitional corridor provision for children's hospitals. Medicare will continue to pay for items such as clinical diagnostic laboratory services, prosthetics and orthotics, take-home surgical and wound care dressings, chronic dialysis, mammogram screening, outpatient rehabilitation services, and the 10 cancer hospitals are eligible for hold harmless payments under the TOP.

OPPS applies to all hospital outpatient departments, except those that only provide Medicare Part B services to their inpatients; Critical Access Hospitals (CAHs); Indian Health Service hospitals; and hospitals located in American Samoa, Guam, Saipan, and the Virgin Islands. This also applies to partial hospitalizations furnished by CMHCs and services provided by certain hospitals in Maryland that are paid under the Maryland waiver provision (CMS, 2012, p. 14).

Payment Status Indicators

An **OPPS payment status indicator** is assigned to every HCPCS code and this indicator identifies whether the service identified by the HCPCS code is paid under OPPS. Moreover, this indicator identifies whether or not the payment is made separately or as a packaged payment. According to Casto & Forrestal (2013), the 10 types of indicators are Payment Status Indicator V that is for clinic or emergency departments, Payment Status Indicator T that represents a significant procedure and multiple reductions, Payment Status Indicator S that is for significant procedure that is not discounted when

TABLE 8.1 HOPPS payment status indicator.

Payment Status Indicator	Description
G	Pass-through for drugs and biologicals
H	Pass-through for device categories
K	Non-pass-through drugs and non-implantable biological agents
P	Partial hospitalizations
R	Blood and blood products
S	Significant procedure that is not discounted with multiple procedures apply
T	Significant procedure and multiple reductions
U	Brachytherapy
X	Ancillary services

multiple procedures apply, Payment Status Indicator X for ancillary services, Payment Status Indicator K that is for non-pass-through drugs and nonimplantable biological agents such as therapeutic radiopharmaceuticals, Payment Status Indicator G for pass-through drugs or biologicals, Payment Status Indicator H covers pass-through device categories, Payment Indicator P for partial hospitalizations, Payment Status Indicator R for blood and blood products, and Payment Status Indicator U for brachytherapy sources (Casto & Forrestal, 2013, p. 182). A full listing of Payment Status Indicators are available in the Addendum D1 of the OPPS/ASC proposed final rules each year.

APC Payment Groups

Each HCPCS code is assigned to only one Ambulatory Payment Classification (APC), however there can be an unlimited number of APCs per encounter for a single beneficiary. The number of APC assignments are based on the number of reimbursable procedures provided to that patient (Casto & Forrestal, 2013, p. 182). However, multiple surgical procedures performed on a patient on the same day are subject to a reduction or discount on the additional procedures.

All services that fall into an APC are similar in both the clinical aspect and resource consumption at the facility. The law requires that the median cost for the highest cost service in an APC may not be more than 2 times the median cost of the lowest cost service in the APC. This is referred to as the "2 times rule" (CMS, 2012, p. 15). Since the costs are determined by the hospital cost reports, the APC assignment of a service may change from year to year due to the change in costs and the "2 times rule." Moreover, this will have an impact on billing and reimbursement for a facility.

Composite APCs

As with a DRG, an APC will provide a single payment for a comprehensive diagnostic treatment or service that may be reported with multiple HCPCS codes. When this takes place, a facility that provides services that fall into a Composite APC, the facility will be paid on payment for all the services that have HCPCS codes that fall under the Composite APC. For example, composite APC 8000 Cardiac Electrophysiologic Evaluation and Ablation Composite will cover at least one unit of CPT code 93619 or 93620 and at least one unit of CPT code 93650 on the same date of service; or, at least one unit of CPT codes 93653, 93654, or 93656 (no additional concurrent service codes required) (CMS, 2012, p. 15). There is no financial incentive to report these procedures together or separately, as the payment is almost identical either way. Hospitals should continue to follow the correct coding guidelines and report these services as supported by clinical documentation in the health record (Casto & Forrestal, 2013, p. 184).

Calculation of APC Payment Rates

Payment rates for APCs, outside of drugs and biologicals, are products of the relative weight of the APC and the OPPS conversion factor. The ultimate payment comes after the application of any adjustments for things such as multiple procedures or rural adjustments. Then the wage index that applies to the area is factored in and the payment is adjusted based on the rate of the location of the facility. The scaled relative weight is based on the median cost, including capital and operating costs, of all the services that are in a particular APC. These median costs are derived from the most recent filing of cost report data.

The process in which OPPS payment rates are determined is by hospital-specific cost-to-charge ratios to convert the billed amount to a cost for each HCPC code billed. For most APCs, since they are single procedures, all of the procedures within a particular APC are used to find the median cost for the APC payment weight. If there is a Composite APC, then the calculations are a little different in that these are for multiple procedures that meet the criteria for the Composite APC payment. Then the wage adjustment is calculated where it takes 60 percent of the total cost and then adjusts it based on the wage adjustment for the area and the other 40 percent is not adjusted. There are no token charges for devices, interrupted procedures, and no cost or full credit devices used to set the median cost for APCs. The median costs are then converted to a relative weight by dividing the median cost of the APC by the median cost for a Level 3 Hospital Clinic Visit APC. Then the relative weights are scaled for budget neutrality and then it is ready for payment calculation. This next step is taking the relative weight and multiplying it by the conversion factor and any other adjustments such as cost of outlier payments and annual market basket update factors to come up with the APC payment.

Packaging

Packaged services under OPPS include items and services that are considered to be an important or critical part of another service that is paid under the OPPS program. If the payment is for a packaged service, no other payments are made for the additional services or items. For example, routine supplies, anesthesia, recovery room use, and most drugs are considered to be an integral part of a surgical procedure, so payment for these items are packaged into the APC payment for the surgical procedure (CMS, 2012, p. 20).

If there is a payment made for an OPPS APC that contained packaged services, a separate payment would not be made to the provider for those services. Healthcare facilities need to make sure that they are following Coding Clinic and Best Practices to ensure that all HCPCS codes are consistent in their descriptions, CPT codes, and CMS instructions along with correct coding principles for all charges to payers regardless of if the claim is a separate or packaged claim.

Packaging Types under the OPPS

There are different types of packaging for services under OPPS. The payment status indicators that will be referenced are "N," which is not reimbursed under OPPS; "S," which is for significant procedures that do not involve multiple procedure reductions; "T" for surgical procedures where multiple procedure reductions apply; "V" is for medical visits; and "X" for ancillary services.

There are unconditionally **packaged services** that a separate payment is never made on claims with a status indicator of "N." The next group is for status indicators STVX packaged services. For the status indicator of S, T, V, and X there is not an additional payment made to the provider. If there is a STVX packaged claim there can't be another payment made for this packaged product. The "T" packages service is where a separate payment is made only if there is not another service reported for the same day that falls into the "T" status indicator. The T-packaged service is assigned the status indicator Q2. A service that is assigned a composite APC is a major component of a single **episode of care payment**. The facility only receives one payment through a composite APC for when there are multiple major separately identifiable services (CMS, 2012, p. 22).

Discounting

There are several areas where a discount is taken by CMS on a facility. One instance is a procedure where anesthesia is planned but then discontinued, as this type of service will have the facility receive 50 percent of the full OPPS payment. The discounting process goes on in that 50 percent of the full amount is paid if a procedure is used for which anesthesia is not planned. Then multiple surgical procedures furnished during the same hospital stay will generate a payment based on the highest reimbursement.

If there are multiple surgical procedures performed on a patient on the same operative session, then they will be discounted. The full amount is paid for the surgical procedure with the highest cost-weight, and 50 percent is paid for any other surgical procedure(s) that are performed at the same time.

Payment Adjustments

Payments under the OPPS structure are impacted by geographic differences in labor-related costs. In addition to the differences in labor-related costs, there are adjustments for rural hospitals, cancer hospitals, and outlier adjustments.

OPPS incorporates an outlier payment to make sure that all outpatient services with potentially significant costs do not pose excessive financial risk to providers. A service or group of services that are billed become eligible for outlier payments when the cost-to-charge ratio (CCR) separately exceeds each relevant threshold.

Outlier payments are determined by calculating the cost-related portion of the OPPS line item, including all charges such as pass-through devices, and multiplying this amount by the hospitals overall CCR and then determining whether the total cost for a service exceeds 1.75 times the OPPS payment and if the cost for the service exceeds both thresholds, the outlier payment is 50 percent of the amount by which the cost exceeds 1.75 time the OPPS payment (CMS, 2012, p. 28).

To demonstrate the line item portion of packaged services and revenue codes, the cost of the claim is $100 and there are three APC payment amounts paid for OPPS services on the claim that are $200, $300, and $500 for a total payment of $1,000. The first OPPS service line item will be allocated $20 or 20 percent of the total cost of the packages services as this line item accounts for 20 percent of the total payment on the claim. Then the next line that is for $300 is allocated $30 and the third line is allocated $50 as it was 50 percent of the total cost of the packaged services (CMS, 2012, p. 29).

For a composite payment and pass-through device the outlier payments are calculated as follows. The composite payment takes all costs and rolls them up into one line to establish a single cost for the composite APC and then the packaged cost is allocated proportionately to the separate line items. For the pass-through device the payment for this device is added to the payment for the related procedures, less any offset, in determining if the procedure is eligible for an outlier payment.

OPPS Coinsurance

OPPS has frozen the outpatient hospital coinsurance at 20 percent of the national median charge for the services within each APC, but the coinsurance amount for an APC cannot be less than 20 percent of the APC payment rate. According to Casto & Forrestal (2013), CMS wanted to move to a PPS to ensure that beneficiary copayment amounts from hospital to hospital would be consistent. Prior to this, Hospital A could charge $3,000 for a colonoscopy and the beneficiary would be responsible for $600, but if Hospital B charged $3,500 for the same colonoscopy, the beneficiary would be responsible for $700 (Casto & Forrestal, 2013, p. 182).

The sequence for calculating payment for a Medicare payment and coinsurance by applying the appropriate wage index adjustment to the payment for each APC group, subtract from the adjusted APC rate any deductible, multiply the adjusted APC payment (APC rate less deductible) by the program payment percentage or 80 percent (whichever is lower) to determine the Medicare payment amount. Then you take this amount and subtract it from the adjusted APC payment rate. If this amount is less than the inpatient deductible for the calendar year, the amount is the beneficiary's coinsurance amount. If the amount exceeds the deductible for the calendar year, the beneficiary coinsurance amount is limited to the inpatient hospital deductible amount and Medicare will pay the difference to the provider (CMS, 2012, p. 64).

Pass-Through Payments

The list of devices that are eligible for pass-through payments changes as new device categories are approved for pass-through payment status on an ongoing basis. The Medicare, Medicaid, and SCHIP Benefits Improvement and Protection Act (BIPA) of 2000 requires establishing categories for purposes of determining transitional pass-through for devices. Each category is defined as a separate code in the C series, or occasionally, a code in another series of HCPCS (CMS, 2012, p. 85).

Devices that qualify may be billed using the currently active category codes for pass-through payments as long as they meet the definition of a device that qualifies it for this type of payment and are described by the long descriptor associated with a currently active pass-through device category HCPCS code and are describe according-ing to the definitions of terms and other general explanations issued by CMS (CMS, 2012, p. 86).

Ultimately, the hospital is responsible for the content of the bills they present to Medicare. If hospital administrators have any questions regarding the appropriate coding processes they can review the HCPCS codes available for the year of service in question. Many device manufacturers will make information available to hospitals with coding information for the devices that they manufacture. This can be helpful but does not supersede federal requirements (CMS, 2012, p. 87).

New Technology

New technology APCs were created to allow procedures and services to enter OPPS quickly, even though their complete cost and payment information is not known. New technology APCs house modern procedures and services until enough data are col-lected to properly place the new procedure in an existing APC or to create a new APC. A procedure or service can remain in a new technology APC for an indefinite amount of time (Casto & Forrestal, 2013, p. 183).

Transitional Corridor Payments

The Medicare, Medicaid, and SCHIP Balanced Budget Refinement Act of 1999 (BBRA) established transitional payments to limit providers' losses under the OPPS; the additional payments are for 3.5 years for community mental health centers (CMHCs) and most hospitals, and permanent for cancer hospitals effective August 1, 2000. Section 405 of BIPA provides that children's hospitals are held harmless permanently and some rural hospitals are held harmless for several years after the implementation of OPPS (CMS, 2012, p. 97).

Eligible facilities receive a quarterly interim hold-harmless payment that provides additional reimbursement when the payment received under OPPS is less than the payment the facility would have received for the same services under the prior reasonable cost-based system in 1996 (Casto & Forrestal, 2013, p. 187). The calculation for payment is done by taking the OPPS reimbursement for the facility for the current quarter less the Pre-OPPS reimbursement will equal the hold-harmless payment. If the OPPS payment exceeds the Pre-OPPS payment, there will be no hold-harmless payment made to the facility.

■ Home Health Prospective Payment System (HH PPS)

History

The **Home Health Prospective Payment System (HH PPS)** was initially mandated by law in the Balanced Budget Act of 1997. **Home health care** agencies provide skilled nursing care to patients that are considered to be homebound. The services that are provided are skilled nursing care, physical therapy, occupational therapy, speech therapy, social work, and home health aide services. In addition, a nursing agency can provide durable medical equipment (DME) to their patients. To process claims an agency has two options to process claims for payment. For most agencies, they are to submit claims electronically by using the electronic HIPAA standard institutional claim transaction called 837I. The other option for some of the agencies is to submit a claim via the paper form CMS-1450, or otherwise known as a UB-04.

Medicare beneficiaries have no cost sharing for home health services except for a 20 percent coinsurance for any durable medical equipment that is provided to the patient during the time the home health agency is servicing the patient. Since DME is covered under HH PPS, services are covered by Medicare Part A for nursing and Medicare Part B for DME. In the beginning, homecare was established for short-term care for a patient that was discharged from an acute care facility. The case would be opened by a registered nurse and if clinical need was present, a Plan of Care (POC), or certification would be created and sent to the patient's physician for signature. These POCs can be made by a home health physician, a nonphysician practitioner

(NPP) working with the certifying physician, or after a stay in an acute care facility or post-acute facility. The POC is for a 60-day time frame.

The certification must state that a face-to-face encounter took place within 90 days prior to the start of homecare or within 30 days after the start of care. Then the patient must be considered to be confined to their home environment and in need of intermittent care. A POC needs to be established and reviewed by a physician and all services need to be furnished while under the care of a physician. The number of 60-day POCs were unlimited as long as the patient was considered to be meeting the criteria for care from the agency.

Certifications, or POCs, must be completed at the time of care being established or as soon as possible after the start of care. After the first POC, the physician must recertify services for the patient for each 60-day POC thereafter. The POC will identify how long the physician feels the patient will be in need of care from the homecare agency.

Homecare agencies are paid by an episode-of-care method of payment. This payment is considered to cover all services rendered to the patient during the current 60-day period or POC. This one payment will cover all skilled nursing, physical therapy, speech therapy, home health aide services, medical social work services, and medical supplies that include nonroutine medical supplies such as supplies that are needed to fulfill the orders from the physician and the particular needs of the patient as related to the POC.

Outcomes Assessment Information Set

Home health agencies collect data in six major domains, which are as follows (Casto & Forrestal, 2013, p. 241):

1. Sociodemographic
2. Environment
3. Support system
4. Health status
5. Functional status
6. Behavioral status

The data is collected at the following times:

1. Start of care (SOC)
2. Significant changes in condition (SCIC)
3. Transfer to inpatient facility
4. Resumption of care (ROC) after inpatient hospitalization situation occurs
5. Discharge from care of HHA
6. Death at home

Payment of Episodes

Typically a split percentage payment is made to the homecare agency. The payments consist of an initial payment and final payment. The initial payment is in response to a **Request for Anticipated Payment** (RAP) and the final payment is in response to a submitted claim. The total of the RAP and the final payment will total to 100 percent of the allowed payment for the episode (CMS, 2013b, p. 10).

There are multiple PPS for Medicare for different provider types. Each system operates differently and has variation how payments are made and how units are calculated. For the HH PPS program the payments are for a 60-day period (or less) as the payment unit. The payment itself is not made totally in advance, but the amount of the payment is known before the start of care. With HH PPS, the majority of the payment is made after the first visit is completed or delivered.

Case-mix is an underlying component of prospective payment. HH PPS is built on the prospective payment system similar to the inpatient prospective system works with the use of DRGs. In HH PPS, the resource groups are called home health resources groups (HHRGs) instead of DRGs. The 60-day POC payment is calculated and there are case-mix adjustments identified through the patient assessment. The POC payment is adjusted through this case-mix process in that the adjusted payment is based on the elements of the OASIS data set that includes the therapy visits over the course of the episode. The number of therapy visits will be projected at the time of the patient starting services. The initial payment is based on the case-mix adjustment based on the Grouper software (CMS, 2013b, p. 11).

The 60-day episode of care payment is case-mix adjusted by using one of 153 HHRGs. These HHRGs are represented in the HIPPS codes and allows the HHRG to be reported more efficiently and include additional information for things such as payments for nonroutine supplies. There are five positions in this alphanumeric home health HIPPS codes and described as follows:

1. The first position is for the grouping step that applies to the three domain scores that follow.

2. The second, third, and fourth positions of the code are a one-to-one crosswalk to the three domains of the HHRG coding system and these characters are alphabetical only in HH PPS.

3. The fifth position indicates the severity group for nonroutine supplies.

Billing Process under HH PPS

Home health agencies are required by Medicare to assess potential patients and reassess existing patients using the Outcome and Assessment Information Set (OASIS). The information is entered and formatted and transmitted to state agencies and HAVEN software, that is available through CMS, supports the OASIS data and the transmission. The HAVEN software is not mandatory and some home health agencies have chosen their own software applications for this purpose.

Grouper software determines the appropriate case-mix group for payment of a HH PPS 60-day episode from the results of an OASIS submission for a patient. This process groups everything into a CMS HIPPS. Grouper will also output a Claims-OASIS Matching Key that will link the HIPPS code to a particular OASIS submission. Under HH PPS, both HIPPS code and the Claims-OASIS Matching Key will be entered on RAPs and claims. If an adjustment is done after the initial submission or the claim is rejected by the state agency and a corrected claim is sent, the RAP and final claim for the episode must be rebilled using the updated or correct HIPPS code (CMS, 2013b, p. 16).

Submitting a Request for Anticipated Payment

The home health agency can submit a Request for Anticipated Payment (RAP) after the OASIS assessment is complete, export ready, or finalized for transmitting to the state, and after a physician's verbal orders for home care have been received and documented. Next, a POC is established and sent to the physician for signature. Finally, the first service visit has been completed by the home health agency (CMS, 2013b, p. 16).

Once an episode is opened on the Common Working File (CWF) with the processing of a RAP. Initial claims, subsequent claims or episodes, and transfer cases should be submitted as soon as possible after care is started so as to ensure being established as the primary home health agency for the patient/beneficiary. The initial RAP is submitted in a standard claim format, however, it is not treated as a home health claim and is not subject to many of the claims regulations. After a submission for a RAP payment is made, the next submission will be a final bill or the bill at the end of the 60-day period. The home health agency cannot submit this claim until all services have been delivered and are completed. Home health claims must be submitted with type of bill (TOB) 329. The HH PPS claim will include the elements originally submitted on the RAP and all other line item details for the entire episode. If the home health agency provided durable medical equipment, oxygen, or prosthetics and orthotics, these services will be paid in addition to the episode of payment (CMS, 2013b, p. 17).

RAPs can be adjusted and/or cancelled by the home health agency. An adjustment is submitted to correct any information that was submitted in error and that may change the payment amount to the provider. A cancellation of a claim is used to change the beneficiary HICN or the home health agency's provider number if it was submitted in error. This is due to the fact if the beneficiary number is wrong, the patient that is being billed in error may cause a denial for the home health agency that might be starting up care. If the wrong home health agency number is transmitted, then the wrong agency will be receiving payment for care that they are not providing.

Transfer Cases

Transfer of a patient in home care is when a beneficiary chooses to change home health agencies during a 60-day period that they are currently with another home healthcare provider. By law, patients have the right to change or transfer from one home health agency to another home health agency. For this process to go smoothly, the receiving home health agency must submit a RAP with a transfer indicator placed in the condition code field. This will identify that an episode of care payment may already be open for the patient with another home health agency. Then the receiving home health agency will document, in writing, that the patient has been informed that the initial home health agency will no longer be receiving Medicare payments on behalf of the patient and will no longer be the agency that will be delivering services after the transfer date.

The previously open episode will automatically be closed in the Medicare claims processing system as of the date the patient begins service with the new home health agency. The payment will be prorated for the shortened length of care provided by the transferring agency that is less than 60 days. Sometimes a patient may choose to transfer to another home health agency the day after the previous POC ends with the other home health agency. In this instance, the transferring from agency may not have submitted the RAP for the upcoming 60-day POC and the home health agency that the patient is being serviced going forward will need to identify that their POC will be adjacent to the previous agency's POC. The agency that the patient has transferred to will need to educate the patient (and family or caregivers) that the previous agency will not be billing for services after the transfer/discharge date and they will not be providing services after that date.

Discharge and Readmission

A **discharge planning** for a patient that is on service for a home health agency is when a patient completed the POC through the 60-day window and all goals have been met on or by the 60th day. This is a clean admission and discharge, as the home health agency has started the POC and submitted the RAP at the start of care and received payment and then delivered care up to the 60th day before discharging the patient on the 60th day and submitting their final bill. As perfect as this sounds, it is not always the case in home care. Sometimes the patient can be discharged during the 60-day episode and then readmitted back to the same agency. In this case, the same agency cannot bill for another episode during the same 60-day period. The agency will need to have the first period prorated to reflect the time spent with the agency. Then the new POC for the most recent admission will be a new episode for the home health agency once the first visit is delivered and completed. In situations where a patient is currently with a home health agency and they are admitted to an inpatient facility, the servicing home health agency can discharge the patient if they feel that the patient will not return within the 60-day POC. At this point, the patient was discharged early in the POC and the agency will receive full payment. If the home health agency decides not to discharge the patient when they are sent to a hospital or skilled nursing facility, and the patient returns to the agency during the 60-day POC, the care will simply continue where they left off.

Partial Episode Payment

When a patient is discharged, readmitted, and transferred to the same agency in a 60-day period, it results in a shortened episode of care payment given by the agency. In this instance, the payment to the home health agency will need to be prorated for the shorter episode. These adjustments are called **Partial Episode Payments** (PEP). This situation will occur when (CMS, 2013b, p. 20):

- A patient has been discharged and readmitted to home care within the same 60-day episode. This will be indicated by putting a Patient Discharge Status code of 06 on the final claim for the first part of the 60 day episode; or

- When a patient transfers to another home health agency during a 60-day episode. This is also indicated with a Patient Discharge Status code of 06 on their final claim.

After January 1, 2008, the nonroutine supply (NRS) payment amount is also subject to this prorated PPE.

Low Utilization Payment

The normal episode of care payment covers a 60-day period. However, there are times that a shorter length of stay, or episode, is experienced for a patient. If a home health agency provides four visits or less in an episode, they will be paid a standardized per visit payment instead of an episode payment for a 60-day period. Such payments, adjustments, and episodes themselves are called **Low Utilization Payment Adjustments** (LUPAs).

On a LUPA claim, nonroutine supplies will not be reimbursed in addition to the per visit payment. This is due to the fact that the total annual supply payments are already calculated into all payment rates. Since home health agencies in such cases are likely to have received one split-percentage payment, which would likely be greater than the total LUPA payment, the difference between these visit payments and the payment already received will offset against future payments when the claim for the episode is received. If at a later date the patient receives five or more visits, the payments will be adjusted to an episode basis rather than a visit basis (CMS 2013b, p. 21).

If the home health agency anticipates that the episode of care payment will be four visits or less, they can elect not to submit a RAP at the start of care. This will avoid the home health agency from experiencing an adjustment, or recouping of funds, for receiving the initial payment and not exceeding four visits.

Therapy Thresholds

When the home health agency reports data on the episode for a patient in OASIS, the amount of visits that are estimated will be verified from the line item detail on the claim form for the episode. The HH PPS adjusts the Medicare payment based on 3 therapy thresholds of 6, 14, or 20 visits being met. Due to the complexities of the payment system regarding therapies, the Pricer software in the Medicare claims processing system will recode the claim based on the actual number of visits completed by the home health agency. Since the number of therapy visits provided can change the payment equation under the refined four-equation case mix model, in some cases it will changes several positions in the HIPPS code. The electronic remittance advice (RA) will show the original code submitted on the claim at the beginning of the episode and the code actually used for payment so as to keep things clearly identified for the home health agency (CMS, 2013b, p. 22).

Adjustment of Episode of Payment – Early and Late Episodes

HH PPS uses a 4-equation case-mix model that recognizes and differentiates payment for early episodes of care that are the first or second episode in a sequence of adjacent covered episodes or a later episodes that is in the third episode and beyond in a sequence of adjacent covered episodes. An adjacent episode is one that is not separated by more than a 60-day period between claims.

Adjustment of Episode of Payment – Outlier Payments

HH PPS payment groups are based on averages of home care experience. When cases are considered to be outside the expected experience by involving an unusually high level of services in 60-day periods, Medicare will provide for extra or outlier payments in addition to the case-mix adjusted episode payment. Outlier payments can be a result of medically necessary high utilization of any or all of the service disciplines. A claim is determined to be an outlier eligible claim if the number of visits of each discipline on the claim and each wage-adjusted national standardized per visit rate for each discipline with the sum of the episode payment and a wage-adjusted standard fixed loss threshold amount (CMS, 2013b, p. 24).

If the total product of the number of visits and the national standardized visit rate is greater than the case-mix specific payment amount plus the fixed loss threshold amount, a percentage of the difference may be payable to the home health agency. This amount will be a percentage of the amount that exceeds the case-mix payment and threshold. This outlier calculation is done automatically and the home care agency does not have to submit anything to have a claim to be eligible. Due to the fact that the outlier payment will show up on the electronic remittance advice in a separate segment, the type of outlier does not need a long stay outlier payment because the number of continuous episodes of care for eligible beneficiaries is unlimited (CMS, 2013b, p. 25).

■ Home Health Prospective Payment System Consolidated Billing

Section 1842 (b)(6)(F) of the Social Security Act requires consolidated billing of all home health services while a patient is under a POC for a home health agency that is authorized by a physician. The home health agency is considered to be overseeing the care for the patient, and any items or services are to be paid to a single home health agency overseeing the patient. The home health agency will be responsible for making payment to the other providers.

The types of service that are subject to the home health consolidated billing provision are skilled nursing care, home health aide services, physical therapy, speech-language pathology, occupational therapy, medical social services, routine and nonroutine medical supplies, medical services provided by an intern or resident-in-training of a hospital, and care for homebound patients involving equipment too cumbersome to take to the home (CMS, 2013b, p. 29). In some instances, if a home health agency is not aware of a vendor providing services either directly or under arrangement would not be responsible for payment to another provider when there was no knowledge of these services being rendered to the patient.

Under the Medicare Home Health Services Conditions of Participation: Patient Rights (42CFR§484.10 [c] [i]), the home health agency must advise the patient, in advance, of the disciplines (e.g., skilled nursing, physical therapy, home health aide, etc.) that will furnish care, and the frequency of visits proposed to be furnished. It is the responsibility of the home health agency to fully inform beneficiaries that all home health services, including therapies and supplies, will be provided by his/her primary home health agency (CMS 2013b, p. 31).

In addition, under the Conditions of participation: Patient liability for payment, (42 CFR, §484.10[e]), home health agencies are responsible for advising the patient, in advance, about the extent to which payment is expected from Medicare or other sources, including the patient (CMS, 2013b, p. 31).

Responsibilities of Providers

Medicare makes payments to one home health agency under the consolidated billing process. With that in mind, it is the responsibility of the home health agency to determine if any other services or providers are in a patient's home prior to starting care with that patient. Therapy providers or suppliers can speak with the patient or caregivers to see if there are any providers of care presently giving care to the patient and document this in the medical record. This documentation does not shift any liability for payment to Medicare or the patient. Home health agencies can also check the Common Working File to see if any documentation exists showing that the patient is currently under the care of another agency.

Discharge Planning and Transfer Patients

Under the Medicare Conditions of Participation for Hospitals: Discharge planning, (42 CFR, §482.43 [b] [3] and [6]), hospitals must have a discharge process in place that applies to all patients and must include the evaluation or likelihood of the patient needing post-hospital services and of the availability of the services. The discharge planning evaluation must be present in the patient's medical record and the hospital must discuss the planning process and evaluation with the patient and/or family members. In addition, under 42 CFR, § 482.43 (c) (5), the patient and family or caregivers need to be counseled to prepare them to be able to handle post-acute care and 42 CFR, § 482.43 (d) Transfer or referral, the hospital must transfer or refer patients, along with the necessary medical information, to appropriate facilities, agencies, or outpatient services, as needed for follow up or ancillary care (CMS, 2013b, p. 33).

The intent of this process is to make sure that, not only the patient, but the caregivers and family members are aware of which home health agency will be providing care for the patient and what services are going to be provided. In addition, the hospital must give the patient freedom of choice to choose which agency that they would like to be transferred to after the hospital stay. The hospital must transfer all necessary information to the receiving agency so as to prepare properly for the admission of the patient.

Physician and Nonphysician Practitioners

A system that is designed for classifying health services based on the cost of furnishing physician services is called resource-based relative value scale (RBRVS). This system is the federal government's payment system for physicians. RBRVS became effective on January 1, 1992. To avoid major disruptions to physicians' reimbursements, the RBRVS was gradually phased in beginning in 1992 with full implementation by 1996 (Casto & Forrestal, 2013, p. 155).

A relative value scale permits comparisons of the resources needed or appropriate for various units of services. Relative value scale takes into account labor, skill, supplies, equipment, space, and other costs associated with each procedure or service in a physician's office (Casto & Forrestal, 2013, p. 155).

The structure of payment is based on a **relative value unit (RVU)** and has a geographic adjustment, and a conversion factor (CF). This system is based on the HCPCS and each HCPCS/CPT code has been assigned an RVU. An RVU is defined as a unit of measure designed to permit comparison of the amount of resources required to perform various provider services by assigning weights to such factors as personnel time, level of skill, and sophistication of equipment required to render services to a patient (Casto & Forrestal, 2013, p. 155).

The fully implemented resource-based Medicare Physician Fee Schedule is calculated as follows:

$$\text{MPFS Amount} = [(\text{RVUw} \times \text{GPCIw}) + (\text{RVUpe} \times \text{GPCIpe}) + (\text{RVUm} \times \text{GPCIm})] \times \text{CF}$$

- The RVUw equals a relative value for physician work
- The RVUpe equals a relative value for practice expense
- The RVUm refers to a relative value for malpractice (MP)
- The GPCIw is for physician work
- The GPCIpe is for practice expense
- The GPCIm is for malpractice

The GPCI stands for **Geographic Practice Cost Indices** and this is the means in which each payment is adjusted based on the geography or payment locality. The last part of the equation is the CF or Conversion Factor. The CF is used in the computation of every MPFS amount. The current CF is $34.0230 (CMS, 2013a).

WORK is the component that covers the physician's salary. This includes the work time that the physician spends working with the patient and the intensity in which that time is spent. The parts of intensity are mental effort and judgment, technical skill, physical effort, and psychological stress (Casto & Forrestal, 2013, p. 156).

Practice Expense (PE) is the overhead and costs to operate the practice. CMS conducts a survey called the Socioeconomic Monitoring System (SMS) to obtain data to calculate the overhead costs of running a physician practice. The SMS includes six categories of costs. The first one is for clinical payroll that includes physician assistants, nurse practitioners, but does not include the physician's payroll. The second expense category is administrative payroll, which covers the non-physician administrative payroll for office manages and secretaries. The third category is for office expenses, which covers rent, mortgage, interest, depreciation, and utilities such as telephone and electricity. The fourth category is for medical material and supply expenses that covers drugs, x-ray films, and disposable medical products. The fifth category is medical equipment expenses that includes depreciation, leases, and rental for medical equipment. The sixth category is all other expenses that coves legal services, accounting, office management, professional association membership, and any professional expenses (Casto & Forrestal, 2013, p. 156).

The GPCI is an adjustment that adjusts for costs that vary in different parts of the country. This adjustment will take the relative differences in costs of a **market basket** of goods and normalize them to the area in which the practice is located.

The conversion factor is an across the board multiplier. This is a constant that applies to the entire calculation into a payment. There are two categories that a physician can bill in and they are Facility and Nonfacility. For a facility setting, the physician is paid a facility rate in the inpatient hospital setting, outpatient hospital setting, emergency room setting, Medicare participating ambulatory surgical center, skilled nursing facility, ambulance (land or air), inpatient psychiatric facility, community mental health center, psychiatric residential treatment center, and comprehensive inpatient rehabilitation facility. A nonfacility setting is a pharmacy, school, homeless shelter, prison, office, home or private residence, group home, assisted living facility, mobile unit, temporary lodging, walk-in retail health clinic, urgent care facility, birthing center, nursing facility, custodial care facility, independent clinic, federally qualified health center, end-stage renal facility, rural health clinic, and independent lab to name a few.

■ Ambulatory Surgical Center

History

Ambulatory Surgical Centers (ASC) before 2008 handled certain surgical procedures under Medicare Part B. These procedures were those that generally did not exceed 90 minutes in length and did not require more than 4 hours of recovery time. Prior to 2008 Medicare did not pay an ASC for those procedures that required more than an ASC level of care. Beginning in January 2008, payment is made to ASCs under Medicare Part B for all surgical procedures except those that CMS determines may pose a significant safety risk. In addition, certain drugs and biologicals, OPPS pass-through devices, brachytherapy sources, and radiological procedures were covered at an ASC (CMS, 2010, p. 3).

In 2008, CMS started publishing updates to the list of procedures that an ASC can get paid for each year. This is also updated quarterly for new surgical procedures and covered ancillary services to establish payment indicators and payment rates for newly created Level II HCPCS and Category III CPT Codes. To be paid under this provision, a facility must be certified and meet the requirements for ASC and accept Medicare's payment as payment in full for the services covered at an ASC. Certain other lab services or nonimplantable DME may be performed when billed using the appropriate certified provider/supplier UPIN/NPI (CMS, 2010, p. 4).

An ASC for Medicare is defined as an entity that operates exclusively for the purpose of furnishing outpatient surgical services. The ASC must have in effect an agreement with CMS in accordance with 42 CFR 416 subpart B. An ASC is either independent or operated by a hospital. A hospital-operated facility has the option of being considered by Medicare either to be an ASC or to be a provider-based department of a hospital (CMS, 2010, p. 4).

ASC Listing

ASC services are those surgical procedures that are identified by CMS and on a list that is updated annually. For surgical procedures not covered in ASCs, the related professional services may be billed by the rendering provider as Part B services and the beneficiary is liable for the facility charges, which are not covered by Medicare.

■ Conclusion

The Hospital Outpatient Prospective Payment system (OPPS) that started in 2000 has evolved to a complex prospective payment system. The outpatient environment includes outpatient services, home health, physician and nonphysician practitioners, and ambulatory surgical settings. Each area has a specific set of procedures and requirements to be compliant with regulations involving billing. Since 1992, the system that we call Medicare has evolved, and to remain competitive and to continue to deliver quality patient care with a margin, the prospective payment system is needed to be understood by all levels of management and caregivers. This new way of reimbursing a healthcare facility has shifted the responsibility of profit and loss directly to the provider. Much as the Inpatient Prospective Payment System has done on the acute care side. As hospitals continue to struggle with understanding this type of reimbursement, this chapter has introduced the many parts of the payment system which will assist the healthcare professional in navigating through this payment system in the current state and future changes that may happen along the way.

References

Casto, A.B., & Forrestal, E. (2013). *Principles of healthcare reimbursement* (4th ed.). Chicago: AHIMA.

Centers for Medicare and Medicaid Services. (2013a). CY 2013 Physican fee schedule final rule with comment period. Retrieved from http://www.cms.gov/Medicare/Medicare-Fee-for-Service-Payment/PhysicianFeeSched/index.html?redirect=/physicianfeesched/

Centers for Medicare and Medicaid Services. (2010a). Chapter 14: Ambulatory surgical centers. In: *Medicare claims processing manual*. Retrieved from http://www.cms.gov/Regulations-and-Guidance/Guidance/Manuals/Downloads/clm104c14.pdf

Centers for Medicare and Medicaid Services. (2012). Chapter 4: Part B hospital (including inpatient hospital part B and OPPS). In *Medicare claims processing manual*. Retrieved from http://www.cms.gov/Regulations-and-Guidance/Guidance/Manuals/Downloads/clm104c04.pdf

Centers for Medicare and Medicaid Services. (2013b). Chapter 10: Home health agency billing. In *Medicare claims processing manual*. Retrieved from http://www.cms.gov/Regulations-and-Guidance/Guidance/Manuals/Downloads/clm104c10.pdf

9 | Coding for the Non-HIM Professional

Learning Outcomes

After reading this chapter, the student will be able to:

- Define the health record and the components that make up the record.
- List the requirements for timely and accurate documentation in completing medical record entries.
- Define the meaning and structure of ICD-9-CM, ICD-10-CM, and HCPCS.
- Differentiate the coding found in ICD-9-CM, ICD-10-CM, and HCPCS.

■ Introduction

This chapter is focused on the development and use of the health record. In today's healthcare environment the history, care, and treatment of the patient is documented in the patient health record. This record is a paper or electronic document of the care provided and outcomes of care. Based on the health record data, a coding process occurs to organize the data into a form to generate payment as well as generate reports. The coding is currently completed using ICD-9-CM. In 2015 the system will begin to change to ICD-10-CM. This chapter will provide the foundation for understanding the health record and coding processes for the non-HIM professional.

■ The Health Record

History of the Health Record

Over the years, the medical record was basically one-dimensional, as the content was paper and various x-ray and other imaging films that formed what we came to know as the medical record. This medical record was considered the legal business record and the patient did not own the record, but had certain rights to the content of the medical record. According to Kuehn (2013), the health record is the source of information on all aspects of an individual's health care. The health record is vital to patient care as it includes demographics, reasons for visits, results of tests, treatments ordered, and plans for follow-up. In short, the health record explains who, what, when, where, why, and how of patient care (Kuehn, 2013, p. 2).

The legal health record is a subset of the entire patient database, which serves as the legal business record for the organization. The roles of the legal health record are to (NDHIT, 2010, p. 1):

- support the decisions made in a patient's care;
- support the revenue sought from the third-party payers; and
- document the services provided as legal testimony regarding the patient's illness or injury, response to treatment, and caregiver decisions.

The legal health record contains documentation on all the services provided to a patient during their stay in a hospital or while receiving treatment at a physician's office, ambulatory care center, or other healthcare facility. This record must meet the standards defined by the Centers for Medicare and Medicaid Services Conditions of Participation, any other federal regulations, state laws, and accrediting agencies such as the Joint Commission on Accreditation of Healthcare Organizations. In addition, the record must meet the standards of the healthcare provider and that of the third-party payer.

Making an Entry in the Health Record

All entries in the medical record must be legible. These entries include written progress notes, nursing notes, physical therapy, occupational therapy, speech therapy, consultations, and other notes that are handwritten in the patient's medical record to support the treatment provided during the visit or stay.

All entries must be complete. To be able to effectively code a medical record for a hospital stay or visit to a facility, the entries must be complete and contain sufficient information to identify the patient, support the diagnosis and condition, justify the care, treatment and services, document the course and results of care, treatment, and services; and promote continuity of care among providers (DHHS, 2009, p. 2).

All entries in the medical record must be dated, timed, and authenticated, in written or electronic form, by the person responsible for providing or evaluating the services provided. This includes the time and date of each entry, which must be accurately documented. The timing establishes when the order was given and when the activity is to take place. The timing and dating of entries is necessary for patient safety and quality of care and establishes a baseline for future actions or assessments and creates a timeline of events. There are many patient interventions or assessments that based on time intervals or timelines of various signs, symptoms, or events (DHHS, 2006a, p. 68687).

The facility must have a method to establish the identity of the author of each entry in the patient's file. This includes verification of the author or the order that comes into the facility through a fax or a computer entry. In addition, the facility will need to have a method that requires each author to take a specific action to verify that the entry they are making is authenticated by their entry or that they are responsible for the entry and that the entry is accurate (DHHS, 2009b, p. 2).

EXHIBIT 9-1   PARTS OF A MEDICAL RECORD

Face sheet

Demographics

History and physical

Consents for treatment/care

Laboratory

Radiology

Progress notes

Physicians' orders

Nurses' notes

Medication sheets

Flow records

Operative reports

Pathology

Copies of other facility records

Release of information section

The requirements for dating and timing do not apply for any orders or prescriptions that are initiated outside the hospital. Only when they are presented to the facility at the time of service will they need dating and timing on the order. For preprinted ordering systems, the healthcare practitioner will need to sign and date the last page of the order and note how many pages they are signing off on. If there are sections that are inside the preprinted order where a change was made, the practitioner will need to initial or sign any areas where changes were made and then initial or sign the top or bottom of the page where the changes were made. If there were no changes made and the practitioner checked the boxes as wanted, the practitioner does not need to initial the checked boxes as long as there were not any changes made to the text beside the box. The same principles would apply for an electronic order. The practitioner will need to date, time, and authenticate the order.

Authentication of medical record entries may include written signatures, initials, computer key, or other code. For authentication, a method must be established to identify the author in both written and electronic forms. When rubber stamps or electronic authorizations are used for authentication, the hospital must have policies and procedures to ensure that such stamps or authorizations are used only by the individuals whose signature they represent. There can be no delegation of stamps or authentication codes to another individual. It is important to note that some insurers and other payers may have a policy prohibiting the use of rubber stamps as a means of authenticating the medical records that support a claim for payment. Medicare payment policy no longer allows the use of rubber stamps. Although use of a rubber stamp for a signature may not be against the rules found in the Conditions of Participation (CoP) or be against any survey policy, a healthcare facility may want to discontinue the use of rubber stamps in the process of validating orders or authentication of a document that is used in the medical record (DHHS, 2009, p. 3).

When an electronic medical record is in use, the facility must demonstrate how it will prevent alterations of an entry in a medical record after it has been authenticated. During a survey, the facility must make available all pertinent codes and security features that are needed to review an electronic medical record.

There will be times during or after a patient's hospital stay where a practitioner dictates a report or gives an order and needs to authenticate the document. The use of auto-authentication, in which a practitioner dictates a report or order and wants to authenticate it without reading the document, is not permitted. This is not allowed, as every facility needs to have in place a process that can determine that a practitioner authenticated an entry or report after it was created. More importantly, the use of an exception rule (in which the document is created and if after 48 hours the physician has not disapproved the entry or report that it will automatically be authenticated) is also not permitted. Practices such as this one is not allowed. The report or order must be transcribed or entered into the system and be physically read by the practitioner making the order or dictating the report and then authenticated.

The practitioner must separately date and time his/her signature authenticating an entry, even though there may be a date and time already on the document, since the latter may not reflect when the entry was authenticated (DHHS, 2009, p. 4). When the electronic medical record (EMR) system documents the date and time that the practitioner viewed the document, then the practitioner does not need to separately authenticate the document with the date and time that they viewed the document. When the EMR system only puts the date and time that the document was created, but does not date- and time-stamp when the practitioner viewed it, then the practitioner will need to authenticate the document or acknowledge that the document was reviewed in another document, which would then authenticate the document. An example would be to state in a progress note that the lab results were viewed and note the date and time that this took place in the note; at this point, the lab results will be authenticated, dated, and timed by the practitioner.

A sample survey tool will include several areas of focus. First, the tool will check to see if all entries in the medical record are legible. Second, it will determine if all orders, progress notes, nursing notes, physical therapy, occupational therapy and other discipline entries are complete. The documentation must support the services delivered to the patient, which allows the facility to bill the payer. Third, it will ensure that all entries in the medical record are dated, timed, and appropriately authenticated by the person responsible for the entry. Fourth, it will verify that the orders in the record, including telephone verbal orders (TVO), are written or entered into the record by the practitioner who is caring for the patient and who is authorized by hospital policy and in accordance with state law to write orders. Fifth, it will make sure that the facility has the means to verify the signatures in the chart, both written and electronic, by signature verification for paper and security features for electronic signatures and authorizations. Sixth, it will make sure that all documents are being authenticated after they are being created (DHHS, 2009, p. 5).

Hybrid Medical Records

As the progression over the years from a completely paper file to a **hybrid medical record** file containing that consisted of paper that was scanned into a file that was combined with electronic images that created this hybrid format. Hospital systems, ambulatory surgery centers, home health, and other medical providers are moving to a completely electronic health record.

Formats of Medical Records

There are three types, or formats, of medical records, and the first type is a source-oriented medical record. The **Source-Oriented Health Record** consists of a conventional or traditional method of maintaining paper-based health records. In this method, health records are organized according to the source or originating department that provided the service to the patient (LaTour & Eichenwald Maki, 2013, p. 255).

The second type is the **Problem-Oriented Health Record**. This format was developed by Lawrence Weed in the 1970s. The problem-oriented health record is comprised of a problem list, the database or the history and physical exam and initial lab findings, the initial plan of what tests or treatments the patient will receive during their stay, and progress notes that are organized so that every member of the healthcare team can easily follow the course of the patient's treatment (LaTour & Eichenwald Maki, 2013, p. 256).

The third type is called the **Integrated Health Record**. The content of the integrated health record is arranged in strict chronological order. The order of the record is determined by the date the information was entered or the date of the service that gives the sequence of the care that the patient received during their stay (LaTour & Eichenwald Maki, 2013, p. 257).

When the record comes to the Health Information Management Department from the floor or nursing unit, it will be assembled if the facility is still on a paper record or hybrid system. The order will be changed to a reverse-chronological order, in which the first date of service in every section of the medical record is on top and the most recent date of service is the last page.

Record Retention

Health records are legal business records and must be maintained following federal and state regulations to ensure that the information, if accessed, is accurate and complete. Individual states generally govern how long medical records are to be retained. HIPAA rules require a Medicare Fee-For-Service provider to retain required documentation for 6 years from the date of its creation, or the date when it last was in effect, whichever is later. CMS requires that providers submitting cost reports to retain all patient records for at least 5 years after closure of the cost report. If your facility is a Medicare Managed Care program provider, CMS requires that you retain the patient records for 10 years. Medicare does not have a specific format in which the records are to be maintained or stored. The records can be in the original form or a legally reproducible form and that can be electronic or digital. Whichever format is chosen, it is important to use a system that protects and ensures the security and integrity of all records. It is very important that records should be accurately written, promptly completed, properly filed, and readily accessible (Medicare Learning Network, 2010, 1).

■ ICD-9-CM

Currently in use in the United States is the *International Classification of Diseases, Ninth Revision, Clinical Modification (ICD-9-CM)*; it remains in use until October 2015, when ICD-10-CM is proposed to replace ICD-9-CM. The ICD-9-CM was developed by the National Center for Health Statistics (NCHS) and has been in use since 1979. Although the international version of ICD focuses on acute illnesses and mortality, ICD-9-CM was expanded to include morbidity or chronic conditions and procedure reporting (Casto & Forrestal, 2013, p. 27).

ICD-9-CM serves several uses as follows (Casto & Forrestal, 2013, p. 28):

- Classifying diagnosis and procedure information for epidemiological and clinical research
- Indexing hospital records by disease and surgical procedure
- Reporting information to various healthcare reimbursement systems
- Analyzing resource consumption patterns
- Analyzing adequacy of reimbursement for health services

Providers use the ICD-9-CM coding to determine payment categories for various Prospective Payment Systems (PPS). Hospital Inpatient uses Medicare-severity diagnosis-related groups (MS-DRG), Hospital Rehabilitation uses case-mix groups

(CMGs), Long-term Care uses long-term care Medicare-severity diagnosis-related groups (LTC-MS-DRGs), and Home Health uses home health resource groups (HHRGs) (Casto & Forrestal, 2013, p. 28).

ICD Volumes and Code Format

The ICD-9-CM book is divided up into three volumes and they include Volume I which is a tabular list of diseases and injuries, Volume II which is an alphabetic index to diseases, and Volume III consists of a classification for procedures.

ICD-9-CM diagnosis codes vary in length anywhere from 3 to 5 digits. There is a decimal point placed after the third digit. The first 3 digits consist of a category code. The fourth and fifth digits are subcategory and subclassification codes that provide the detailed information to better describe a patient's clinical condition. For example, 428 is the category Heart Failure. The code 428.0, with the additional fourth digit, shows that the heart failure is considered Congestive Heart Failure, unspecified. To further specify this diagnosis a fifth digit can be added. So the code 428.21, for example, now shows that the condition is specified as Acute Systolic Heart Failure.

Similar to the diagnosis codes, a procedure code will also vary in length anywhere from three to four digits. The first two digits of the procedure code comprise the category of the procedure being performed. The third and fourth digits are subcategory and subclassification codes that provide the detailed information on the procedure. For example, an operation on the gallbladder and the biliary tract is a category 51. If the patient has Laparoscopic Cholecystectomy, the code would be 51.23.

Maintenance of the ICD-9-CM is by the ICD-9-CM Coordination and Maintenance Committee which is made up by the NCHS and CMS and handle the United States clinical modification of the code set. The committee holds public meetings every year in March and September. At that time they take suggestions for any new codes needed, modifications to existing codes, and any codes that need to be discontinued or deleted. These submissions come from the public and private sectors. Any requests for changes must be made in writing and submitted prior to one of the semiannual meetings.

ICD-9-CM Coding Guidelines

The ICD-9-CM Coding Guidelines have been approved by the four organizations that make up the Cooperating Parties for the ICD-9-CM: the American Hospital Association (AHA), the American Health Information Management Association (AHIMA), CMS, and NCHS. These guidelines are included in the official government version of the ICD9-CM, and also appear in "Coding Clinic for ICD-9-CM" published by the AHA (DHHS, 2010a, p. 1).

The ICD-9-CM guidelines are a set of rules that have been developed to accompany and complement the official conventions and instructions provided within the ICD-9-CM itself. These guidelines are based on coding sequencing instructions found in the three volumes of the ICD-9-CM, but provide additional instruction. Adherence to these guidelines when assigning ICD-9-CM diagnosis and procedure codes is required under the Health Insurance Portability and Accountability Act (HIPAA). A joint effort between the healthcare provider and the coder is essential to achieve complete and accurate documentation, code assignment, and reporting of diagnoses and procedures. The importance of consistent, complete documentation in the medical record cannot be overemphasized. Without such documentation, the level of accuracy needed cannot be achieved. Basically, the entire record should be reviewed to determine the specific reason for the encounter and the conditions treated (DHHS, 2010a, p. 1).

The coding guidelines are published by the AHA in Coding Clinic for ICD-9-CM. This is the only official publication for ICD-9-CM coding guidelines and advice. The Coding Clinic is published quarterly and includes the following information (Casto & Forrestal, 2013, p. 29):

- Official coding advice and official coding guidelines
- Correct code assignments for new technologies and newly identified diseases
- Articles and topics that offer practical information and improve data quality
- Coding changes and/or corrections
- "Ask the Editor" questions with practical examples

Each healthcare facility should use the Coding Clinic as an integral part of all continuing education for the coding staff and for development of the compliance program for their healthcare facility.

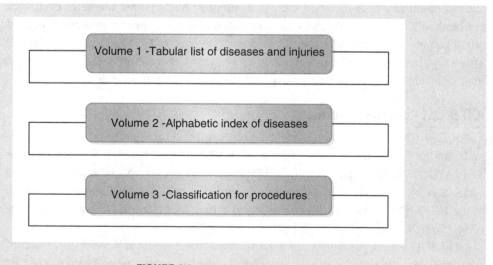

FIGURE 9.1   ICD-9-CM Volumes.

■ ICD-10-CM

History of ICD-10-CM

The current version of ICD is version 9 in the United States, but it is version 10 everywhere else in the world. The United States adopted the ninth version and modified it clinically and continues to use it as the method for communicating diagnosis and inpatient procedures for public and private reimbursement systems. ICD-10 will come into effect on October 1, 2015 for ICD-10-CM and ICD-10 procedure coding system (ICD-10-PCS) (Casto & Forrestal, 2013, p. 27).

The ICD-10-CM is a morbidity classification published by the United States for classifying diagnoses and reason for visits in all healthcare settings. The ICD-10-CM is based on the ICD-10, the statistical classification of disease published by the World Health Organization. These guidelines have been approved by the four organizations that make up the Cooperating Parties for the ICD-10-CM: the American Hospital Association (AHA), the American Health Information Management Association (AHIMA), CMS, and NCHS (DHHS, I-10, 2010b, p. 1).

ICD-10-CM Guidelines

The guidelines have been approved by the four organizations that make up the Cooperating Parties for the ICD-10-CM and these guidelines are a set of rules that have been developed to accompany and complement the instructions provided in the ICD-10-CM. The instructions and conventions of the classification take precedence over the guidelines.

The guidelines are based on the coding and sequencing instructions contained in Volume I and Volume II of the ICD-10-CM and provide additional instruction. Under HIPPA, the adherence to the guidelines is required. The diagnosis codes in Volume I and Volume II have been adopted under HIPAA for all healthcare settings. An excellent relationship between the healthcare provider and the codes is essential to achieve complete and accurate documentation, code assignment, and reporting of diagnoses and procedures. These guidelines are designed to assist both the healthcare provider and the coder to identify the diagnoses and procedures that are to be reported. The importance of consistent, complete, and legible documentation, cannot be overemphasized. Without accurate documentation, complete review of the medical record, and an excellent relationship between the healthcare provider and the coder, accurate coding cannot be achieved (DHHS I-10, 2010b, p. 1).

The term encounter is used for all settings and is a professional, direct personal contact between a patient and a physician or other person who is authorized by state licensure law, and if application by medical staff bylaws to order or furnish healthcare services for the diagnosis or treatment of the patient; face-to-face contact between a patient and a provider who has a primary responsibility for assessing and treating the condition of the patient at a given contact and exercise (LaTour & Eichenwald Maki, 2013, p. 498). In the context of the guidelines, the term provider will mean a physician or any healthcare provider that is qualified and legally accountable for establishing the patient's diagnosis.

The guidelines are organized into sections. Section I includes the structure and the classification and general guidelines that apply to the entire classification. Section II includes guidelines that pertain to the selection of **principal diagnosis** for non-outpatient settings. Section III includes guidelines for reporting additional diagnoses in nonoutpatient settings. Section IV is for outpatient coding and reporting (DHHS, 2010a, p. 1).

Conventions for the ICD-10-CM

The conventions for the ICD-10-CM are general rules used in the classification independent of the guidelines and are incorporated within the Index and Tabular of the ICD-10-CM as instructional notes (DHHS, 2010b, p. 2). ICD-10-CM has an Alphabetic Index that is an alphabetical list of terms and their corresponding code and is divided into the Index of Diseases and Injury and the Index to External Causes of Injury. The Tabular List is a chronological list of codes divided into chapters based on body symptoms or conditions. The format of the Tabular List contains categories, subcategories, and codes. All categories have three characters and subcategories have either four or five characters. Codes may end up being four, five, six, or seven characters long. The only codes that are permissible are complete codes with all category and subcategory codes and the seventh character if applicable.

General Coding Guidelines

To select a code in ICD-10-CM that corresponds to the diagnosis or reason for the visit that is documented in the medical record, the coder will locate the term in the Index and then verify the code in the Tabular List. The coder will be guided by the instructional notations that appear in both the Index and the Tabular List. The ICD-10-CM diagnosis codes are composed of codes with three, four, five, six, or seven digits and the coder needs to report the diagnosis code at the highest number of digits.

Codes that describe symptoms and signs, as opposed to diagnoses, are acceptable for reporting purposes when a related definitive diagnosis has not been established or confirmed by the provider. There are conditions that are an integral part of the disease process and those that are routinely associated with a disease process should not be assigned additional codes. The conditions that are not an integral part of a disease process should be coded when present. There are some conditions that require more than one code. The coder will see "Use additional code" notes in the Tabular for codes that are not part of an etiology/manifestation pair where a secondary code is useful to fully describe a condition. The coder will also come across "Code first" where they will code a condition first even if it is an underlying condition. They may also come across "Code, if applicable, any causal condition first" that identifies that this code may be assigned as a principal diagnosis when the causal condition is unknown or not applicable (DHHS, 2010b, p. 13).

Coders will come across situations where there are both acute and chronic conditions presented in the medical record that represent the same condition and they will come across the need to use a combination code that can represent more than one code. If the coder comes across a situation where the same condition is described in the medical record as being both acute and chronic and separate subentries exist in the Alphabetic Index at the same indentation level, the coder will code both and sequence the acute (subacute) code first. There are also times where a coder will come across a situation where there is a need to use a combination code that will result in the use of a single code that can be used to classify two diagnoses, or a diagnosis with an associated secondary process (manifestation) or a diagnosis with an associated complication (DHHS, 2010b, p. 13).

The term Late Effect is a residual effect, or a condition produced, after the acute phase of an illness or injury has terminated. There is no time limit on when a late code can be used as the residual may be apparent early, such as in cerebral infarction, or it may occur months or years later in instances due to a previous injury. The condition is sequenced first and the late effect code is sequenced second (DHHS, 2010b, p. 14). An example of a late effect of a patient that has a burn and they develop a contracture of a muscle at any time after the burn.

Each ICD-10-CM code is unique and cannot be reported more than one time per encounter. This also applies to bilateral conditions where there are no distinct codes identifying laterality or two different conditions classified to the same ICD-10-CM code (DHHS, 2010b, p. 14).

Selection of a Principal Diagnosis

For each encounter the coder will take into account the circumstances of the inpatient admission in the selection of the principal diagnosis. The principal diagnosis is defined in the Uniform Hospital Discharge Data Set (UHDDS) as "that condition established after study to be chiefly responsible for occasioning the admission of the patient to the hospital for care." UHDDS definitions have been expanded to include, but not limited to, all nonoutpatient settings such as acute care, short-term care, long-term care, psychiatric hospitals, home health agencies, rehab facilities, and nursing homes (DHHS, 2010b, p. 90).

The importance of complete, consistent documentation in the patient's medical record cannot be overemphasized and without this level of documentation the ability for the coder to effectively code a patient's medical record, following the guidelines, would be very difficult, if not impossible. There are guidelines to follow in determining the principal diagnosis such as the following (DHHS, 2010b, p. 91):

- Codes for symptoms, signs, and ill-defined conditions can't be used as a principal diagnosis when a related, definitive diagnosis has been established.

- If there are two or more interrelated conditions, such as diseases in the same ICD-10-CM chapter, potentially meeting the definition of a principal diagnosis, either condition may be sequenced first, unless the circumstances of the admission, the therapy provided, the Tabular List, or the Alphabetic Index indicates otherwise.

- Where there are two or more diagnoses that equally meet the definition for a principal diagnosis and the coding guidelines do not provide sequencing direction, any one of the diagnoses may be sequenced first.

- If the original treatment plan is not carried out the coder will sequence the principal diagnosis as the condition that caused the admission to the hospital.

- Where there are complications of surgery and other medical care that result in an admission to the hospital, the complication code is sequenced as the principal diagnosis.

- If the diagnosis documented at the time of discharge is qualified as "probable," "suspected," "likely," "questionable," "possible," or "still to be ruled out," or other terms indicating uncertainty, the coder will code the condition as if it existed or was established.

Admission from Observation Unit

If a patient is admitted to an observation unit in a hospital for a medical condition and the patient either does not improve or the condition worsens, at which point the patient is then admitted to the hospital as an inpatient, the coder will use the principal diagnosis as the condition that led to the actual hospital admission.

An admission following a Post-Operative Observation where a patient is in the observation unit so that their condition can be monitored and develops a complication that requires an inpatient admission at the same hospital, the hospital should apply the UHDDS definition of principal diagnosis which states that the condition established after study to be chiefly responsible for the admission to the hospital (DHHS, 2010b, p. 92).

Admission from Outpatient Surgery

If a patient receives outpatient surgery and is admitted to the same hospital as an inpatient, the principal diagnosis for the admission will be based on the reason for the inpatient admission. If no complications or other condition is documented as the reason for the inpatient admission, then the coder will assign the reason for the outpatient surgery as the principal diagnosis. Finally, if the reason for inpatient admission is another condition that is unrelated to the surgery, the coder will assign the unrelated condition that caused the admission as the principal diagnosis (DHHS, 2010b, p. 92).

Reporting Additional Diagnoses

Other diagnoses that are interpreted as additional conditions, that affect patient care, are in terms of clinical evaluation, therapeutic treatment, diagnostic procedures, extended length of hospital stay, increased nursing care, and monitoring. Other diagnoses are conditions that coexist at the time of admission or develop subsequently or that affected the treatment received or the **average length of stay**. If there is a diagnosis that is related to an earlier stay or encounter, and has no bearing on the current hospital admission, then these codes are to be excluded (DHHS, 2010b, p. 93).

If there are abnormal findings where the coder picks up on lab, x-ray, pathologic, or other diagnostic results, these are not coded unless the provider indicates their clinical significance. If the coder sees these results and the tests were ordered to evaluate the condition or prescribed treatment, it would be appropriate for the coder to query the physician whether the abnormal findings should be reported. In the situation where there is an uncertain diagnosis, such as "probable," "suspected," "likely," "questionable," "possible," or "still to be ruled out," the coder will code the condition as if it existed or was established. This guideline is applicable only to inpatient admissions to short-term, acute, long-term care, and psychiatric hospitals (DHHS, 2010b, p. 94).

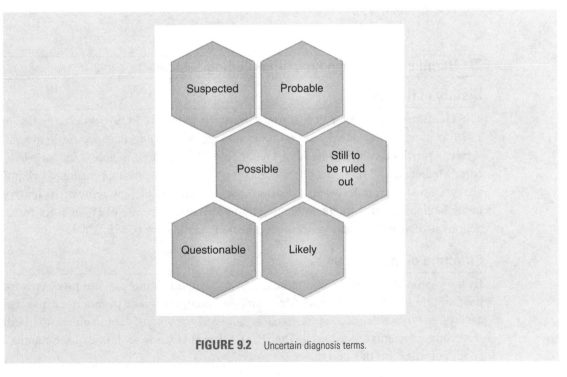

FIGURE 9.2 Uncertain diagnosis terms.

Guidelines for Outpatient Services

In the outpatient setting, the term used for principal diagnosis is first-listed. When a patient is presented to the outpatient surgery center for same day surgery, the coder will code the reason for the surgery as the first-listed diagnosis or reason for the encounter. When a patient is admitted for an observation stay after outpatient surgery in which the patient developed complications, the coder will assign the reason for the surgery as the first-listed diagnosis followed by secondary codes for the complications the patient is experiencing.

Overall, the coder should report accurately the ICD-10-CM diagnosis codes and make sure that the codes describe the symptoms and signs that are documented in the medical record. The coder will be aware of the level of detail in the coding and make sure that the ICD-10-CM codes are complete and the full number of digits required for a code are used. For patients that are receiving treatment for chronic diseases the coder can report the chronic disease as many times as the patient receives treatment and care for the condition. In addition, the coder will code all documented conditions that coexist at the time of the encounter or visit if they require or affect patient care treatment or management. The coder will not code conditions that were previously treated and no longer exist. For patients receiving diagnostic or therapeutic services, the coder will sequence the diagnosis, condition, problem, or other reason for the encounter shown in the medical record to be chiefly responsible for the outpatient services provided (DHHS, 2010b, p. 97).

◼ Healthcare Common Procedure Coding System

History of HCPCS

The **Healthcare Common Procedure Coding System (HCPCS)** was established in 1978 to provide a standardized coding system for describing the specific items and services provided in the delivery of health care. Such coding is necessary for Medicare, Medicaid, and other health insurance programs to ensure that insurance claims are processed in an orderly and consistent manner. The HCPCS system was voluntary in the beginning, but with the implementation of HIPAA, the use of HCPCS for transactions involving healthcare information became mandatory (CMS, 2004, p. 1).

Structure of the HCPCS

Every year in the United States there are over 5 billion claims that are processed for payment. In order for Medicare, Medicaid, and other insurance payers to ensure that each one of these claims are processed in an orderly and consistent manner, standardized coding systems are required. The HCPCS **Level II Code** set is one of the standard codes sets used for this purpose.

The HCPCS is divided into two principal subsystems, referred to as Level I and Level II of the HCPCS. Level I of the HCPCS is comprised of **Current Procedural Terminology** (CPT) codes that are comprised of a numeric coding system maintained by the American Medical Association (AMA). The CPT is a uniform coding system that is made up of descriptive terms and codes that are primarily used to identify medical services and procedures that are furnished by physicians and other healthcare professionals (CMS, 2013). Healthcare professionals use the CPT to identify the services that they provide to a beneficiary so that they can bill a third-party payer for reimbursement. All decisions for additions, deletions, and edits are made by the AMA. All CPT codes are published annually and this includes existing and updated codes. The CPT code consists of five numeric digits. An example of a CPT code for nerve conduction studies; one to two studies would be CPT Code 95907 (AMA, 2013, p. 535).

The terminology is divided into six main sections known as Category I codes that include two types of supplementary codes that are Category II and Category III, and modifiers. Category I CPT codes consist of six sections that are:

- Evaluation and Management
- Anesthesia
- Surgery
- Radiology
- Pathology and Laboratory
- Medicine

Category II codes contains a set of supplemental tracking codes that can be used for performance measurement. This use of the Category II codes is designed to reduce the need for abstraction and chart review that will reduce the administrative burden on physicians and other healthcare professionals and facilities. These codes are intended to facilitate data collection about the quality of the care rendered by coding certain services and test results that support nationally established performance measures and that have an evidence base as contributing to quality patient care. Category II codes make use of alphabetical characters as the fifth character in the string (AMA, 2013, p. 561).

An example of a Category II code used in Patient History to describe measures for select aspects of patient history or review of symptoms during a patient visit or assessment would be code 1000F. This code is defined as the following: 1000F-Tobacco use assessed (CAD, CAP, COPD, PV) (DM) (AMA, 2013, p. 564).

Category III codes are a set of temporary codes for emerging technology, services, and procedures. Category III codes allow data collection for these services and procedures. If a Category III code is available, this code must be reported instead of a Category I code. This activity is critically important in the evaluation of healthcare delivery and the formation of public and private policy. The use of Category III codes allows physicians and other qualified healthcare professionals, insurance companies, health service researchers, and health policy experts to identify emerging technology, services, and procedures for clinical efficacy, utilization, and outcomes (AMA, 2013, p. 579). An example of a Category III code is 0318T. The description for this is as follows: 0318T-Implantation of catheter-delivered prosthetic aortic heart valve, open thoracic approach (AMA, 2013, p. 593).

Level II of the HCPCS is a standardized coding system that is used primarily to identify products, supplies, and services not included in the Level I CPT codes. These codes can identify services/products such as ambulance services, durable medical equipment (DME), prosthetics, orthotics, and supplies when used outside of a physician office setting. Level II codes were established because not all the supplies and services that are provided to a beneficiary are covered in the Level I CPT codes. The Level II codes are used to allow a provider to bill for these services by entering the codes on a healthcare claim form and submitting to the third party for payment. Level II codes are made up of alpha numeric codes. The format of the code is one alphabetical letter followed by four numeric digits. An example of a Level II HCPCS code is E0601 which is for a Continuous Positive Airway Pressure (CPAP) device.

HCPCS Level II codes have permanent and temporary codes, along with the use of modifiers. The Level II permanent codes may be used by public and private health insurers. In addition to permanent codes, there are temporary codes. Temporary codes are used to meet the immediate and short-term operational needs of individual insurers, public and private (Casto & Forrestal, 2013, p. 33).

Modifiers are two-digit alpha or alphanumeric codes. A modifier is designed to give Medicare and other third-party payers additional information needed to process a claim. An example of a modifier used on the HCPCS code E0601 would be NU for new. Another example of a modifier to show that the procedure that is being performed is a bilateral procedure would be to use the modifier 50.

Coding guidelines for HCPCS Level II codes is the *AHA Coding Clinic for HCPCS*. This is a quarterly newsletter that was first introduced in March 2001 and is published by the Central Office of ICD-9-CM. The newsletter includes an Ask the Editor section with actual examples, correct code assignments for new technologies, articles, and a bulletin of coding changes and/or corrections (Casto & Forrestal, 2013, p. 34).

Medicare National Correct Coding Initiative

The **Medicare National Correct Coding Initiative (NCCI)** or the Correct Coding Initiative (CCI) was implemented to promote a national correct coding methodologies and to control improper coding that can lead to inappropriate payments. NCCI code pair edits are automated prepayment edits that prevent improper payment when certain codes are submitted together for Part-B covered services. NCCI also includes a set of edits known as Medically Unlikely Edits (MUEs). A MUE is a maximum number of Units of Service (UOS) allowable under most circumstances for a single HCPCS or CPT code billed by a healthcare provider on a date of service (DOS) for a single beneficiary (Medicare Learning Network, 2013, p. 3).

If a service is denied based on the NCCI code pair edits or MUEs, the provider cannot bill the Medicare beneficiaries. The use of an Advanced Beneficiary Notice (ABN) is not permitted to seek payment from the Medicare beneficiary. The NCCI does not include all possible combinations of correct coding edits or all types of unbundling that exist. It is the responsibility of the healthcare provider to code correctly even if edits do not exist to prevent the use of an inappropriate code or combination of codes (Medicare Learning Network, 2013, p. 3).

■ Evaluation and Management

Documentation is the basis for all coding, including Evaluation and Management (E/M) services. In 1995 the American Medical Association (AMA) and the Centers for Medicare and Medicaid Services (CMS) implemented documentation guidelines to clarify E/M code assignment for both physician and claims reviewers. In 1997, CMS and the AMA collaborated on a revised edition of the documentation guidelines that delineated specific elements to be performed and documented for general multisystem and selected single-specialty examinations. Both the 1995 and 1997 guidelines are acceptable for use in determining an E/M code. The 1997 guidelines can be more beneficial to physicians in specialties that have a specific exam identified such as ophthalmology, orthopedics, dermatology, or psychiatry. For physicians in primary care, the 1995 guidelines may be simpler and much easier to understand and memorize (Kuehn, 2013, p. 40).

New Patient

New Patient is a patient that has not received any professional services from the physician or qualified healthcare professional or another physician or qualified healthcare professional of the exact same specialty and subspecialty who belongs to the same group practice, within the past 3 years.

Established Patient

An **Established Patient** is one who has received professional services from the physician or qualified healthcare professional or another physician or qualified healthcare professional of the exact same specialty and subspecialty who belongs to the same group practice within the past 3 years (AMA, 2013, p. 4).

Levels of E/M Services

The levels of E/M services include examinations, evaluations, and treatments, conferences with or concerning patients, preventive pediatric and adult health supervision, and similar medical services such as the determination of the need and/or location for appropriate care. For medical screening the services include the history, examination, and medical decision-making required to determine the need and/or location for appropriate care for the patient such as office, outpatient, emergency department, or nursing facility (AMA, 2013, p. 6).

The levels of care that are recognized by E/M services consist of seven components. Of these seven components there are six of which are used in defining the levels of E/M services. The first three are considered key components in selecting a level of E/M services and they are history, examination, and medical decision making. The next three components that are counseling, coordination of care, and nature of presenting problems are considered contributory factors in the majority of encounters. The final component is time and the specific times in the CPT book are considered to be a range of time or an average. Some visits will run shorter and some longer, so the time allotments are considered to be an average.

Office or Other Outpatient Services (99201–99205)

The codes in this section are for services provided in the office or in an outpatient or other ambulatory facility for a New or Established Patient. The patient is considered to be an outpatient until they are admitted to an inpatient setting in a healthcare facility.

The codes range for a New Patient from code 99201 that is a patient with a problem-focused history and a problem-focused examination and a straightforward medical decision-making process that takes about 10 minutes to code 99205 that entails a comprehensive history and a comprehensive examination with medical decision making of a high complexity that can take up to 60 minutes (AMA, 2013, p. 12).

For an Established Patient, the codes range from code 99211 for an office or other outpatient visit of an established patient that may not require a physician or other qualified healthcare professional and code 99212 that requires two of the following: a problem-focused history, a problem-focused examination, and a straightforward medical decision-making process and can take about 10 minutes to a more complex code of 99215 that requires two of the following: a comprehensive history, a comprehensive examination, or the medical decision making of a high complexity that can take up to 40 minutes (AMA, 2013, p. 13).

Hospital Observation Services (99218–99226)

Hospital observation services are provided to patients that are designated as admitted to an "observation status" in a hospital. It is not necessary that the patient be located in the observation unit or area designated by the hospital. If an observation area is not present in the hospital then the coder will assign these codes as if they were placed in such a unit.

Initial Observation Care is for a New Patient or Established Patient. For a New Patient, the codes range from 99218 for initial observation care where the following three components of a detailed or comprehensive history, a detailed or comprehensive examination, and medical decision making that is straightforward or of low complexity to a code of 99220 that require the three components of a comprehensive history, a comprehensive examination, and a medical decision making process of high complexity (AMA, 2013, p. 14).

Subsequent Observation Care for a patient can range from the code 99224 that requires two of the following three components are met that are a problem-focused interval history, a problem-focused examination, or a medical decision making process that is straightforward or of low complexity to a code of 99226 that requires that two of the following three components are met that are a detailed interval history, a detailed examination, and a medical decision-making process of high complexity (AMA, 2013, p. 15).

Hospital Inpatient Services (99221 to 99233)

This section covers E/M services that are provided to hospital inpatients and includes those services that are provided to a patient that is in a partial hospital as well. Initial hospital care for a New Patient ranges from code 99221 that requires the following three components of a detailed or comprehensive history, a detailed or comprehensive examination, and medical decision making that is straightforward or of low complexity and takes about 30 minutes of face-to-face time be completed to a code of 99223 that requires a comprehensive history, a comprehensive examination, and medical decision making of a high complexity that takes around 70 minutes of face-to-face time be completed (AMA, 2013, p. 16).

Subsequent hospital care includes review of the medical record and diagnostic studies and changes since the last visit from code 99231 where at least two of the following three components of a problem focused interval history, a problem focused examination, or medical decision making that is straightforward or of low complexity are completed and typically spend 15 minutes with the patient face-to-face to a code of 99233 that requires two of the following three components of a detailed interval history, a detailed examination, or the medical decision making of a high complexity is met and about 35 minutes is spent face-to-face with the patient (AMA, 2013, p. 17).

Hospital Observation and Discharge Planning (99234–99239)

These codes are to be used when a patient is admitted and discharged on the same date of service. The codes range from a 99234 for observation or inpatient hospital care that requires that a detailed or comprehensive history, a detailed or comprehensive examination, and the medical decision-making process that is straightforward or of low complexity is met and physician spends about 40 minutes of face-to-face time to a code of 99236 that needs a comprehensive history, a comprehensive examination, and medical decision making of a high complexity be met and the physician spends about 55 minutes of face-to-face time with the patient. For hospital discharge planning, the codes 99238 hospital discharge management for a visit less than 30 minutes or code 99239 hospital discharge management more than 30 minutes should be used (AMA, 2013, p. 18).

Office Consultations (99241–99245)

A consultation is a type of E/M service provided at the request of another physician or appropriate source to recommend care for a specific condition or to take on responsibility of managing the patient's care for the specific problem or condition. The New Patient codes range from 99241 office consultation that requires the following three components of a problem-focused history, a problem-focused examination, and straightforward medical decision making are met and the physician spends about 15 minutes of face-to-face time with the patient to a code of 99245 office consultation that requires a comprehensive history, a comprehensive examination, and medical decision making of high complexity be met and the physician spends about 80 minutes of face-to-face time with the patient (AMA, 2013, p. 20).

Inpatient Consultations (99251–99255)

Inpatient consultations include inpatients, residents of nursing facilities, or patients in a partial hospital setting. Only one consultation should be reported by a consultant per admission. Subsequent services during the same admission should be reported under Subsequent Hospital Care (99231–99233) or for subsequent nursing facility care the codes to use are (99307–99310). Inpatient consultations for a new patient range from code 99251 inpatient consultation that requires the three components of a problem-focused history, a problem-focused examination, and straightforward medical decision making be met and spend about 20 minutes of face-to-face time with the patient to the code of 99255 inpatient consultation where a comprehensive history, a comprehensive examination, and medical decision making of high complexity is met and the physician spends about 110 minutes of face-to-face time with the patient (AMA, 2013, p. 21).

Emergency Department (99281–99288)

Emergency services are provided in an organized hospital-based facility for the provision of unscheduled episodic services to patients who are in need of immediate medical attention. The facility must be open and services available 24 hours a day. The codes range from code 99281 emergency department visit that requires a problem-focused history, a problem-focused examination, and straightforward medical decision making be completed to code 99285 emergency department visit for a patient that requires a comprehensive history, a comprehensive examination, and medical decision making of high complexity (AMA, 2013, p. 23).

Other Services Covered

The other areas that are covered in the CPT book are (AMA, 2013, p. 23–46):

- Critical Care Services (99291–99292)
- Nursing Facility Services
  - Initial Nursing Facility Care (99304–99306)
  - Subsequent Nursing Facility Care (99307–99310)
  - Nursing Discharge Services (99315–99316)
  - Other Nursing Facility Services (99318)
- Domiciliary, Rest Home, or Custodial Care Services (99234–99337)
- Domiciliary, Rest Home, or Home Care Plan Oversight Services (99239–99340)
- Home Services (99341–99350)
- Prolonged Services (99354–99360)
- Case Management Services (99363–99368)
- Care Plan Oversight Services (99374–99380)
- Preventive Medicine Services (99381–99397)
  - Counseling Risk Factor Reduction and Behavior Change Intervention (99401–99412)
  - Other Preventative Medicine Services (99420–99429)
- Non-Face-to-Face Services
  - Telephone Services (99441–99443)
  - On-Line Medical Evaluation (99444)
- Special Evaluation and Management Services
  - Basic Life and/or Disability Evaluation Services (99450)
  - Work Related or Medical Disability Evaluation Services (99455–99456)
- Newborn Care Services (99460–99463)
  - Delivery/Birthing Room Attendance and Resuscitation Services (99464–99465)
- Inpatient Neonatal Intensive Care Services and Pediatric and Neonatal Critical Care Services
  - Pediatric Critical Care Patient Transport (99466–99486)
  - Inpatient Neonatal and Pediatric Critical Care (99468–99476)
  - Initial and Continuing Intensive Care Services (99477–99480)

- Complex Chronic Care Coordination Services (99487–99489)
- Transitional Care Management Services (99495–99496)
- Other Evaluation and Management Services (99499)

■ Conclusion

The non-HIM professional utilizes the information from the **health record** to provide a legal document of care provided, provide coding for billing, and to retrieve data from coded material to research and measure quality. The health record is important and needs to meet the requirements as reviewed in this chapter. Coding processes are based on specific coding definitions and rules as identified by ICD-9-CM, ICD-10-CM, and HCPCS. The health record is a critical document in healthcare delivery.

References

American Medical Association. (2013). *Current procedural terminology*. Chicago: AMA.

Casto, A.B., & Forrestal, E. (2013). *Principles of healthcare reimbursement* (4th ed.). Chicago: AHIMA.

Centers for Medicare and Medicaid Services. (2013). HCPCS-General information. Retrieved from http://www.cms.gov/Medicare/Coding/MedHCPCSGenInfo/index.html?redirect=/MedHCPCSGeninfo/

Department of Health and Human Services. (2004). New CMS coding changes will help beneficiaries; improvements will speed use of technology. *Medicare news*. Retrieved from http://www.cms.gov/Medicare/Coding/MedHCPCSGenInfo/Downloads/HCPCSReform.pdf

Department of Health and Human Services. (2006). Medicare and Medicaid programs; Hospital conditions of participation: Requirements for history and physical examinations; Authentication of verbal orders; Securing medications; and postanesthesia evaluations. *Federal Register 71*, 68687.

Department of Health and Human Services. (2009). CMS Manual System. *State Operations Provider Certification* Pub. 100–07.

Department of Health and Human Services. (2010a). *ICD-9-CM official guidelines for coding and reporting*. Retrieved from http://www.ucdmc.ucdavis.edu/compliance/pdf/icdguide11.pdf

Department of Health and Human Services. (2010b). *ICD-10-CM official guidelines for coding and reporting*. Retrieved from http://www.cms.gov/Medicare/Coding/ICD10/downloads/7_Guidelines10cm2010.pdf

North Dakota Health Information Technology. (2010). *Guidelines for defining the legal health record for disclosure purposes*. Retrieved from http://www.healthit.nd.gov/files/2010/07/hit_legal_health_record_considerations.pdf

Kuehn, L. (2013). *Procedural coding and reimbursement for physician services: Applying current procedural terminology and HCPCS.* Chicago: AHIMA.

LaTour, K.M., & Eichenwald Maki, S. (2013). *Health information management: Concepts, principles, and practice* (4th ed.). Chicago: AHIMA.

Medicare Learning Network. (2010). Medical record retention and media format for medical records. Retrieved from http://www.cms.gov/Outreach-and-Education/Medicare-Learning-Network-N/MLNProducts/downloads/MLN_Podcast_Medical_Record_Retention_and_Media_Format.pdf

Medicare Learning Network. (2013). How to use the Medicare national correct coding initiative (NCCI) tools. Retrieved from http://www.cms.gov/Outreach-and-Education/Medicare-Learning-Network-MLN/MLNProduexcts/Downloads/How-To-Use-NCCI-Tools.pdf

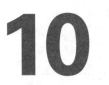

Revenue Cycle Management

■ Introduction

With the transition from fee-for-service payment environment to a prospective payment environment **Revenue Cycle Management (RCM)** has become a very important part of managing a healthcare facility. In the past, while in the fee-for-service environment, the healthcare facility simply billed for every service that was performed on the patient. With the shift to a prospective payment environment, the focus is no longer on managing the revenue from the beginning of care in the preadmissions process where providers can get the services that are going to be rendered to the patient from an office visit to an outpatient procedure all the way up to a hospital admission. The management of this process is to now ensure that the practice or facility will be paid for their services. This process of RCM, in conjunction with the prospective payment systems that are in place, may differ from facility to facility or treatment type to treatment type, but the one constant is that now more than ever the revenue for a healthcare facility is now managed from before the visit to ensure payment after the visit. Along the way there are changes as to what the patient is responsible for and how the healthcare provider is to go about collecting this amount from the patient. In combining the clinical management of the patient along with the management of the revenue cycle, and all the things in between show that the approach to health care has now come full circle and managing the patient's stay has now become a comprehensive multidisciplinary approach to the overall care of the patient in both the clinical and financial arenas. Revenue Cycle Management can be defined as "a complex process that involves balancing people, processes, technology, and the environment in which the process takes place" (LaTour & Eichenwald Maki, 2013, p. 460).

Comprehensive and Integrated Approach

The reimbursement approach in health care has gone from a simple fee-for-service to a more complex approach called Revenue Cycle Management. In the past in the fee-for-service approach to managing the financial side of healthcare reimbursement, it was fragmented and departmentalized. Every department worked independently to achieve the financial goals of the organization and individually contributed to its own revenue cycle for its department. In the fee-for-service the provider and the payer all acted in a retrospective manner with regards to managing their revenue cycle. In a retrospective environment both the provider and payer worked after the fact, in that the provider would bill for all services rendered but not really know if all the work was covered but would find out when the payment came into the facility. Another example is that if a home care agency was billing for services and the provider found that there were things not being documented accurately then the agency may be put on a retrospective review. This means that the agency would submit all their bills and after the payer reviewed for accuracy and documentation, then they would pay the home care company. From a provider's point of view, in a retrospective environment, the payer would not know what they were going to be charged for a hospital stay until they received the bill. Then they would work after the fact to make sure that everything was done properly. One area of concern was that even though they knew that the patient was having a surgery, they would not know what they were going to be billed by the facility for the care delivered to the patient. In the fee-for-service arrangement where the revenue management function is fragmented, working after the fact in this retrospective manner, all the departments could work independent of each other and it was not necessary to work as a team.

Now in the prospective environment as the complexity of reimbursement has come to light, it has become necessary that all the individual departments work together and form a strong team to manage the revenue for a facility or provider in a RCM approach. In a prospective environment it is entirely up to the healthcare facility to manage their profit or loss with regards to a particular patient's hospital stay. This approach has become a RCM team approach and it requires all departments from registration and admissions to the servicing department, inpatient or outpatient, and the surgery or medicine departments, care management, finance, health information management, and the clinical staff to all work together to effectively initiate, implement, and manage the revenue for a healthcare facility in the RCM approach.

■ Components of the Revenue Cycle

The revenue cycle is a critical element to the reimbursement processes of a healthcare facility. There are several areas or parts of the cycle that have responsibility of their own functions and how those functions blend in to the overall goal of submitting a clean claim for services rendered at the healthcare facility. The major **components of the revenue cycle** vary by organization and can be a three-tiered approach or a four-tiered approach. This is a more complex model of reimbursement and the more effective model is where the RCM is divided up into three categories: front-end process, middle process, and the back-end process.

The first part of the revenue cycle is the front-end, and this entails payer negotiation that happens outside the patient encounter, the patient access component that includes the scheduling of the patient for inpatient or outpatient services, registration, insurance verification, obtain a prior authorization or a precertification if necessary, and patient financial counseling. During this part of the revenue cycle the provider can verify the patient demographics and payer information to secure the source of payment and identify any requirements from the insurance company prior to services being rendered. In addition to this part that involves the patient and the payer, prior to this the provider will have completed contract negotiations with the payer and have agreed upon pricing and requirements necessary to treat their members and this pricing will be loaded into the billing system and charge description master (CDM). Without this process being complete for all payers, the provider is at risk for being out-of-network and possibly not being eligible for payment if they don't do all the parts of this process.

The middle process in the revenue cycle is where case management is involved, charge capture, hard coding and soft coding of diagnoses and procedures that are all based on clinical documentation. Overall, during this process the clinical team will deliver the services required for this admission or encounter and during all of this, make sure that all necessary clinical documentation is present in the chart so that the Health Information Management Department can code what was documented in the patient's chart.

The back end of the revenue cycle usually resides in the patient financial services or business office area. This area will handle processing bills, posting payments, correcting any claims that were denied for errors, appeal any denials that are incorrect, supply additional documentation when needed, and make corrections to the charge description master if needed. The success of this process "is achieved through a balance of people, processes, the technology used to support the process, and the environment in which the processes are done" (HIMSS, 2009, p. 3).

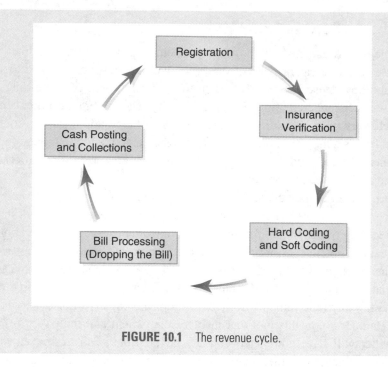

FIGURE 10.1   The revenue cycle.

■ Front-End Process

In this section of the RCM model all of the "front-end" processes are completed to ensure that the revenue that the facility is going to book will be collectable. This portion of the RCM model entails Scheduling and Registration, Insurance Verification and Preauthorization, Patient Financial Counseling and Patient Responsibility, Medical Necessity Requirements, **Contract Management**, and Technology.

Patient Scheduling is the first point of contact with the patient. At this point, the staff is responsible for capturing all possible demographics and other data that will support the care provided and the billing process for the encounter. The staff should be well-versed in services that they are scheduling for and be very knowledgeable of all the insurance carrier requirements for providing services to the patient. For a new patient, the information that the staff will gather, by a patient interview or by having the patient fill out various forms, will be the patient's name, address, city, state, zip code, physician name or referring doctor, date of injury (if applicable), date of birth, social security number, emergency contact, insurance company, insurance identification number and group number, place of employment along with address of the employer and phone number, and secondary insurance if applicable. For an existing patient, the staff will verify that all information they have on file has not changed. If there are any changes, such as address or insurance company, the staff can update their file and verify the information again before proceeding. Once all data is complete the staff will ask for the patient's photo identification and/or insurance cards to make copies of them and then they will print out forms for the patient to sign such as authorization to treat, bill for services, and release of information.

Insurance Verification

Insurance verification is the next step in the registration process and is a critical element in the RCM model. The staff can come across two types of verifications and they are scheduled and unscheduled patient visits. For the scheduled visits where the patient has been seen before and all of the information is in the system, the staff can run an insurance verification prior to the patient arriving for services. Moreover, for this patient the staff will already know if there are any special requirements from the insurance company such as referral or prior authorization needed for the visit. For a new patient, the staff will take the insurance information provided by the patient and verify with the insurance carrier, electronically or by phone, that the patient is an active member of the insurance plan, what are the co-pays and coinsurance, and if any special documentation is necessary such as prior authorization or referral needed for this patient.

CMS uses an electronic verification process to allow the provider to inquire about a patient's eligibility, the coverage that they have, and any benefits associated with the health plan that they have and can be used inform the provider or practitioner of any changes that may have occurred to the patient's coverage or benefits that they currently have in place. The provider will have to fill out a CMS 270/271 form electronically and submit it to the Medicare Eligibility Integration Contractor (MEIC) for security authentication. Then the provider will be directed to fill out a MDCN form that will allow the provider the ability to get connected to the system. Once this form is completed, it will be forwarded to the MEIC for completion and the provider will then receive a submitter identification number. At this point the provider will have to obtain the necessary telecommunication software from an AT&T reseller (CMS, 2014a).

If the insurance verification process is not complete, the things that can go wrong are the patient's claim is denied, the wrong co-pay amount was collected, the proper forms were not collected, and all of this will happen weeks after the patient's visit. Insurance verification is the first point, and the most important point, to secure payment from the insurance carrier for the practice or facility. In addition, if this process is not accurate and timely, it will result in a denied claim and a delay in payment anywhere from an additional 30–90 days on top of the original payment turnaround time of 14–45 days.

Prior Authorization and Precertification

Prior authorization is a requirement of the insurance carrier and may also be referred to as authorization, precertification, predetermination, or simply prior approval.

As suggested by the word, preauthorization, this must be done before rendering services to the patient. If the approval is not obtained prior to providing services the insurance carrier can deny the claim. Moreover, the insurance carrier is not obligated to assign a prior authorization or authorization to the provider after the services are rendered. This process is spelled out in the provider contract from the insurance carrier which will give the provider the information such as when a prior authorization or precertification is needed, the contact information for the prior authorization department at the insurance carrier, the time frame in which to request a prior authorization and to receive it back from the carrier. This process can be via telephone, fax, e-mail, or electronic. Moreover, with the rising cost of health care and the type of plan that the patient has, this process may require a lot of focus from the staff to obtain the necessary prior authorizations necessary for the services to be rendered and the payment of the claim.

Financial Counseling

The healthcare organization is required to educate the patient on their responsibility for his or her encounter with the healthcare provider. This can be accomplished by using Financial Counselors. They are staff members that are dedicated to helping the patient and the provider to secure a means of payment for the services that are going to be rendered to the patient. The Financial Counselors need to have a complete understanding of the patient's financial position with regards to assets and be fully aware of the patient's responsibility according to their plan for the services that are being rendered and to discuss payment options with the patient so that they can ensure or secure a method of debt resolution for services provided.

Some patients that do not have health insurance or the financial ability to pay for the services that are being rendered to them by the provider may qualify for **Charity Care** from the provider. Charity Care is a way in which the facility can choose to help a patient that is in need of services from the provider. This is not designed as a tool for people who refuse to pay, but a tool in which people who have unplanned or unforeseen medical needs and do not have insurance or a means to pay for those services at the time of treatment. For a patient to qualify for Charity Care, the Financial Counselor will review the patient's financial ability to pay through verifying their income through their W-2, bank statements to demonstrate cash on hand, and any available credit to pay the facility for their care. If it is determined through the application process and verification of the patient's income, household expenses, employment, assets, and other forms of potential payment sources that the patient, or responsible party, and it is determined that they are unable to pay, they may qualify for Charity Care. At the point of approving the patient for Charity Care, the services will be rendered, or may have already been provided, to the patient and there will be no charge to the patient or responsible party. Each facility should have an Indigent Care or Charity Care policy that will help guide the staff and keep everything consistent across the board for every patient that enters the practice or facility.

Any charity or indigent care, along with discounts based on a patient or family's ability to pay, is typically based on the current federal poverty level guidelines. Some facilities can set limits for the Financial Counselors to follow in a written policy and should outline the percentage that the patient's income must be under the Federal Poverty Guidelines. For example, a facility can state in their policy that total household income must be less than 400 percent of the current published Federal Poverty Income Guidelines. Moreover, this process in determining if a patient, or responsible party, is eligible for Charity Care should be on case-by-case basis and have detailed policies to support the process.

Patient Pay at the Time of Service

Patients have taken on an increasing amount of financial responsibility for their healthcare costs through the different healthcare insurance options the patient has to choose from. They range in a variety of levels of co-insurance and co-payments, along with yearly maximums of out-of-pocket expenses for the patient and/or their family. "Insurance companies determine that the annual co-payments and deductibles for which the patient is responsible account for 5–6 percent of total net revenue and 16–17 percent of outstanding receivables" (LaTour & Eichenwald Maki, 2013, p. 2010).

Point-of-Service (POS) collections are defined as "the collection of the portion of the bill that is likely the responsibility of the patient prior to the provision of services" (LaTour & Eichenwald Maki, 2013c, p. 461). This process works in the environment of scheduled and nonemergency care. In the situation of an emergency, the discussion of payment should not be entered into by the Financial Counselor as the goal of the program is to collect revenues at the time of service, but not to deter patients from receiving emergency care by discussing payment. The decision for the patient's family in the time of an emergency should be involving what treatment is needed to take care of their loved one in an emergency and not to be one of payment of a co-pay. Outside of an emergency, the Financial Counselors should discuss and document the patient's responsibility for payment of any co-payment or deductible at the time of service and how they plan on paying the amounts that they are personally responsible for.

Medical Necessity

Medicare and various insurance companies have standards that need to be met in the delivery of healthcare services. In the home care environment Medicare requires a Plan of Care to be filled out to demonstrate the patient's need for homecare and that they meet the requirements such as the patient is homebound and leaving his or her place of residence would be medically contraindicated, leaving home must require a considerable taxing effort, the patient must be under the care of a physician, the services that the patient will receive must be periodically reviewed by a physician, and the intermittent care delivered is provided fewer than 7 days per week or less than 8 hours a day (CMS, 2013, p. 25).

Other areas where **medical necessity** must be met are in areas such as joint replacement surgery. Medicare requires that a history that includes the description of the pain from onset and duration, the limitations on Activities of Daily Living (ADLs), safety issues, and a listing of treatments that have taken place that were nonsurgical in nature such as medications, weight loss, braces, orthotics, and physical therapy. Finally, in the clinical judgment of the physician the need for surgery is documented in the medical record such as osteoarthritis, inflammatory arthritis, and failure of previous knee replacement (MLN, 2011, p. 3–5).

Medical necessity is needed for home medical equipment and requires that certain criteria be met such as in the example of a Continuous Positive Airway Pressure (CPAP) unit the physician must document if the device is being ordered for the treatment of obstructive sleep apnea, the date of the sleep test, the patient's Apnea-Hypopnea Index (AHI) or Respiratory Disturbance Index (RDI), documentation if the patient has had excessive daytime sleepiness or impaired cognition or insomnia, has there been a face-to-face evaluation (initial and follow-up), and has the patient demonstrated improvement in their symptoms with the use of the CPAP. Without this documentation the claim for the equipment stands a good chance of being denied by Medicare as Not Medically Necessary (CMS, 2014, CMS-10269).

The American College of Medical Quality has defined Medical Necessity as "accepted health care services and supplies provided by health care entities, appropriate to the evaluation and treatment of a disease, condition, illness or injury and consistent with applicable standard of care" (ACMQ, 2010, p. 1).

ACMQ has developed Policy 8 that is titled Definition and Application of Medical Necessity that has the following nine principles for the application of medical necessity. The nine principles cover the determinations of medical necessity, must adhere to the standard of care, is the standard terminology that healthcare professionals and entities will use in the review process, must reflect the efficient and cost-effective application of patient care, should include discussions with the attending provider relating to the current medical condition, must be unrelated to the payers monetary benefit, be made on a case-by-case basis, approval of medical necessity may be made by a nonphysician but a negative determination must be made by a physician advisor who has clinical training in the area under review, is the process used in evaluating medical necessity should be made known to the patient, and all organizations involved in the determination of medical necessity have uniform policies and procedures for the appeals of denied services (ACMQ, 2010, p. 1).

Medicare's National Coverage Determinations (NCDs) and Local Coverage Determinations (LCDs) define specific ICD-9-CM diagnosis codes or conditions that will support coverage for the service or equipment. There is not a NCD or LCD or form for every service or piece of equipment, but the provider should have on hand payer billing manuals for all payers and any other carrier policies that can help to determine if payment for the services or equipment may be made by the insurance company.

System Tools

There are various tools that can support the front-end part of the Revenue Cycle that will help to capture data to aid in the securing of payment from the payers. These tools include enterprise-wide scheduling system, order tracking and management system, telephone system tracking in order to measure call activity, registration quality assurance tools, online third party eligibility and coverage limitations, workflow drivers, estimation tools for patient out-of-pocket, and electronic financial assistance applications (HIMSS, 2009, p. 5).

■ Middle Process

The Middle Process is defined as it "represents the intersection of clinical practice and billing" (HIMSS, 2009, p. 5). In addition, the key focus in this part of the Revenue Cycle is to balance clinical practice guidelines and to document services completely and accurately and to ensure the coding of documented service is accurate to ensure reimbursement (HIMSS, 2009, p. 5).

Case Management and Utilization Management

Case Management is defined by the Case Management Society of America as "a collaborative process of assessment, planning, facilitation, care coordination, evaluation and advocacy for option and services to meet an individual's and family's comprehensive health needs through communication and available resources to promote quality, cost-effective outcomes (CMSA, 2014).

The Case Manager helps the patient to identify appropriate providers that fit the patient's needs and to make sure that the provider fits the patient's insurance company provider listing to ensure the continuum of care for the patient that is uninterrupted by having to change providers as one may not be in network or accept the payer that the patient is a member with currently.

The overall goal of the Case Manager is to improve quality, provide access to care and services, all the while balancing the needs of the patient and the payer to find the optimum situation for all. Today's Case Manager role has evolved to include partnering with physicians during rounds and participate in treatment plan progress reporting, questioning duplicate services that are not in line with evidence-based protocols, collaborating with other nurses to identify any obstacles to keep the treatment plan moving forward, initiate communication between primary care physicians and consultative physicians, advocating for the patient and family, initiating the planning discussion for transitioning the patient from one level of care to the next (LaTour & Eichenwald Maki, 2013, p. 464).

The Case Manager is charged with coordinating care between the current place of care to the next place of care, keeping in mind the needs of the patient and family, all the while balancing those needs with the clinical team involved and the payer guidelines. The Case Manager looks to expedite all parts of the care process to make sure that there are no delays in care, delays in discharge, delays in admission to the next provider or facility, and no delays to the patient receiving the necessary treatment to continue progressing in their healing or management of symptoms.

Utilization Management is defined as "the evaluation of the medical necessity, appropriateness, and efficiency of the use of healthcare services, procedures, and facilitates these under the provisions of the applicable health benefits plan" (URAC, 2014).

Utilization Management is sometimes called Utilization Review (UR) where staff is responsible "for the day-to-day provisions of the hospital's utilization plan as required by the Medicare Conditions of Participation" (LaTour & Eichenwald Maki, 2013, p. 464).

The UR personnel are required to perform a review of the medical record and use this information to make a decision based on UR, apply all criteria objectively for admission, during the stay, and discharge readiness, provide around the clock all services needed in the UR field, review all patient medical records within 24 hours of being placed in an inpatient bed, screen and coordinate elective and emergency admissions, transfers, outpatient observation beds, and any conversions, and provide UR services to all admissions regardless of the payer that the patient has, review on a scheduled basis all continued stays/admissions, screen for the timeliness and appropriateness of all hospital services, meet weekly on all complex or high-dollar cases, and complete all retrospective or focused reviews as directed (LaTour & Eichenwald Maki, 2013, p. 464).

CMS requires that hospitals that have the requirement to issue Hospital-Issued Notices of Noncoverage (HINNs) to Medicare patients either prior to admission, during the admission, or at any point if the care that the patient is receiving is not covered due to medical necessity, care not delivered in the most appropriate setting, or if the care is custodial. With regards to commercial insurance, they generally notify the patient, their family, and the department that they are being treated in that is responsible for utilization review or adverse determinations. Generally, the UR staff will take the lead on all communications with the patient of any adverse determinations from the payer (LaTour & Eichenwald Maki, 2013, p. 465).

Charge Capture

Charge Capture is defined as "a method of recording services and supplies or items delivered to a patient and then directing them to be billed on a claim form"

(LaTour & Eichenwald Maki, 2013, p. 465). Moreover, it is a process in which all charges are documented, posted, and reconciled for all patients for all services and supplies that they may have received. This process has one main element, consistency. If this process is not consistent and accurate then charges will be off, bills to insurance companies will be incorrect, and inventory may not be accurate. Moreover, if the bills are incorrect they stand a chance of being either too high or too low, either way it compromises the cash flow of the facility. It also lends itself to being fraudulent if the bills are consistently higher and the services were not actually given to the patient. The following are some reasons why Charge Capture is so critical to the success of a facility and they are, payments are related to charges, charges drive prices and rates for reimbursement, charges reflect utilization, charges assist in measuring labor cost and overall productivity, and errors in charge capture can lead to rework and errors that can negatively impact the cash flow of the facility and overall profitability (LaTour & Eichenwald Maki, 2013, p. 465).

The charge capture may be managed by individual departments, but this process impacts the entire facility and there needs to be policy and procedures in place for all to follow. Consistency is a key because if all of the departments are not following policy then it will skew the numbers and create errors and rework. Medicare will use something that is called a "scrubber." This scrubber is part of the claims process when they receive the claim from the provider for processing. The scrubber will pick up errors in the billing and return it as an incomplete claim and not a denial. This delay in processing can have a severe impact on the cash flow of the facility.

In the Health Information Management (HIM) department the coders perform a process that is called "Soft Coding." This is where the coder reviews the chart for documentation and assigns the appropriate coding for the bill. Once the chart is completed, the bill will drop and be sent to the payer. Before all of this takes place there is something that is called a "Bill Hold." A bill hold is where the facility waits several days, usually three, for all documentation and reports to make it to the patient's chart. This bill hold is sometimes referred to as a "Discharged But Not Final Billed," or DNFB.

Other areas of this process are to make sure all diagnoses and procedures are captured and appropriately coded by the HIM coder. Most payers, if not all, will not pay a claim unless it has all appropriate ICD-9-CM or CPT codes that represent the services and procedures that were delivered to the patient. Not included in this coding when the care involves outpatient clinical visits using Evaluation and Management (E/M) coding. This coding represents the physician time spent with the patient and is not reflected in the resources that are captured in the CPT codes for the facility.

Charge Description Master

The **Charge Description Master (CDM)** is "an electronic file that represents a master list of all services, supplies, devices, and medications that are charged for inpatient or outpatient services (LaTour & Eichenwald Maki, 2013, p. 467). The CDM contains all necessary information that will identify the item used, the charge associated with it, and the code that is associated with it that will enable the system to place the information on the claim form that will be sent to the payer. This process is called "Hard Code" where all the coding is done as the information is hard coded into the system. There are additional pieces of information in the CDM and the first one is the charge code that can be associated with the General Ledger and is an internal code that will identify the department that the charges are associated with for revenue and Cost of Goods Sold. The second one is the charge code description that is a narrative of what supply or service was rendered. Third, there is the CPT or HCPCS code that is associated with the item so that the item can be placed on the bill with the correct coding. Fourth, there is a modifier, which is a two digit numeric or alphanumeric extension that is added to the CPT or HCPCS code that will give additional information on the code and the reason for its use. Fifth, there is a Revenue Code that is nationally recognized that is four digits in length and will tell the payer what the item charge represents. This Revenue Code is required on each line item of the bill from the facility and can be for inpatient and outpatient. Finally, there is the price category and this is the billed amount from the facility after the standard markup rates for the item are applied (LaTour & Eichenwald Maki, 2013, p. 467).

The CDM must continually be updated to make sure that the most up-to-date information is present in this system. If there are updates to the ICD-9-CM or CPT or HCPCS codes the system needs to be updated. It is not good practice to delete old items out of the CDM as there may be previously submitted claims that are tied to the old data and may need to be resubmitted.

The maintenance of the CDM is a multidisciplinary activity and requires the team to have experience in coding, clinical procedures, health record or clinical documentation, and billing regulations. The HIM department have experts on coding and the finance department has staff that are experts in the general ledger and revenue codes along with contracting that impacts pricing and the pharmacy department are experts in the drugs and costs associated with them and the associated coding. Other departments such as radiology, physical therapy, nursing, and others are all good members to have on this multidisciplinary team (LaTour & Eichenwald Maki, 2013, p. 468).

Correct Coding Initiative

The CDM also provides a process in which direct entry of charges to the billing system can be accomplished that will support the optimum revenue cycle performance. There also needs to be checks and balances in this process to guard against improper coding, incorrect charges, and omissions. The Correct Coding Initiative (CCI), along with the Local Medical Review Policy (LMRP) and National Coverage Determination (NCD) edits need to be applied at the time of the original transaction taking place in the billing system and CDM. These edits require coded diagnosis or procedures and in the EHR system the clinician that is involved with the entry should be notified immediately of the edit so it can be corrected. If the clinician is alerted that the edit has occurred, once the documentation is present to allow the clinician to correct or fix the edit, then the edit should be corrected so as to not delay the entry of the claim into the billing cycle (HIMSS, 2009, p. 7).

Clinical Documentation Improvement

The **Clinical Documentation Improvement (CDI)** is a program to assure that the health record accurately reflects the condition of the patient. According to the American Health Information Management Association (AHIMA) the definition of the CDI program is "to initiate concurrent and, as appropriated, retrospective reviews of inpatient health records for conflicting, incomplete, or nonspecific provider documentation" (AHIMA, 2010, p. 4).

The goal of these reviews is to ensure that the ICD-9-CM codes are supported by the clinical documentation in the health record. The reviews of the records usually occur in the patient care units or via the EHR. If any items are found that are deficient in any way, the clinician that is responsible for the documentation will be queried by the CDI team member. The use of a CDI team has been primarily used in the inpatient setting, but has recently been moving towards other points of care in settings such as acute rehabilitation and skilled nursing facilities (AHIMA, 2010, p. 4).

CDI staff can include HIM coding professionals or Registered Nurses, or a combination of both types of professionals. Sometimes there will be a physician that can act as a liaison that can help with reviews and communicating the needs of the CDI team to the physicians on the documentation issues present in the patient's chart. The CDI team members need to have excellent written and oral communication skills. They need to be completely knowledgeable in the clinical environment, coding concepts, coding guidelines, regulatory and compliance, know their way around a clinical setting, and payment systems and methodologies (AHIMA, 2010, p. 5).

The key stakeholders for the CDI include HIM Management and Coders, Case Management and UR, Medical Staff, Executive Team, Patient Financial Services, Finance, RCM Team, Quality Management, Nursing Staff, and Compliance (AHIMA, 2010, p. 6).

According to AHIMA the CDI Goals are identifying and clarifying missing or conflicting documentation, support accurate diagnostic and procedural coding and DRG assignment along with severity of illness, promote health record completion in a timely manner during the patient's stay, improve communication between physicians and other members of the team, provide education to all departments as needed, improve documentation to reflect quality outcomes and scores, and improve the coder's clinical knowledge (AHIMA, 2010, p. 6).

Coding

The HIM Coding Team is responsible for assigning the appropriate codes that reflect the level of care documented in the patient record. The coder will assign ICD-9-CM for inpatient stays, and CPT or HCPCS codes for outpatient services. Coders must be skilled at reading the entire medical record from the history and physical to the discharge summary, lab reports, radiology, pathology, surgical reports, verbal orders, and progress notes. When the documentation is not consistent to the reports or otherwise, the coder must query the physician to help them to come to the correct code assignment. If a query takes a long time, this will delay the Revenue Cycle if the coder cannot drop the bill in a reasonable amount of time.

Case Mix Index

The **Case Mix Index (CMI)** is measurable and analyzable and allows the organization to compare the cost of providing services to its DRG mix and compare it to other like or similar hospitals. The CMI is calculated by summing up the Medicare DRG's weight for the number of patients in the DRG. Then the sum of the weights is divided by the total number of discharges. The lower the CMI the lower the overall resource consumption of the facility and the higher the CMI the higher the resource consumption the facility is experiencing.

■ Back-End Process

Claims Processing

Claims processing involves the totaling of charges for all services that a patient has incurred during their encounter. Once a patient has been discharged, the goal of the facility is to get a complete and accurate claim generated and submitted for payment to the payer. An organization will routinely measure the success of the collections process by looking at the Accounts Receivable Days, which is an average number of days that a claim for services rendered is paid by the payer. The amount of days it takes to collect on a claim submitted to a carrier for payment is a direct reflection on how well the Revenue Cycle is working. An efficient Revenue Cycle Management team will have a lower number for the days a claim is on the Accounts Receivable list and therefore improve the facilities cash flow.

Payment Posting

Payment posting is where the insurance company pays the claim that was submitted and then once the facility receives payment they can post the payment to the open accounts receivable. This posting reduces the accounts receivable and increases the cash account for the facility. The goal is for the patient's account to be at a zero balance. This shows that the entire claim was paid by the payer and the patient, if there were co-pays, coinsurance, or deductibles. There are times where there are payments made on an account that exceed the amount in the patient's account. This will create a negative balance and the team will have to research the payments to verify the accuracy and refund any amounts that were overpaid by the payer or patient.

Denial Management

Denials are responses by the payer that the claim is either incorrect or the billed amount is not representative of the services documented in the patient record. Sometimes it is as simple as a missing modifier or incorrect patient identification number. In this process, there are other reasons for denial such as the patient's insurance was not in effect at the time the services were rendered to the patient. In this instance, the team will have to contact the patient and secure the correct payment information and do a complete insurance verification and inform the patient of their potential responsibility. The claim will need to be dropped to the new payer and followed up on regularly until payment is made.

Some of the more common reasons for denial are beneficiary not covered, lack of medical necessity, lack of precertification, noncovered services, incorrect charges or unbundled code, incorrect coding, and late or untimely filing (LaTour & Eichenwald Maki, 2013, p. 472).

■ Quality Measures for Improvement

Increasing the RCM performance will have a positive impact on the overall health of the organization's financial condition. There are Key Performance Indicators (KPIs) that allow a facility to measure or benchmark their data against best practices. The KPIs are not the only way to allow for success in managing the revenue cycle. There needs to be a focus on revenue cycle improvement along with a dedicated team, root cause analysis done on any changes needed in the revenue cycle of the organization, a shared sense of accountability across the RCM team, collaboration with other departments, a comprehensive approach to uncompensated care given by the facility, continuous improvement in customer service, and commitment from the executive team all the way down to the line staff on improving the patient's overall experience (LaTour & Eichenwald Maki, 2013, p. 473).

■ Conclusion

Revenue Cycle Management is a critical process in the financial health of an organization. It enables the organization to manage revenue from the time the order is processed and the patient is registered until the actual posting of the bill and if necessary managing the denial of payment. This is a multidisciplinary process, no longer a silo approach, with the focus on effective procedures and management of the revenue cycle. Effective Revenue Cycle Management will improve the patient's overall experience and ensure that the facility has paid for all resources consumed in the process of caring for the patient. This is becoming even more important as the patients are moving towards a high-deductible health plan where the monthly premiums are low but the annual deductible is very high. This will force the healthcare facility to be more integrated with a solid RCM model to ensure that all revenues are collected at the time of service. This way the only accounts that actually age out will be insurance claims and not patient claims. These patient claims, if not collected up-front, will be much more difficult to collect in the future as they get older.

The effectiveness of the facility's RCM model will be directly related to the overall financial stability of the facility. The more that a facility can manage this process and avoid the silo, or fragmented approach, the better their cash flow and various key indicator reports will be on a regular basis.

References

American College of Medical Quality. (2010). Policy 8: Definition and application of medical necessity. Retrieved from http://www.acmq.org/policies/policy8.pdf

American Health Information Management Association. (2010a). Clinical documentation improvement toolkit. Retrieved from http://library.ahima.org/xpedio/groups/public/documents/ahima/bok1_047236.pdf

Casto, A.B., & Forrestal, E. (2013). *Principles of healthcare reimbursement* (4th ed.). Chicago: AHIMA.

Case Management Society of America. (2014). What is a case manager? Retrieved from http://www.cmsa.org/Home/CMSA/WhatisaCaseManager/tabid/224/Default.aspx

Centers for Medicare and Medicaid Services. (2013). Chapter 7: Home health services. In *Medicare benefit policy manual*. Retrieved from https://www.cms.gov/Regulations-and-Guidance/Guidance/Manuals/downloads/bp102c07.pdf

Centers for Medicare and Medicaid Services. (2014a). Eligibility inquiry. Retrieved from http://www.cms.gov/Medicare/Billing/ElectronicBillingEDITrans/Eligibility.html

Centers for Medicare and Medicaid Services. (2014b). CMS-10269: Positive airway pressure (PAP) devices for obstructive sleep apnea. Retrieved from https://www.cms.gov/Medicare/CMS-Forms/CMS-Forms/downloads/cms10269.pdf

Healthcare Information and Management Systems Society (HIMSS). (2009). Revenue cycle management: A life cycle approach. Retrieved from https://www.himss.org/files/HIMSSorg/content/files/20090909RCMTFwhitepaper.pdf

LaTour, K.M., & Eichenwald Maki, S. (2013). *Health information management; Concepts, principles, and practice* (4th ed.). Chicago: AHIMA.

Medicare Learning Network. (2011). Documenting medical necessity for major joint replacement. Retrieved from http://www.cms.gov/Outreach-and-Education/Medicare-Learning-Network-MLN/MLNMattersArticles/downloads/se1236.pdf

URAC. (2014). About URAC. Retrieved from https://www.urac.org/about-urac/about-urac/

Healthcare Fraud and Abuse

Learning Outcomes

After reading this chapter, the student will:

- Define Medicare fraud and abuse.
- Differentiate Medicare fraud and abuse.
- Identify tools for detection of Medicare fraud and abuse.
- Describe at least three acts related to Medicare fraud and abuse.
- Identify penalties for Medicare fraud and abuse.
- Describe processes to use in an organization to prevent Medicare fraud and abuse.
- Establish an effective and comprehensive compliance program for a healthcare facility.

■ Introduction

According to the Medicare Learning Network, Medicare fraud and abuse is a serious problem and requires your attention. There is no precise measure of healthcare fraud and the majority of the healthcare providers are honest and well-intentioned, but there is a minority of providers that are not honest and are intent on abusing the system and costing the taxpayers billions of dollars. The overall impact of these losses and risks is now magnified by the growing numbers of people served by Medicare which in turn places an increased strain on federal and state budgets (MLN, 2012a, p. 1). This chapter will take the student through defining fraud and abuse to prevention initiatives, integrity programs, the False Claim Act, antikickback and physician self-referral, and the Office of the Inspector General (OIG) and their view on fraud and abuse and the work plans that they develop each year.

In addition, the chapter will outline an effective compliance plan for the student and cover areas in the plan such as auditing and monitoring, practice standards, and specific risk areas that an administrator needs to be made aware of upfront. At the conclusion of the chapter the student will understand fraud and abuse and will be able to develop and implement a formal compliance program for a healthcare facility.

■ Medicare Fraud

Medicare defines fraud as an occurrence where someone intentionally falsifies information or deceives Medicare. And abuse is when a healthcare provider or supplier does not follow good medical practices that results in unnecessary costs, improper payment, or services that are not medically necessary (DHHS, 2013a, p. 10).

Fraud can range from an individual or single practitioner to a group of individuals or practitioners to an institution or corporate entity. Fraud is not only limited to practitioners, it is now becoming involved with organized crime where they are masquerading as Medicare providers and suppliers. Fraud can be committed by a healthcare provider, such as a doctor or healthcare practitioner, or supplier such as a Durable Medical Equipment (DME) company, business owners such as physicians and employees of physician's offices, employees of companies that manage Medicare billing, and people with Medicare, or people with Medicaid (DHHS, 2013a, p. 13). A few examples of **Medicare fraud** may include knowingly billing for services that were not furnished or supplies that were not provided and billing Medicare for the services or supplies that were not furnished. In addition, if a provider or supplier knowingly alters a claim form to receive a higher payment amount it is considered fraud. Punishment for this crime against the federal government may involve imprisonment, significant fines, or both. Criminal penalties for healthcare fraud reflects the serious harms associated with the healthcare fraud and the need for aggressive and appropriate prevention (MLN, 2012b, p. 2).

CMS estimates that the federal government distributed about $65 billion in improper payments, or payments that should not have been made or were for the incorrect amount, through Medicare and Medicaid combined in fiscal year 2011. Through the Affordable Care Act and its programs, CMS recovered more than $10 billion in the last 3 years (DHHS, 2013a, p. 14).

Quality of care concerns are not considered fraud. These are concerns that can be addressed by a Quality Improvement Organization. Some examples are medication errors when a patient is given the wrong medication or given the right medication at the wrong time. Other quality issues are inappropriate or unnecessary surgery where the surgery did not need to be done and the symptom or condition could have been treated by medications or physical therapy. Another area is being discharged from the hospital too soon or being discharged from the hospital too soon with incomplete discharge instructions. In these instances, Medicare Quality Improvement Organizations will help the patient with the issues they have experienced (DHHS, 2013a, p. 17).

■ Medicare Abuse

Medicare **abuse** is when a supplier or practitioner either directly or indirectly has practices that result in unnecessary costs to the Medicare Program. This abuse includes any practice that is not consistent with the goals of providing patients with quality services that are medically necessary or meet professionally recognized standards and are fairly priced. Examples of **Medicare abuse** may include misusing codes on a claim, charging excessively for products or services, and billing for services that were not medically necessary. Both Medicare fraud and Medicare abuse can expose providers to criminal and civil liability (MLN, 2012a, p. 2).

■ CMS Fraud Prevention Initiative

Over the past few years the Centers for Medicare and Medicaid Services (CMS) has implemented some powerful tools that shift the focus from a "pay and chase" approach to a prospective approach that looks to prevent fraud, not only in CMS, but collaboratively with state and law enforcement partners that work on detecting and preventing fraud. The results of the efforts of CMS have been positive. In 2012 the federal government recovered a record $4.2 billion dollars from people who attempted to defraud seniors and taxpayers. The Accountable Care Act provided additional resources that allowed CMS to have the success they had in 2012. CMS also uses predictive analytic technology that is called the Fraud Prevention System that will identify high-risk claims for fraud in real time that has stopped, prevented, or identified $115 million in payments. The success of a program like this one is realized in dollars in that for every $1 dollar spent resulted in $3 dollars saved in the first year of this program. In addition, Medicare has redesigned the Medicare Summary Notice to make it easier for the beneficiary to spot fraud or errors (DHHS, 2013a).

CMS has also started a campaign called "Help Prevent Fraud" which educates people on how they can protect themselves against fraud. This education process includes telling people to never give their Medicare or Social Security number to anyone other than an authorized person that is part of their provider of care's staff. More importantly, to report any suspicious activity such as being asked for their Medicare or Social Security number or banking information. Medicare states that they will never call for this information (DHHS, 2013a).

■ Health Care Fraud Prevention and Enforcement Action Team (HEAT)

The **Health Care Fraud Prevention and Enforcement Action Team (HEAT)** is a joint initiative between the Department of Health and Human Services and the Department of Justice. This was to improve interagency collaboration on reducing fraud in federal healthcare programs. This was achieved by increased coordination, data sharing, and training among investigators, agents, prosecutors, analysts, and policymakers. Moreover, the HEAT Team expanded to nine Fraud Strike Force cities (DHHS, 2013a, p. 27).

The mission of the HEAT Team is to gather resources across government agencies to help prevent waste, fraud, and abuse in the Medicare and Medicaid programs. To reduce the skyrocketing healthcare costs and improve the quality of care by ridding the system of perpetrators who are preying on Medicare and Medicaid beneficiaries. In addition, to highlight best practices by providers and public sector employees who are dedicated to ending waste, fraud, and abuse along with building upon existing partnerships between the Department of Justice and the Department of Health and Human Services to reduce fraud and recover taxpayer dollars (DHHS, 2013a, p. 27).

The results of the HEAT Team initiatives in 2012 were 91 people, including doctors and nurses and other professionals, being charged with criminal activity that resulted in a total of $432 million in false billing that encompassed $230 million in home health care, $100 million in community mental health care, and $49 million in ambulance transportation. There were more than 500 law enforcement agents from the Federal Bureau of Investigations (FBI), HHS-OIG, multiple Medicaid Fraud Control Units, and other state and local law enforcement agencies taking part in this takedown. This Strike Force operation in the 9 cities resulted in 117 indictments, information and complaints against 278 defendants who allegedly billed Medicare more than $1.5 billion in fraudulent schemes. In fiscal year 2012, there ended up being 251 guilty pleas and 13 jury trials were litigated with guilty verdicts against 29 defendants. The average prison sentence in these cases was more than 48 months (DHHS, 2013a, p. 27).

■ Zone Program Integrity Contractors

The **Zone Program Integrity Contractors (ZPICs)** were created to perform program integrity functions in zones for Medicare Part A and Part B, Durable Medical Equipment (DME), Prosthetics, Orthotics, and Supplies, Home Health and Hospice, and Medicare–Medicaid data matching. The responsibilities of the ZIPCs is to investigate leads generated by the new Fraud Prevention System (FPS), perform data analysis to identify cases of suspected fraud, and make recommendations to CMS for appropriate administrative actions to protect the Medicare Trust Fund dollars. In addition, responsibilities included making referrals to law enforcement for potential prosecution, support ongoing investigations, provide feedback and support to CMS, and identify improper payments to be recovered (DHHS, 2013a, p. 30–31).

■ National Benefit Integrity and Medicare Drug Integrity Contractor

The **National Benefit Integrity Medicare Drug Integrity Contractor** (NBI MEDIC) program supports CMS Center for Program Integrity, monitors fraud and abuse in Medicare Part C and Part D programs in all 50 states, the District of Columbia, and U.S. territories. In addition, they have investigators throughout the country and work with federal, state, and local law enforcement agencies. NBI MEDIC key responsibilities include investigating potential fraud, waste, and abuse. NBI MEDIC will also receive complaints, resolve beneficiary fraud complaints, perform proactive data analyses, identify program vulnerabilities, and refer potential fraud cases to law enforcement (DHHS, 2013a, p. 34).

Some examples of cases that NBI MCDIC handles are when someone pretends to represent Medicare or SSA and ask for a beneficiary's Medicare number. They also investigate if someone is asking a beneficiary to sell their Medicare prescription drug card. Moreover, if someone is trying to get a beneficiary to take cash from someone to visit a specific provider, supplier, or pharmacy and if the beneficiary was billed for drugs that they did not receive (DHHS, 2013a, p. 35).

■ Medicare Fraud and Abuse Laws

The mid-1980s through the late 1990s brought about a wave of legislation targeted at fighting Medicare and Medicaid fraud and abuse. In an effort to eliminate erroneous healthcare spending for Medicare and Medicaid programs, Congress passed several acts that target the fraud and abuse that is present in the Medicare and Medicaid systems. In addition, not only did the new legislation show a commitment to protecting the Medicare Trust Fund by Congress, but it gave CMS the resources necessary and the penalties necessary to battle healthcare fraud and abuse (Casto & Forrestal, 2013, p. 35).

There are several laws that govern Medicare Fraud and they are The False Claims Act, Anti-Kickback Statute, Physician Self-Referral Law (**Stark Law**), Social Security Act, and the U.S. Criminal Code. Violations of these laws can result in nonpayment of healthcare claims, Civil Monetary Penalties (CMPs), exclusion from the Medicare Program, and criminal and civil liability. In addition to these laws covering Medicare Part A and Medicare Part B, they cover Medicare Part C and Medicare Part D along with those who are dual eligible for Medicare and Medicaid (MLN, 2012b, p. 2).

■ The Center for Program Integrity

The **Center for Program Integrity (CPI)** was created in 2010 and brought together the Medicare and Medicaid program integrity groups under one management structure to strengthen and better coordinate existing activities and to detect fraud, waste, and abuse. The CPI created a more rigorous screening process for providers and suppliers enrolling in Medicare, Medicaid, and CHIP. It also required a cross-termination among federal and state health programs where if a provider lost privileges under Medicare that the provider would also lose privileges under Medicaid and CHIP. CPI temporarily stopped enrollment of new providers and suppliers in high-risk areas of healthcare fraud and abuse. Lastly, CPI stopped payments to providers and suppliers in cases of suspected fraud if there has been a credible fraud allegation. Payments in this type of situation would be stopped to the provider while the investigation is underway (DHHS, 2013a, p. 20).

■ Top Ten Ways Consumers Can Help Fight Medicare Fraud

The consumer is the first line of defense when it comes to fighting Medicare fraud. This is due to the patient, or consumer, being between the provider providing a service and the provider actually submitting a claim for the services rendered. So this makes the patient the first person to identify if anything fraudulent has taken place on their account. The top ten ways are as follows (DHHS, 2011, p. 1–2):

1. When the patient has a doctor's appointment or receives healthcare services, the patient should record the date(s) on a calendar. In addition, the patient should note the tests or services received on those dates on the calendar. Finally, the patient should keep a file of the receipts and statements that they get from their providers.

2. Patients need to review their Medicare claims, Medicare Summary Notices (MSN), and compare them to the services listed on their calendar and the receipts that they have on file. They should compare the services listed on the MSN with the receipts and notes on the calendar and make sure that the dates match and the services received listed on the MSN match those of their notes. If there are items listed on the MSN and not in their calendar or matches their receipts, this could be a possible false claim that was filed on their account.

3. The patient can review their Original Medicare claims, once they have been processed, by visiting www.MyMedicare.gov or by calling 1-800-MEDICARE (1-800-633-4227, TTY 1-877-486-2048) and using the automated phone system. For Medicare Prescription Drug Plan, the patient may call their plan for more information about a claim.

4. The patient may request the assistance of their local Senior Medicare Patrol program in reviewing their Medicare claims statement or MSN. If the patient

identifies any errors or if fraud is suspected, they can also call upon the Senior Medicare Patrol program.

5. The patient should be aware of or recognize any potential sources of fraud, including unrecognized claims on their MDS, suspicious advertisements from companies offering Medicare-covered items or services that may not be legitimate.

6. Patients should not use another person's Medicare card, nor allow anyone else to use their Medicare card to access benefits or for any other reason.

7. Patients should protect their Medicare identification number, and only give it out to their doctor or other Medicare providers. Most importantly, patients should not give out their Medicare number in exchange for a special offer.

8. Patients need to report suspected instances of fraud by calling 1-800-MEDICARE.

9. Patients should consider becoming a member of the Senior Medicare Patrol (SMP) so that they may assist other beneficiaries and their caregivers in identifying and reporting any suspected Medicare fraud and abuse. The patient may call 1-877-808-2468 or go to the SMP locator at www.smpresource.org.

10. Patients can learn more about Medicare fraud and ways to protect themselves against fraud and abuse by visiting www.stopmedicarefraud.gov.

■ False Claims Act

The **False Claims Act** (FCA) of the United States Code Sections 3729–3733 protects the government from being overcharged or sold substandard goods or services. The FCA will impose civil liability on any person who knowingly submits, or causes to be submitted, a false or fraudulent claim to the federal government for payment. The term "knowing" is a standard that includes acting in deliberate ignorance or reckless disregard of the truth relating to the claim. An example is where a practitioner, or provider of services, submits a claim to Medicare for a visit for medical services that they know was not provided. The civil penalties for violating the FCA may include fines up to three times the amount of damages sustained by the government as a result of these false claims being submitted. In addition, there can also be criminal penalties for submitting the false claims that may include fines, imprisonment, or both (MLN, 2012b, p. 2).

■ Criminal Health Care Fraud Statute

The **Criminal Health Care Fraud Statute** is found in 18 U.S.C. Section 1347 and prohibits knowingly and willfully executing or attempting to execute and scheme or artifice to defraud any healthcare benefit program or to obtain by means of false or fraudulent pretenses, representations, or promises any of the money or property owned by or under the custody or control of any healthcare benefit program that is in the connection with the delivery of or payment for healthcare benefits, items, or services. Proof of actual knowledge or specific intent to violate the law is not required. Penalties may include fines, imprisonment, or both (MLN, 2012b, p. 3).

■ Anti-Kickback Statute

The **Anti-Kickback Statute** is found in 42 U.S.C. Section 1320a–7b(b) and makes it a criminal offense to knowingly and willfully offer, pay, solicit, or receive any remuneration to induce or reward referrals of items or services reimbursable by a federal healthcare program. The Anti-Kickback Statute is violated when remuneration is paid, received, offered, or solicited purposefully to induce or reward referrals of items or services payable by a federal healthcare program. If the activity satisfies the Safe Harbor Regulations in 42 Code of Federal Regulations (CFR) Section 1001.952 it is not treated as an offense of the code. Criminal penalties for violating the Anti-Kickback Statute may include fines, imprisonment, or both (MLN, 2012a, p. 3).

■ Physician Self-Referral Law (Stark Law)

The Physician Self-Referral Law, known as the Stark Law, is found in 42 U.S.C. Section 1395nn, and this law prohibits a physician from making a referral for certain designated healthcare services to an entity in which the physician, or an immediate member of his or her family, has an ownership or investment interest, or with which he or she has a compensation arrangement, unless an exception applies. Penalties for physicians who violate the Physician Self-Referral Law include fines as well as exclusion from participation in all federal healthcare programs (MLN, 2012a, p. 3).

■ Exclusion from Participation in Federal Healthcare Programs

In 1977, in the Medicare-Medicaid Anti-Fraud and Abuse Amendments, Congress first mandated the exclusion of physicians and other practitioners convicted of program-related crimes from participation in Medicare and Medicaid. In 1981, the Civil Monetary Penalties Law (CMPL) was enacted that took additional steps to better address healthcare fraud and abuse. The CMPL authorizes the Department of Health and Human Services and the OIG to impose Civil Monetary Penalties (CMPs), assessments, and program exclusions against any person that submits false, fraudulent, or other types of improper claims to Medicare or Medicaid for payment (DHHS, 2013b, p. 5).

The enactment of the Health Insurance Portability and Accountability Act (HIPAA) and the Balanced Budget Act (BBA) of 1997 further expanded the OIG's sanction authorities. These statutes extended the application and scope of the current CMPs and exclusion authorities beyond programs funded by the Department of Health and Human Services to all Federal Healthcare Programs. In addition to this, the BBA authorized a new CMP authority to be imposed against healthcare providers or entities that employ or enter into contracts with an excluded person to provide items or services for which payment may be made under a Federal Healthcare Program. The Health Care Education Reconciliation Act of 2010 (ACA) expanded the OIG's waiver authority and exclusion waiver authority by adding a new provision that subjects an excluded person to liability if the person orders or prescribes an item or a service while excluded and knows or should know that a claim for the item or services may be made to a Federal Healthcare Program (DHHS, 2013b, p. 6).

When a provider is excluded from all Federal Healthcare Programs, this provider cannot receive any payment for any items or services furnished by the excluded person; nor can services be provided at the direction of or on the prescription of an excluded person. This exclusion will follow the excluded healthcare provider even if he or she changes from one healthcare profession to another while excluded. The payment prohibition applies to any form or method of Federal Healthcare Program payment. An excluded provider, since they are unable to treat the patient, may refer a patient to a nonexcluded provider if the excluded provider does not furnish, order, or prescribe any services for the referred patient. In addition, the nonexcluded provider must treat the patient and independently bill the Federal Healthcare Program for the services that they provided. All covered items will be payable to the nonexcluded provider even if the referral came from an excluded provider (DHHS, 2013b, p. 7).

The prohibition on the Federal Healthcare Program payment for items or services furnished by an excluded individual includes items and services that are provided beyond direct patient care. In other words, if an excluded individual works under an arrangement with a hospital, nursing home, home health agency, or managed care entity to perform services such as preparation of surgical trays or review of treatment plans, regardless of the payment arrangement the facility has with the Federal Healthcare Program. An example in a pharmacy is when there is an excluded pharmacist, this pharmacist is not permitted to input prescription information for pharmacy billing or be involved in any way in filling prescriptions. Moreover, if there is an excluded person, this individual is not permitted to provide transportation services that are paid for by a Federal Healthcare Program such as an ambulance driver or even a dispatcher for an ambulance company (DHHS, 2013b, p. 8).

Excluded persons are not permitted to furnish administrative and management services that are payable by Federal Healthcare Programs. Some levels of management are any executive leadership such as Chief Executive Officer (CEO),

Chief Financial Officer (CFO), general counsel, Director of Health Information Management, Director of Human Resources, or a Physician Practice Manager for a provider that furnishes items or services that are payable by a Federal Healthcare Program. In addition, this person cannot provide any other types of administration such as information technology (IT), strategic planning, billing and accounting, staff training unless the facility is totally unrelated to Federal Healthcare Programs (DHHS, 2013b, p. 8).

A healthcare provider or organization must do their due diligence with regards to who is ordering or prescribing items or services for patients. For example, if a physician has a valid Drug Enforcement Agency (DEA) number in a state it does not necessarily mean that the provider is not on the excluded list for Federal Healthcare Programs.

■ Violation of OIG Exclusion by an Excluded Person

If an excluded person violates the exclusion that was imposed upon him or her, and furnishes items or services to a Federal Healthcare Program beneficiary and submits a claim for payment of these services, the excluded person may be subject to CMP of $10,000 for each claimed item or service furnished during the period that the person was excluded. The excluded person may also be subject to an assessment of up to three times the amount claimed for each item or service. In addition, the OIG may deny reinstatement when requested by the excluded person due to the additional violation. The excluded person may also be liable under the False Claims Act for knowingly presenting or causing to be submitted/presented a false or fraudulent claim for payment from the Federal Healthcare Program (DHHS, 2013b, p. 10).

A person that is excluded by the OIG may own a provider that participates in the Federal Healthcare Program, but there are several risks to this type of ownership. First, the OIG may exclude the provider if circumstances regarding the ownership are present. This includes where the OIG, at their discretion, can exclude any provider that is owned in part, 5 percent or more by an excluded person. Second, an excluded individual may be subject to CMPL liability if he or she has an ownership or controlling interest in a provider that is participating in Medicare or a state healthcare program if he or she is an officer or managing employee of the entity. Overall, an excluded person may own a healthcare provider, but may not provide any items or services such as administrative and management services if these services or items are reimbursable by a Federal Healthcare Program (DHHS, 2013b, p. 11).

If a provider employs or enters into a contract with an excluded person, the provider is subject to CMPs if they provide items or services that are payable by the Federal Healthcare Program. If the excluded person provides services payable, directly or indirectly, by a Federal Healthcare Program, the OIG may impose CMPs of up to

$10,000 for each item or service furnished by the excluded person, as well as assessment of up to three times the amount claimed, and program exclusion of the provider (DHHS, 2013b, p. 12).

A provider could be subject to CMP liability if an excluded person participates in any way in the furnishing of items or services that are payable by a Federal Healthcare Program. This can include, or apply to, direct patient care, indirect patient care, administrative and management services, items or services furnished at the direction or on the prescription of an excluded person when the person furnishing the services is aware or should be aware of the exclusion. CMP liability could result if the provider's claim to the Federal Healthcare Program any items or services furnished by an excluded person, even if the excluded person does not receive payment from the provider for his or her services when this person is a nonemployed excluded physician who is a member of a hospital's medical staff or an excluded healthcare professional who works at a hospital or nursing home as a volunteer (DHHS, 2013b, p. 12).

A person may not provide services that are payable by a Federal Healthcare Program regardless of whether the person is an employee, a contractor, or a volunteer or has any other relationship with the provider. For example, if a hospital contracts with a staffing agency for temporary or per-diem nurses, the hospital will be subject to overpayment liability and may be subject to CMP liability if an excluded nurse from the contracted staffing agency furnishes items or services to Federal Healthcare Program beneficiaries. In a hospital setting, the facility may reduce or eliminate its CMP liability if the hospital is able to adequately demonstrate that it reasonably relied on the staffing agency to perform a check of the List of Excluded Individuals and Entities (LEIE) for the nurses furnished by the staffing agency through contract language that demonstrates the agency accepted responsibility to provide the LEIE and the hospital exercised due diligence in ensuring that the staffing agency was meeting its contractual obligation (DHHS, 2013b, p. 13).

■ Determining If an Individual or Entity Is Excluded

The Exclusions website where the LEIE can be found is at http://oig/hhs.gov/exclusions.

The LEIE is a searchable online database and has the availability of downloadable data files. In addition to this information, the OIG provides Quick Tips on how to use the LEIE, Frequently Asked Questions (FAQ) regarding the OIG's Exclusion Program, information regarding how an excluded person or entity can apply for reinstatement, video podcasts, and contact information for the OIG Exclusion Program (DHHS, 2013b, p. 13).

The online database contains the following information (DHHS, 2013b, p. 14):

- The name of the excluded person at the time of the exclusion
- The person's provider type
- The authority under which the person was excluded
- The state where the excluded individual resided at the time of exclusion or state where the entity was doing business
- A mechanism to verify search results via a Social Security number (SSN) or Employer Identification number (EIN)
- The OIG will soon update the LEIE to include National Provider Identifier (NPI) for individuals and entities excluded after 2009 that have an NPI

The LEIE Downloadable Data File enables users to download the entire LEIE. The OIG posts supplemental exclusion and reinstatement files on a monthly basis to their website. The Downloadable Data File does not include SSNs or EINs. Therefore, to process a verification of a specific individual or entity, the Downloadable Data File can be reviewed, but to verify that a person or entity is excluded the SSN or EIN will have to be added to the search to verify the entry is accurate. The provider performing this verification should maintain the documentation provided by the OIG website Online Searchable Database by taking a screen-shot and printing it and maintaining it in their files. If the provider or facility decides to use an outside agency to perform the screening on the LEIE, they should be aware that because it is the provider's responsibility to determine whether an employee is excluded or not, the provider or facility retains the potential CMP liability if they employ or contract with an excluded person (DHHS, 2013b, p. 14).

■ Frequency of Screening and Which Individuals to Screen

To avoid any potential liability, providers should check the LEIE prior to contracting or employing a person and then periodically check the LEIE against the current employees and contractors. Since the OIG does not mandate that a provider or entity check the LEIE, providers may determine on their own how frequently to check the Online Searchable Database. The OIG updates the LEIE monthly, so it may be good policy to check all employees and contractors monthly to best minimize any potential overpayment and CMP liability (DHHS, 2013b, p. 15).

The OIG recommends that to best determine which persons should be screened against the LEIE Online Searchable Database, the provider should review each job category or contractual relationship to determine whether or not the item or service being provided is directly or indirectly, in whole or in part, payable by a Federal Healthcare Program. If the answer is yes, then the provider should, in the best interest of the provider to limit CMP liability, screen all persons that perform under that contract or that are in that job category. Providers should determine whether or not to screen contractors, subcontractors, and employees of contractors using the same methodology that they use for their own employees (DHHS, 2013b, p. 16).

System for Award Management (SAM) is another searchable database that is available and includes the OIG exclusions along with debarment actions taken by federal agencies. The OIG recommends that providers use the LEIE as the primary source of information about the OIG exclusions because the LEIE is maintained by the OIG and updated monthly, and provides more details about any person or entity that is excluded than SAM (DHHS, 2013b, p. 17).

Other databases available are the National Practitioner Data Bank (NPDB) and the Healthcare Integrity and Protection Databank (HIPDB). The NPDB was established under the Health Care Quality Improvement Act of 1986 and is an information clearinghouse that originally collected medical malpractice payments paid on behalf of physicians and adverse actions taken by licensing agencies against healthcare practitioners and healthcare entities. In addition, the NPDB tracked adverse privileging actions and any negative actions or findings taken against healthcare practitioners or entities by Quality Improvement Organizations and Private Accreditation Organizations. HIPDB was created by HIPAA to provide information on adverse licensing and certification actions, criminal convictions that were healthcare related, civil judgments, exclusions from federal or state healthcare programs, and other adjudicated actions or decisions. Overall, the OIG recommends that providers use the LEIE as the primary database for the purposes of screening for exclusions of current or potential employees or contractors (DHHS, 2013b, p. 18).

■ Physician Self-Referral

Section 1877 of the Social Security Act (42 U.S.C. 1395nn), also known as the physician self-referral law and is commonly known as or referred to as the "Stark Law." The Stark Law is as follows (CMS, 2013b):

1. Prohibits a physician from making referrals for certain designated health services (DHS) payable by Medicare to an entity with which he or she (or immediate family member) has a financial relationship (ownership, investment, or compensation), unless an exception applies.

2. Prohibits the entity from presenting or causing to be presented claims to Medicare (or billing another individual, entity, or third party payer) for those referred services.

3. Establishes a number of specific exceptions and grants the Secretary the authority to create regulatory exceptions for financial relationships that do not pose a risk of program or patient abuse.

The following are items or services that are considered designated healthcare services (DHS) (CMS, 2013b):

1. Clinical laboratory services

2. Physical therapy services

3. Occupational therapy services

4. Outpatient speech-language pathology services

5. Radiology and certain other imaging services

6. Radiation therapy services and supplies

7. Durable medical equipment

8. Parenteral and enteral nutrients, equipment, and supplies

9. Prosthetics, orthotics, and prosthetic devices and supplies

10. Home health services

11. Outpatient prescription drugs

12. Inpatient and outpatient hospital services

When the Stark Law was enacted in 1989, it only applied to physician referrals for clinical laboratory services. Congress expanded the prohibition to additional DHS and applied certain aspects of this law regarding self-referral to the Medicaid program. Congress added a provision permitting the Secretary to issue written advisory opinions concerning whether a referral relating to DHS, outside of clinical laboratory services, is prohibited under this Act in 1997. In addition, Congress authorized the secretary in 2003 to promulgate an exception to the physician self-referral prohibition for certain arrangements where a physician receives nonmonetary remuneration that is necessary and used solely to receive and transmit electronic prescription information. Moreover, they established a temporary moratorium on physician referrals to certain specialty hospitals in which the referring physician had an ownership or investment interest (CMS, 2013b).

Self-Referral Disclosure Protocol

The CMS Self-Referral Disclosure Protocol (SRDP) enables providers of services and suppliers to self-disclose actual or potential violations of the physician self-referral statute. CMS posts a list of select self-disclosures that were resolved under SRDP and updates the list quarterly. Some of the settlements under SRDP are as follows (CMS, 2013c):

Date: 2011-02-10
Description: CMS settled several violations of the physician self-referral statute disclosed by general acute care hospital located in Massachusetts (the hospital) under the SDRP.
Findings: The hospital disclosed under the SDRP that it violated the physician self-referral statute by failing to satisfy the requirements of the personal services arrangements with certain hospital department chiefs and the medical staff for leadership services and failing to satisfy the requirements of the personal services arrangements exception for arrangements with certain physician groups for on-site overnight coverage for patients in the hospital.
Settlement: All violations disclosed were settled for $579,000.

Date: 2011-09-10
Description: CMS settled violations of the physician self-referral statute disclosed by a physician group practice located in Ohio under the SDRP.
Findings: The practice disclosed under the SDRP that it violated the physician self-referral statute in two instances by prescribing and supplying a certain type of Durable Medical Equipment that did not satisfy the requirements of the in-office ancillary services exception.
Settlement: The violations disclosed were settled for $60.

Date: 2013-11-08
Description: CMS settled several violations of the physician self-referral law disclosed under the SDRP by a nonprofit acute-care hospital located in Oklahoma.
Findings: The hospital disclosed under the SDRP that it may have violated the physician self-referral law, because arrangements with four physicians failed to satisfy the requirements of the personal services arrangements exception for the provision of electrocardiogram interpretation services at the hospital.
Settlement: All violation disclosed were settled for $124,008.

■ Physician Compliance Programs

A **compliance program** is a guide that is intended to assist individual and small group physician practices in developing a voluntary compliance program that promotes adherence to statutes and regulations applicable to the Federal Healthcare Programs. The goal of a voluntary compliance program is to strengthen the efforts of a healthcare provider to prevent and reduce improper conduct. These programs can also benefit physician practices by helping to streamline business operations (DHHS, 2000, p. 59435).

There are seven components that provide a solid basis upon which a physician can create a voluntary compliance program. They are as follows (MLN, 2012b, p. 10):

- Conduct internal monitoring and auditing
- Implement compliance and practice standards
- Designate a compliance officer or contact
- Conduct appropriate training and education
- Respond appropriately to detected offenses and develop corrective action
- Develop open lines of communication with employees
- Enforce disciplinary standards through well-published guidelines

Auditing and Monitoring

Ongoing auditing and monitoring is essential to a successful compliance program. The auditing component of a compliance program will help to evaluate if individuals are properly carrying out their responsibilities and claims are submitted appropriately. Moreover, this is an excellent way for a physician practice to identify, if any, problems that may exist and focus on risk areas that are associated with those problems. There are two types of reviews/audits that can take place and they are a standard procedures review and a claims audit submission audit. The standards and procedures audit is where the practice reviews the standards and procedures to determine if they are current and complete. If they are ineffective or outdated, they should be updated to reflect changes in government regulations. A claims submission audit is where bills and medical records are reviewed for compliance with applicable coding, billing, and documentation requirements. This audit will help to determine whether the bills are accurately coded and reflect the services provided, documentation is completed correctly, services or items provided are reasonable and necessary, and to make sure that no incentives for unnecessary services exist (DHHS, 2000, p. 59437).

Establish Practice Standards

After the internal audits are completed and if they have identified any risk areas, the next step is to develop a method for dealing with those risk areas through practice standards and procedures. Written standards and procedures are a central component of any compliance program. These standards and procedures help to reduce the prospect of erroneous claims and fraudulent activity by identifying risk areas for the practice and establishing tighter internal controls to counter those risks. The OIG believes that written standards and procedures can be helpful to all physician practices, regardless of their size and capability. If a physician practice does not have standards and procedures developed they can start by developing a written standard procedures manual and by updating clinical forms periodically to make sure they facilitate and encourage clear and complete documentation of patient care (DHHS, 2000, p. 59438).

Specific Risk Areas

The OIG recognizes that many physician practices may not have in place standards and procedures to prevent erroneous or fraudulent conduct in their practices. In order to develop effective standards and procedures the practice may want to consider what types of fraud and abuse-related topics are needed to be addressed based on the practice's specific needs. The OIG has identified four potential risk areas affecting physician practices. The first risk area is coding and billing, which determines if the practice is billing for services not rendered. This risk area includes determining if the practice is submitting claims that are reasonable and necessary services, double billing for items that results in double payment, billing for noncovered services as if it was a covered service, unbundling a bundled item to get a higher reimbursement, failing to properly use modifies, and is the practice upcoding the level of service provided to the patient to achieve a higher reimbursement for the services rendered (DHHS, 2000, p. 59439).

The second area the OIG has identified for the practice is focused on the charges and the services provided by the practice are reasonable and necessary. The OIG understands that the physician practice should be able to order tests, including screening tests that they believe are appropriate for the treatment of their patients. With that said, Medicare will only pay for services that meet the Medicare definition of reasonable and necessary. If the treatment is not considered to be reasonable and necessary payment will be denied (DHHS, 2000, p. 59440).

Timely and accurate and complete documentation is important to clinical patient care. This documentation serves a second function when a bill is submitted for payment in that the documentation submitted will support the bill for the services rendered to the patient. One of the most important physician compliance issues is the appropriate documentation of diagnosis and treatment. Physician documentation is necessary to determine the appropriate medical treatment for the patient and the basis for coding and billing determination. In addition, the documentation is a key element to verify and support precisely what services were actually provided. Some examples of internal documentation guidelines include is the medical record complete, documentation of each patient encounter includes the reason for the encounter and history, physical exam and findings, prior test results, assessment and clinical impression, appropriate coding using CPT and ICD-9-CM, and the appropriate health risk factors were identified and documented (DHHS, 2000, p. 59440).

There are standards and procedures that encourage compliance with anti-kickback statutes and physician self-referrals. Remuneration for referrals is illegal because it can distort medical decision making and cause overutilization of services or supplies. This list should be viewed as a starting point for the practice to develop their standards and procedures. Possible risk areas to be aware of are financial arrangements with outside entities to whom the practice may refer Federal Healthcare Program business, joint ventures with entities supplying goods or services to the physician practice or its patients, consulting contracts or medical directorships, office and equipment leases with entities to which the physician refers, and soliciting where the physician or practice accepts a gift or gratuity of more than nominal value to or from those who may benefit from a physician's practice's referral of Federal Healthcare Program business (DHHS, 2000, p. 59441).

■ Conclusion

Healthcare administrators need to know the actions that involve Medicare fraud and abuse. With this knowledge of the programs and processes of an effective compliance program the healthcare administrator may be better prepared to prevent this problem. Fraud and abuse place strains on the finances of health care, not only for the facility, but for the payer such as Medicare and Medicaid along with the other commercial payers. Effectively managing this process contributes to the financial health of the organization. As an administrator, the terms of anti-kickback and physician self-referral may come up once in a while or maybe never. But, if it comes up once, the healthcare administrator needs to be able to immediately identify the problem, isolate it, assess the error or errors and come up with a documented plan of correction, report it immediately to upper management or the board of directors, and then develop a plan that will stop the issue immediately and then stop it from happening again in the future.

Overall, the healthcare administrator needs to be an expert in Revenue Cycle Management, budgeting, finance, operations, and compliance. Without all areas covered, gaps will occur and issues will arise that can threaten the future of the facility and their ability to provide quality care and to be appropriately reimbursed for the care delivered.

References

Casto, A.B., & Forrestal, E. (2013). *Principles of healthcare reimbursement* (4th ed.). Chicago: AHIMA.

Centers for Medicare and Medicaid Services. (2013a). Fraud prevention toolkit: CMS fraud prevention initiative. Retrieved from http://www.cms.gov/Outreach-and-Education/Outreach/Partnerships/FraudPreventionToolkit.html

Centers for Medicare and Medicaid Services. (2013b). Physician self referral. Retrieved from http://www.cms.gov/medicare/fraud-and-abuse/physicianselfreferral/index.html

Centers for Medicare and Medicaid Services. (2013c). Self-referral disclosure protocol settlements. Retrieved from http://www.cms.gov/Medicare/Fraud-and-Abuse/PhysicianSelfReferral/Self-Referral-Disclosure-Protocol-Settlements.html?DLSort=0&DLPage=1&DLSortDir=ascending

Department of Health and Human Services. (2000). Developing a compliance program guidance for individual and small group physician practices. *Federal Register*, *65*(194), 59434–59444.

Department of Health and Human Services. (2011). Top ten ways consumers can help fight medicare fraud. Retrieved from http://www.cms.gov/Outreach-and-Education/Outreach/Partnerships/downloads/FraudCampaignTop10WaysConsumersFightFraudAugust2011.pdf

Department of Health and Human Services. (2013a). 2013 national training program: Module: 10 Medicare and Medicaid fraud prevention. Retrieved from http://www.cms.gov/Outreach-and-Education/Training/CMSNationalTrainingProgram/Downloads/2013-Fraud-and-Abuse-Prevention-Workbook.pdf

Department of Health and Human Services. (2013b). OIG special advisory bulletin on the effect of exclusion from participation in federal health care programs. Retrieved from http://oig.hhs.gov/exclusions/files/sab-05092013.pdf

Medicare Learning Network. (2012a). Medicare fraud & abuse: Prevention, detection, and reporting. Retrieved from http://www.cms.gov/Outreach-and-Education/Medicare-Learning-Network-MLN/MLNProducts/downloads/Fraud_and_Abuse.pdf

Medicare Learning Network. (2012b). Avoiding Medicare fraud & abuse: A roadmap for physicians. Retrieved from http://www.cms.gov/Outreach-and-Education/Medicare-Learning-Network-MLN/MLNProducts/Downloads/Avoiding_Medicare_FandA_Physicians_FactSheet_905645.pdf

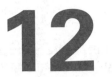

12 | Electronic Health Records and Meaningful Use

Learning Outcomes

After reading this chapter, the student will:

- Define the electronic medical record.
- Define meaningful use and the impact it can have on the healthcare industry.
- Identify the timeline for the different stages of meaningful use.
- Describe the impact of meaningful use on the development and implementation of the electronic medical record.

■ Introduction

The American Recovery and Reinvestment Act of 2009 (ARRA) was signed into law on February 17, 2009. This was an unprecedented effort to jumpstart the U.S. economy, create or save millions of jobs, and put a down payment on addressing long-neglected challenges so our country can thrive in the 21st century. The American Recovery and Reinvestment Act is in response to a crisis unlike any since the Great Depression, and includes measures to modernize our nation's infrastructure, enhance energy independence, expand educational opportunities, preserve and improve affordable health care, provide tax relief, and protect those in greatest need (CMS, 2013a).

There are different programs from the Centers for Medicare and Medicaid Services (CMS) for providers of healthcare services. This chapter will focus on two programs starting with Electronic Health Records and then meaningful use. Since the inception of the EHR the overall adoption of the EHR has doubled among physicians and more than tripled its use in the hospital setting (CMS, 2013e). This program is for providers so that they can demonstrate they are meeting objectives through various stages by, not just having an Electronic Medical Record (EMR) system, but actually using their EMR system in a meaningful way through such things as documentation and access to information. As of October 2013, nearly 85 percent of the eligible hospitals and more than 50 percent of eligible professionals had taken the first step of registering for the Medicare or Medicaid EHR Incentive Program (CMS, 2013e).

■ Electronic Health Record

Introduction to the Electronic Health Record

The **Electronic Health Record (EHR)** is not an easy thing to define. There has been some confusion over the years, but with the introduction of meaningful use, the EHR has taken a more definitive shape in the healthcare arena. Over the years it has been thought that an EHR is a system where pages of a medical record are scanned into a system. This is more in the line of a document imaging system that will lead to a hybrid-style EHR.

The EHR has really moved along as a result of being such an integral part of the meaningful use program and there have been more standards adopted and implemented, new hardware, enhanced access for healthcare professionals and the patient, and increased security to protect the patient and their healthcare information. The EHR is not a simple application, as it represents a complex constructed set of components that are sophistically integrated requiring a significant investment for the provider (Amatayakul, 2013, p. 4).

The definitions of an EHR versus an EMR are:

Electronic Medical Record: "An electronic record of health related information on an individual that can be created, gathered, managed, and consulted by authorized clinicians and staff within one healthcare organization." (Amatayakul, 2013, p. 5)

Electronic Health Record: "An electronic record of health-related information on an individual that conforms to nationally recognized interoperability standards and that can be created, managed, and consulted by authorized clinicians and staff across more than one healthcare organization" (Amatayakul, 2013, p. 5).

A Qualified EHR is an electronic record of healthcare-related information on a patient that includes all pertinent components of a medical record such as demographics, history and physical, and clinical information that allows for the ability of clinical decision support, computer physician order entry (CPOE), the ability to capture and query information in the health record, and to transmit or exchange information with other sources (Amatayakul, 2013, p. 6).

Certified EHR Technology (CEHRT) is a term used to identify EHR products that are certified and meet specific criteria or standards that are required for certification. meaningful use incorporates functionality that is usually more robust than that of typical systems used or implemented in the past and includes important functionality to enable it to meet the standards of meaningful use.

The government recognizes the functionality of the EHR system in two ways. First, it permits the EHR to be certified as "complete" or inclusive of all items necessary to meet the incentives of the meaningful use program. Second, the federal government recognizes the certification as meeting the minimum standards for the meaningful use program and this does not stop the vendor from adding additional capabilities over and above the minimum needed for meaningful use (Amatayakul, 2013, p. 9).

Vision and Benefits of an EHR System

"The Institute of Medicine's contributions to the overall vision of the EHR is significant. They have addressed a specific need for standards development and certification support. They have also defined the scope of the transition to the EHR" (Amatayakul, 2013, p. 13).

Amatayakul goes on to mention about the report by the Institute of Medicine (IOM) that stated that merely automating the forms, content, and procedures of current medical records is not enough. The EHR encompasses a much broader view of the patient record and moving from a device that keeps track of patient care to a device that is involved with and contributes to the effective delivery of patient care as a core of the healthcare system (Amatayakul, 2013, p. 13).

Overall, the EHR should improve quality, enhance patient safety with reminders and alerts, support health maintenance and preventative/wellness care, increase productivity through efficiencies and workflow support, reduce some of the slower process in a manual system such as registration and documentation, support revenue enhancement through eligibility verification, support evidence-based health care, and maintain patient confidentiality during the access and exchange of Protected Health Information (PHI) (Amatayakul, 2013, p. 14).

Components of the EHR

There are four main categories of the EHR and they are source systems that collect data, core clinical systems that enable the use of data that is collected at the point of care, supporting infrastructure that integrates data from applications, and connectivity systems that help to integrate data collected across different organizations, caregivers, and patients (Amatayakul, 2013, p. 18).

Registries

Registries are systems that healthcare delivery organizations contribute specific data or information for subsequent review and analysis. These registries are considered to be disease related and procedure related to include cancer registries, diabetes registries, and immunization registries. These registries are often maintained by medical specialty or a public health department. The capture of information supports aggregation of data for trends and patterns along with statistical analysis (Amatayakul, 2013, p. 23).

Point-of-Care Charting Systems

Point-of-Care (POC) charting systems are also known as clinical documentation systems. This is where a clinician can document what is taking place during the patient visit into the system while they are with the patient in real time. The documentation includes vital signs, chief complaint or reason for the visit, review of recent labs, nursing notes, and now physicians can document while with the patient in the POC.

The data entered into the system includes structured data that is also referred to as discrete data. This data is in a predefined table or checklist for the clinician to use while documenting in the record. The other type of data is unstructured data or a narrative style of input into the system. This unstructured data is more difficult to perform searches on for different types of reports. Some variations in the equipment used are bedside terminals, wireless computers on wheels, and systems in the patient exam room. Some of the different ways a clinician can document is through templates in the EHR and another way is natural language processing that allows narrative text to be structured into data for processing by the computer (Amatayakul, 2013, p. 25).

■ Meaningful Use

Introduction to Meaningful Use

CMS has created an incentive program that will provide financial incentives for the **"meaningful use"** of a certified Electronic Health Record (EHR) for Medicare and Medicaid providers. In order to receive an incentive payment the provider must show, or demonstrate, that they are "meaningfully using" their EHR system by meeting established thresholds. Eligible professionals, hospitals, and Critical Access Hospitals (CAH) must meet the established thresholds in order to receive an incentive payment (CMS, 2013b).

Meaningful use is where a provider uses a certified EHR system to improve quality, safety, efficiency, and to reduce healthcare disparities. In addition, the EHR system will allow the provider to engage patients and their families and to improve care coordination to improve the overall health of the population, all while maintaining privacy and security with regards to Protected Health Information (PHI). CMS defines it as "Meaningful use equals the use of EHRs in a way that positively affects patient care" (CMS, 2013d, p. 4).

The three components of meaningful use are the provider using an EHR in a meaningful manner such as electronic prescribing of prescriptions (e-prescribe), use of an electronic exchange of health information to improve the quality of care given to a patient, and the use of the EHR to submit Clinical Quality Measures (CQM) and any other measures that are required of the healthcare provider (CMS, 2010, p. 3).

There are three stages in the Medicare and Medicaid EHR Incentive Program. Stage 1 starts off with the provider participating for a period of 90 days in the first year and the entire second year to meet the Stage 1 requirements. The next part is Stage 2 and this stage must be met for a full 2 years.

CY	CY 2011		CY 2012		CY 2013		CY 2014		CY 2015		CY 2016	
	Medicare	Medicaid	Medicare	Medicaid	Medicare	Medicaid	Medicare	Medicaid	Medicare	Medicaid	Medicare	Medicaid
2011	$18,000	$21,250										
2012	$12,000	$8,500	$18,000	$21,250								
2013	$8,000	$8,500	$12,000	$8,500	$15,000	$21,250						
2014	$4,000	$8,500	$8,000	$8,500	$12,000	$8,500	$12,000	$21,250				
2015	$2,000	$8,500	$4,000	$8,500	$8,000	$8,500	$8,000	$8,500		$21,250		
2016		$8,500	$2,000	$8,500	$4,000	$8,500	$4,000	$8,500		$8,500		$21,250
2017				$8,500		$8,500		$8,500		$8,500		$8,500
2018						$8,500		$8,500		$8,500		$8,500
2019								$8,500		$8,500		$8,500
2020										$8,500		$8,500
2021												$8,500
Total (if EP does not switch programs)	$44,000	$63,750	$44,000	$63,750	$39,000	$63,750	$24,000	$63,750	$0	$63,750	$0	$63,750

NOTE: Medicare Eligible Professionals may not receive EHR incentive payments under both Medicare and Medicaid.

NOTE: The amount of the annual EHR incentive payment limit for each payment year will be increased by 10 percent for EPs who predominantly furnish services in an area that is designated as a Health Professional Shortage Area.

FIGURE 12.1   Maximum EHR EP incentive payments.

Reproduced from Centers for Medicare and Medicaid Services. CMS Medicare Learning Network, Maximum EHR EP Incentive Payments, ICN #905343, p. 2, (September 2010)

Meaningful Use Eligible Professionals

The Medicare EHR Incentive Program makes available incentive payments to Medicare Eligible (ME) professionals who are taking part in the meaningful use program and using a certified program for their EHR and are one of the following types of providers such as a Doctor of Medicine or Osteopathy, Doctor of Oral Surgery or Dental Medicine, Doctor of Podiatric Medicine, Doctor of Optometry, or a Chiropractor. These providers are eligible for incentive payments only if they meet the criteria of the program. For physicians that are hospital-based EPs, they are not eligible to participate in the program. An EP is hospital-based when he or she furnishes 90 percent of his or her services in a hospital inpatient or emergency department setting.

Participation in Other CMS Programs

An EP who participates in the Medicare EHR Incentive Program may, at the same time, participate in the Physician Quality Reporting System (PQRS). There are some exclusions, such as if the EP is already receiving incentive payments through the Medicare EHR Incentive Program they cannot receive an additional incentive payment from the Electronic Prescribing (eRx) program. If the EP is receiving an EHR payment through the Medicaid EHR Incentive Program they are also eligible for payment through the eRx incentive program as long as they meet the criteria for the eRx program. Another variable is that in 2011 and 2012 an EP was eligible to earn an additional incentive payment equal to 1 percent of the allowed charges, but this has been discontinued. In addition, the EP may be subject to an adjustment under the eRx Incentive Program.

Incentive Payment Calculation and Time Frame

Under the Medicare EHR Incentive Payment Program an EP is eligible for an incentive payment equal to an annual limit and equal to 75 percent of an EP's Medicare Physician Fee Schedule amount for a calendar year. The EP can file claims for the previous calendar year up to 2 months after December 31st. For example, if an EP is eligible for the incentive payment for the calendar year of 2013, the EP's eligible charges are from January 1, 2013 to December 31, 2013 and the EP has until February 28, 2014 to file their claims to their Medicare Contractor.

Maximum Incentive Payments

The EP started having eligibility for Medicare EHR Incentive Program payments beginning in 2011 and it ends in 2016. The maximum payment in the Medicare EHR Incentive Program per calendar year are as follows (CMS, 2013c, p. 3):

- For an EP that starts as Year 1 in 2011 the payment is $18,000
  - Year 2, $12,000
  - Year 3, $8,000
  - Year 4, $4,000
  - Year 5, $2,000
  - With a total potential maximum amount payable to the EP of $44,000
- If an EP starts in 2012 as Year 1 the payment is $18,000
  - Year 2, $12,000
  - Year 3, $8,000
  - Year 4, $4,000
  - Year 5, $2,000
  - With a total potential maximum amount payable to the EP of $44,000

After 2012, any EP that begins the program to receive incentive payments will realize a reduced payment overall and a smaller starting calendar year payment and a shorter time frame and lower total payable amount over the remaining years.

- If an EP starts in 2013 the payments will start as $15,000 for Year 1
  - Year 2, $12,000
  - Year 3, $8,000
  - Year 4, $4,000
  - Giving the EP a total potential amount of $39,000 payable to the EP

- Finally, if an EP starts the program in 2014, the first payment will be $12,000 for Year 1
  - Year 2, $8,000
  - Year 3, $4,000
  - Giving the EP a total potential amount of $24,000

Meaningful Use Stage 1

During Stage 1, the 90 days of year 1 and the entire following year, there are total of 24 objectives that are included in a Core Set and a Menu Set of objectives. Out of these 24 total objectives, 19 of them must be met to successfully qualify for the incentive payment. The objectives are broken down into 14 core objective requirements and 10 Menu Set objectives. The provider must do their reporting through attestation of the Objectives and Clinical Quality Measures. This reporting can consist of yes/no answers and numerator/denominator attestation and to meet the objectives/measures goal the provider must have 80 percent of their patient records in the certified EHR system.

EP and Hospital Core Objectives Stage 1

The Core Objectives for EPs are as follows (CMS, 2013b, p. 9):

1. Computerized provider order entry (CPOE)

   This measure requires that the EP has more than 30 percent of all unique patients have at least one medication in their medication list and at least one medication order entered using the CPOE. If the EP writes less than 100 prescriptions during the reporting period, then they are excluded from this objective.

2. E-Prescribing (eRx)

   For this objective more than 40 percent of all prescriptions written by the EP are transmitted electronically using the EHR technology and not by phone or fax. An EP can be excluded from this objective if they write less than 100 prescriptions during the reporting period.

3. Report ambulatory clinical quality measures to CMS/states

   Ambulatory Clinical Quality Measures must be reported in the manner selected by CMS. This objective has no exclusions.

4. Implement one clinical decision support rule

   The EP must implement one clinical decision support tool that makes sense for the practice and that will trigger alerts or clinical information for the provider when they encounter patients with certain treatments or diagnoses. All EPs must meet this objective as there is no exclusion for this objective.

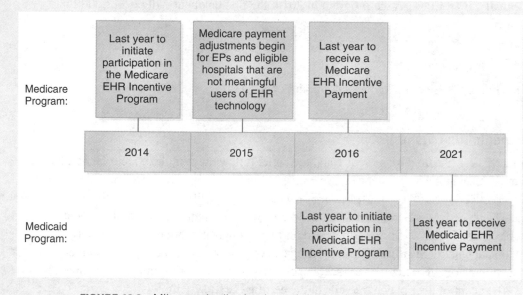

FIGURE 12.2   Milestone timeline for electronic health record incentive program.
Modified from Centers for Medicare and Medicaid Services (2010). EHR Incentive Programs, Milestone Timeline, http:// www.cms.gov/
EHRIncentivePrograms.

5. Provide patients with an electronic copy of their health information, upon request

   The EP must provide more than 50 percent of all patient requests for an electronic copy of their medical records within 3 business days. If there are no requests for an electronic copy of their medical record during the reporting period, the EP will be excluded from this objective.

6. Provide clinical summaries for patients for each office visit

   The EP must provide Clinical Summaries for more than half of the office visits to the patients within 3 days of the visit. If the EP does not provide office visits they will be excluded from this objective.

7. Drug–drug and drug–allergy interaction checks

   The EP must enable this functionality during the entire reporting period and automatically check for potentially adverse drug–drug or drug–allergy interactions. There are no exclusions for this objective.

8. Record demographics

   More than 50 percent of the unique patients that the EP sees must have the patient's demographics recorded as structured data that includes preferred language, race, ethnicity, gender, and date of birth. There is no exclusion for this objective.

9. Maintain an up-to-date **problem list** of current and active diagnoses

The EP must have more than 80 percent of all unique patients that are seen with at least one entry in the EHR indicating that no problems are known for the patient or an actual problem that the patient is experiencing. There are no exclusions for this objective.

10. Maintain active medication list

The EP must have more than 80 percent of all unique patients seen have at least one entry or an entry that the patient is not being prescribed any medications. There are no exclusions for this objective.

11. Maintain active medication allergy list

More than 80 percent of the unique patients seen by the EP have at least one entry indicating that there are no known medication allergies or an entry that the patient does not have any medication allergies. There are no exclusions for this objective.

12. Record and chart changes in vital signs

For more than 50 percent of the patients that the EP sees that are 2 years of age and older have height, weight, and blood pressure recorded in the EHR and available as structured data. The EP can be excluded from this objective if they do not see any patients that are 2 years of age or older or if the EP does not believe that these vital signs are relevant to the scope of their practice.

13. Record smoking status for patients 13 years of age or older

All unique patients that the EP sees that are 13 years of age or older have their smoking status recorded in the EHR. The EP can be excluded from meeting this objective if the EP does not see patients that are 13 years of age or older.

14. Capability to exchange key clinical information among providers of care and patient-authorized entities electronically.

The EP must perform at least one test of the EHR's capability to electronically exchange key clinical information. There are no exclusions for this objective as all EPs have to meet it.

15. Protect electronic health information

The EP must conduct security risk analysis and implement security updates and identify deficiencies through the Risk Management Process. The EP must protect all information as set forth in the HIPAA requirements. There are no exclusions for this objective.

1st Year	Stage of Meaningful Use By Year										
	2011	2012	2013	2014	2015	2016	2017	2018	2019	2020	2021
2011	1	1	1	2	2	3	3	TBD	TBD	TBD	TBD
2012		1	1	2	2	3	3	TBD	TBD	TBD	TBD
2013			1	1	2	2	3	3	TBD	TBD	TBD
2014				1	1	2	2	3	3	TBD	TBD
2015					1	1	2	2	3	3	TBD
2016						1	1	2	2	3	3
2017							1	1	2	2	3

Note that providers who were early demonstrators of meaningful use in 2011 will meet three consecutive years of meaningful use under the Stage 1 criteria before advancing to the Stage 2 criteria in 2014. All other providers would meet two years of meaningful use under the Stage 1 criteria before advancing to the Stage 2 criteria in their third year.

FIGURE 12.3　Stages of meaningful use by year.

Reproduced from Baker & Baker "Health Care Finance, Fouth Edition: Basic Tools for Nonfinancial Managers." Jones & Bartlett Learning, 2014

The 14 Core Objectives for Hospitals are as follows (CMS, 2013b, p. 10):

1. Computerized provider order entry (CPOE)
2. Drug–drug and drug–allergy interaction checks
3. Record demographics
4. Implement one clinical decision support rule
5. Maintain up-to-date problem list of current and active diagnoses
6. Maintain active medication list
7. Maintain active medication allergy list
8. Record and chart changes in vital signs
9. Record smoking status for patients 13 years of age and older
10. Report hospital clinical quality measures to CMS or states
11. Provide patients with an electronic copy of their health information upon request
12. Provide patients with an electronic copy of their discharge instructions at the time of discharge, upon request
13. Capability to exchange key clinical information among providers of care and patient authorized entities electronically
14. Protect electronic health information

Menu Objectives for EPs Stage 1

Eligible Professionals have 10 menu objectives to choose 5 from to complete. They are as follows (CMS, 2013b, p. 14):

1. Drug-formulary checks

    The EP has enabled the drug formulary feature and has access to at least one internal or external formulary and this must be enabled for the entire reporting period. There are no exclusions for this objective for the EP.

2. Incorporate clinical lab test results as structured data

    The EP must have more than 40 percent of all clinical lab results ordered during the reporting period incorporated in the EHR. The EP can be excluded if they did not order any lab tests during the reporting period or if the results did not come back as a number or a positive or negative response.

3. Generate lists of patients by specific conditions

    The EP must be able to create/develop a report for a condition that the EP feels is relevant to their practice. There are no exclusions for this objective.

4. Send reminders to patients per patient preference for preventive/follow-up care

    The EP must send to more than 20 percent of all their patients that are 65 years of age or older or 5 years old or younger a care reminder via mail, e-mail, or telephone. The EP can be excluded if they do not see patients that are 65 years of age or older or if the EP does not see any patients that are 5 years of age or younger.

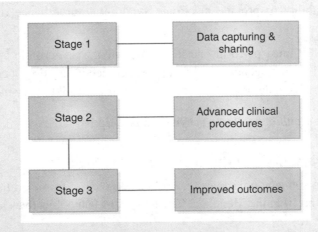

FIGURE 12.4   EHR incentive program: three stages of meaningful use.
Courtesy of J.J. Baker and R. Baker, Dallas, TX.

5. Provide patients with timely electronic access to their health information

At least 10 percent of the patients that the EP sees are provided timely access to their EHR. The EP can be excluded if they do not order or create lab results, problem lists, medication lists, or medication allergy lists.

6. Use certified EHR technology to identify patient-specific education resources and provide to patient if appropriate

More than 10 percent of the patients the EP sees are provided with patient specific education on such things as chronic conditions. There are no exclusions for this objective.

7. Medication reconciliation

The EP performs medication reconciliation for more than 50 percent of patients that are transitioned into their practice. The EP can be excluded from meeting this objective if they did not see or receive any patients from another provider.

8. Summary of care record for each transition of care or referrals

For EPs that transition their patients to other care providers that for 50 percent or more of those transitions a summary of care record is provided. The EP can be excluded from this objective if they do not refer or transfer any patients to other facilities or care settings.

9. Capability to submit electronic data to immunization registries/systems*

The EP must perform at least one test submission of electronic data to immunization registries and a follow up transmission if the initial one is successful. The EP can be excluded if they do not administer immunizations or if there is not an immunization registry available to the EP to transmit to.

10. Capability to provide electronic syndromic surveillance data to public health agencies*

The EP must perform one test submission of syndromic surveillance data to a public health agency. The EP can be excluded if they do not collect any syndromic reportable data or there is not a registry for the EP to transmit to.

At least 1 public health objective must be selected

Menu Objectives for Hospitals Stage 1

There are 10 menu objectives for hospitals to choose from and they need to complete 5 out of the 10 in the Menu Set. The Hospital Menu Objectives are as follows (CMS, 2013b, p. 15):

1. Drug-formulary checks

2. Record advanced directives for patients 65 years of age and older

3. Incorporate clinical lab test results as structured data

4. Generate lists of patients by specific conditions

5. Use certified EHR technology to identify patient-specific education resources and provide to patient, if appropriate

6. Medication reconciliation

7. Summary of care record for each transition of care/referrals

8. Capability to submit electronic data to immunization registries/systems*

9. Capability to provide electronic submission of reportable lab results to public health agencies*

10. Capability to provide electronic syndromic surveillance data to public health agencies*

*At least one public health objective must be selected

Core Set Clinical Quality Measure Stage 1

The EP Core Set of Clinical Quality Measures (CQMs) is as follows (CMS, 2013b, p. 23):

- NQF 0013 – Hypertension: Blood Pressure Measurement
- NQF 0028 – Preventive Care and Screening Measure (Pair: Tobacco Use Assessment and Tobacco Cessation Intervention)
- NQF 0421 and PQRI 128 – Adult Weight Screening and Follow-up

The Alternate Core Set CQMs for EPs are as follows (CMS, 2013b, p. 24):

- NQF 0024 – Weight Assessment and Counseling for Children and Adolescents
- NQF 0041 and PQRI 110 – Preventive Care Screening: Influenza Immunization for Patients 50 Years Old or Older
- NQF 0038 – Childhood Immunization Status

There is an additional set of CQMs that EPs must complete. The total amount of CQMs is 38 and the EP must complete 3 of them. Some of the CQMs are Diabetes, Heart Failure, Coronary Artery Disease (CAD), Breast Cancer Screening, Colorectal Cancer Screening, Asthma Assessment, Prostrate Cancer, and Smoking and Tobacco Use Cessation just to name a few. Eligible Hospitals and Critical Access Hospitals have 15 additional CQMs and all must be completed.

Some things to keep in mind as an EP is that the EHR will calculate the measures for the practice, only choose additional measures that are relevant to the practice, if your EHR reports no activity or a zero on a CQM the practice should select another one from the alternate core listing, and there are no minimum values that the practice must meet as there are no benchmarks with regards to the values, they only have to be reported.

CMS defines an *attestation* as "a legal statement that the EP has met the thresholds and all the requirements of the Medicare EHR Incentive Program" (CMS, 2013b, p. 74). The attestation will cover the EP's reporting of the 15 core objectives, 5 of the 10 menu objectives, 3 core CQMs or 3 alternate CQMs, and 3 out of the 38 additional CQMs. The attestation process is electronic and once the EP has completed this process they will be informed immediately if indicated. The payment will come to the practice about 4–8 weeks after successfully completing the attestation process.

Meaningful Use Stage 2

In meaningful use there are three stages and in Stage 1 it was focused on Data Capture and Sharing whereas Stage 2 the focus now shifts to the Advanced Clinical Processes and Procedures. This includes focusing on Health Information Exchanges (HIE), additional requirements for e-prescribing and integrating lab results, the electronic transmission across multiple settings of patient care summaries, and elevating the level of patient and family engagement (CMS, 2013d, p. 5).

What Stage 2 means to the EP is for those providers that have met meaningful use Stage 1 for the last 2 or 3 years they can now move on to Stage 2 in 2014. The goal of Stage 2 is to take this project and integrate new objectives that will improve patient care by better clinical decision support, improving care coordination, and enhancing patient engagement. In addition, Stage 2 will save money for the healthcare system, save the EPs and hospitals time, and look to save lives through these improvements.

The changes in Stage 2 versus Stage 1 are that the Core Objectives have increased from 13 to 17 in Stage 2, the Menu Objectives have decreased to 6 in Stage 2 and the EP only has to complete 3 of the 6 objectives, and the total objectives have increased from 18 in Stage 1 to 20 in Stage 2. In order to successfully capture all of these new changes CMS and the National Coordinator for Health Information Technology (ONC) have established new standards and criteria for structured data. This new structure requires the existing EHRs to adopt the upgrades and meet the new certification guidelines in order to continue to be in the EHR incentive program. Moreover, the new standards are needed to capture and calculate objectives in Stage 2 (CMS, 2013d, p. 9).

For the calendar year 2014 all providers, no matter what stage they are in, will need to demonstrate for only a 3-month reporting period during the year. This time frame must be fixed to a quarter of the calendar year for the EPs. For any new EP that is entering the meaningful use program in 2014, they can select any 90-day reporting period during the year, as it does not have to be fixed to a quarter of the calendar year. After successfully demonstrating meaningful use for a quarter of the year, the EP will have to report the data for the reporting period no later than February 28, 2015 at 12:00 a.m. ET (CMS, 2013d, p. 10).

EP Core Objectives Stage 2

There are 17 Core Objectives for Eligible Professionals (EPs) for Stage 2 and they are as follows (CMS, 2013d, p. 17–34):

1. Computerized provider order entry (CPOE)

    This measure increased from Stage 1 of only 30 percent of the medication orders to now requiring that the EP has more than 60 percent of all medication orders and in addition, 30 percent of radiology orders are processed through the CPOE by the physician or other licensed staff. If the EP writes less than 100 prescriptions, radiology orders, or lab orders during the reporting period, then they are excluded from this objective.

2. E-Prescribing (eRx)

    For this objective it went from Stage 1 where the EP had to only transmit 40 percent of all prescriptions to where the EP must transmit more than 50 percent of all prescriptions written and now these prescriptions must be compared to at least one formulary and are transmitted electronically using the EHR technology and not by phone or fax. An EP can be excluded from this objective if they write less than 100 prescriptions during the reporting period. In addition, new in Stage 2, if the EP or facility does not have a pharmacy in the organization, or a pharmacy within 10 miles of your location that accepts eRxs they can be excluded.

3. Provide patients with the ability to view online, download, and transmit their health information (New for Stage 2)

    This was moved from Menu Objectives in Stage 1 where it read at least 10 percent of the patients that the EP sees are provided timely access to their EHR. In Stage 2, the EP will have to provide online access to over 50 percent of the unique patients in the practice to access their medical information online within 4 business days. In addition, the EP must have more than 5 percent of their patient's access their medical information online. The EP can be excluded if they do not order any of the required except for Patient Name, Provider Name, and contact information for the office.

4. Use Clinical Decision Support

    In Stage 1 the EP was required to implement one clinical decision support tool that makes sense for the practice and that will trigger alerts or clinical information for the provider when they encounter patients with certain treatments or diagnoses. In Stage 2, the EP must implement 5 clinical support interventions and have them be related to 4 or more clinical quality measures. This must take place, if relevant, at the point in the patient care for the entire reporting period. All EPs must meet this objective as there is no exclusion for this objective.

5. Incorporate clinical lab test results into Certified EHR Technology (New for Stage 2)

This was moved from the Menu Objectives in Stage 1 where the EP was required to have more than 40 percent of all clinical lab results ordered during the reporting period incorporated in the EHR. In Stage 2, the EP must have more than 55 percent of all clinical lab results ordered during the reporting period incorporated in the Certified EHR technology as structured data. The EP can be excluded if they did not order any lab tests during the reporting period or if the results did not come back as a number or a positive or negative response.

6. Provide clinical summaries for patients for each office visit

In Stage 1, the EP was required to provide Clinical Summaries for more than half of the office visits to the patients within 3 days of the visit. In Stage 2 the EP is required to provide clinical summaries for patients for each visit for 50 percent of the visits and now within one day of the visit. If the EP does not provide office visits they will be excluded from this objective.

7. Generate lists of patients by specific conditions (New for Stage 2)

This was moved from the Menu Objectives in Stage 1 and there are no changes made. The EP will need to be able to create/develop a report for a condition that the EP feels is relevant to their practice. There are no exclusions for this objective.

8. Record demographics

More than 80 percent of the unique patients that the EP sees must have the patient's demographics recorded as structured data that includes preferred language, race, ethnicity, gender, and date of birth. There is no exclusion for this objective.

9. Identify patients who should receive reminders for preventive or follow-up care (New for Stage 2)

This was moved from the Menu Objectives in Stage 1 and edited. In Stage 1 the EP was to send to more than 20 percent of all their patients that are 65 years of age or older or 5 years old or younger a care reminder via mail, e-mail, or telephone. In Stage 2 the EP needs to send reminders to more than 10 percent of the unique patients that had 2 or more office visits with the EP over the prior 24 months before the beginning of the current reporting period and per patient preference when possible with no age requirements. The EP can be excluded if they did not have any office visits in the 24 months before the reporting period.

10. Identify patient-specific education resources and provide to the patient (New to Stage 2)

This was moved from the Menu Objectives in Stage 1 where more than 10 percent of the patients the EP sees are provided with patient-specific education on such things as chronic conditions. For Stage 2 this remains the same measure and requirement. There are no exclusions for this objective.

11. Perform medication reconciliation (New to Stage 2)

This was moved from the Menu Objectives in Stage 1, where the EP needed to perform medication reconciliations for more than 50 percent of patients that are transitioned into their practice. In Stage 2, the EP will need to compare more than 50 percent of the transferred in patients' medical record to an external list of medications from the patient, the transferring hospital, or transferring provider. The EP can be excluded from meeting this objective if they did not see or receive any patients after they received care from another provider.

12. Record and chart changes in vital signs

In Stage 1 the EP was required that for more than 50 percent of the patients that the EP sees that are 2 years of age and older have height, weight, and blood pressure recorded in the EHR and available as structured data. In Stage 2, it goes to 80 percent of the unique patients that are 3 years of age and older, and the EP only has to collect blood pressure. The EP can be excluded from this objective if they do not see any patients that are 3 years of age or older or if the EP does not believe that these vital signs are relevant to the scope of their practice.

13. Record smoking status for patients 13 years of age or older

In Stage 1, the EP was required to record smoking status for all unique patients that the EP sees that are 13 years of age or older. In Stage 2, the EP must record only 80 percent of the patients that are 13 years of age or older and have their smoking status recorded in the EHR. The EP can be excluded from meeting this objective if the EP does not see patients that are 13 years of age or older.

14. Provide summary of care record for each transition of care or referrals (New to Stage 2)

This was moved from the Menu Objectives in Stage 1 where if the EP transitions their patients to other care providers that for 50 percent or more of those transitions a summary of care record is provided. In Stage 2 the EP will still have to provide a summary of care for over 50 percent of the patients that were transferred out of their care and will now have to provide a summary of the care provided for over 10 percent of the patients transferred out by electronically transmitting using a Certified EHR Technology (CEHRT) to a recipient, or through an exchange that the transferring provider is a participant. Moreover, the EP must conduct more than one successful electronic exchange of the summary of care and conduct at least one or more test with the CMS designated test EHR during the reporting period. The EP can be excluded from this objective if they do not refer or transfer any patients to other facilities or if the provider transfers less than 100 times during a reporting period.

15. Protect electronic health information

In Stage 1 the EP was required to conduct security risk analysis and implement security updates and identify deficiencies through the Risk Management Process. Moreover, the EP needed to protect all information as set forth in the HIPAA requirements. In Stage 2 the EP is now required to not only do a security risk analysis, but they also need to address the encryption and security of data and implement security updates and correct any deficiencies identified through the risk assessment process. There are no exclusions for this objective.

16. Submit electronic data to immunization registries (New to Stage 2)

This was moved from the Menu Objectives in Stage 1 where the EP needed to perform at least one test submission of electronic data to immunization registries and perform a follow-up transmission if the initial one is successful. In Stage 2 the EP needs to transmit electronic immunization data from a CEHRT to an immunization registry on an ongoing basis during the reporting period. The EP can be excluded if they do not administer immunizations, or if there is no immunization registry available to the EP to transmit to, or if there is no immunization registry that provides timely information or can receive data from the EP, or if the EP operates in an area that there is no registry that is capable of accepting the standards required by the EP's EHR or can enroll additional EPs.

17. Use secure electronic messaging to communicate with patients (New to Stage 2)

For more than 5 percent of the unique patients of the EP must have a secure message sent using the electronic messaging function of the CEHRT to the patient or their authorized representative that were seen by the EP during the reporting period. An EP can be excluded if they had no office visits during the reporting period. In addition, the EP can be excluded if they practice in an area with low or no broadband availability to perform this function.

Menu Objectives Stage 2

There are six Menu Objectives for EPs for Stage 2 and they are as follows (CMS, 2013d, p. 35–41):

1. Submit electronic syndromic surveillance data to public health agencies

In Stage 1 the EP needed to perform at least one test submission of syndromic surveillance data to a public health agency. In Stage 2 the EP must perform ongoing submissions of electronic syndromic surveillance data from a CEHRT to the public health agency during the reporting period. The EP can be excluded if they do not collect ambulatory syndromic surveillance information, the EP operates in a jurisdiction where no public health agency is capable of receiving the data, or the EP operates in a jurisdiction where no public health agency provides information or is capable of receiving the data, or the EP operates in a jurisdiction where there is no public health agency that is capable of receiving data or can enroll additional EPs.

2. Record electronic notes in patient records (New for Stage 2)

   The EP is required to have over 30 percent of the patient base have progress notes entered into the EHR system and the notes must be able to be text searchable. There are no exclusions for this Menu Objective, as all EPs must meet this objective.

3. Imaging results need to be accessible through the CEHRT (New for Stage 2)

   The EP must have all tests that have an image available through the EHR. The images can be stored or have a live or direct link to the EHR that gives the viewer access to the image or test result. An EP can be excluded if they order less than 100 tests that produce an image during the reporting period. The EP can also be excluded if at the start of the reporting period they don't have access to electronic imaging results.

4. Record the patient family health history (New for Stage 2)

   For over 20 percent of the patient base for the EP there must be over 20 percent of the patients that have the family health history that includes one or more first-degree relatives. The EP can be excluded if there are no office visits during the reporting period.

5. Report cancer cases to a public health central cancer registry (New for Stage 2)

   The EP must have an EHR that is equipped with the ability to submit cancer case information electronically on a continual basis to a public health center cancer registry. An EP can be excluded if they don't directly treat or diagnose cancer, operate in a jurisdiction where there is not a public health agency capable of receiving electronic cancer case information or not having a public agency providing timely information, or the EP operates where there are no public health agencies that are capable of receiving electronic cancer case information or not able to enroll additional EPs.

6. Report specific cases to a specialized registry

   The EP must successfully submit specific case information to a specialized registry from the EP's EHR system. A specialized registry is, for the most part, associated with a specific disease, associated with a national society or associated with a public health agency. An EP can be excluded if they don't directly treat any disease associated with a specialty registry, operate in a jurisdiction where there is no public health agency capable of receiving electronic case information or no public agency that provides timely information, or the EP operates where there are no public health agencies that are capable of receiving electronic case information or not able to enroll additional EPs.

Clinical Quality Measures Stage 2

For an EP they must report on 9 CQMs out of a possible list of 64 approved CQMs for the EHR incentive program. In addition, the EP must report in 2014 on a minimum of 2 of the 6 available National Quality Strategy (NQS) domains. These represent the Department of Health and Human Services priorities for quality improvement in health care. The six domains are patient and family engagement, patient safety, care coordination, population and public health, efficient use of healthcare resources, and clinical processes and effectiveness (CMS, 2013d, p. 45).

There is also a recommended core set of CQMs for EPs that primarily focus on high-priority health conditions and best practices. There are nine CQMs for both the adult and the pediatric populations that meet all of the program requirements. These CQMs contribute to the morbidity and mortality of most Medicare and Medicaid beneficiaries and if one of these sets is applicable to the EP's patient population then CMS recommends choosing these nine CQMs (CMS, 2013d, p. 46).

Meaningful Use Stage 3

Since the start of the American Recovery and Reinvestment Act, there has been unprecedented growth in the implementation of EHRs in both physician offices and hospitals. The timeline for meaningful use has been revised, and Stage 2 will now go through 2016 and Stage 3 will begin in 2017. To be eligible for Stage 3, the EPs and hospitals need to have completed at least two years in Stage 2. This revision of the timeline will allow Stage 2 to experience the full implementation of this stage, which includes enhanced patient access and engagement and interoperability of information and exchange requirement that are part of Stage 2. Stage 3 is developing as a stage that is focused on healthcare delivery outcomes and other considerations that will develop in Stage 2 (CMS, 2013c).

■ Conclusion

Meaningful use has stimulated the growth of the electronic medical record throughout the U.S. healthcare system. The benefits include the impact of meaningful use on financial incentives but also the quality of patient care. Facilities and professionals are able to recoup financial investments in the meaningful use payments. To achieve this, the facility and/or provider must demonstrate that they have met all requirements of the stage in order to receive the associated incentive payment. The outcome, outside a financial one, is access to documented information has improved along with the ability of a healthcare facility or provider to actually report the quality data on the patients that they serve. The stages allow incremental changes to occur, keeping in mind that the evolution of the electronic record will play a big part on the overall impact of the delivery of quality care.

References

Amatayakul, M. K. (2013). *Electronic health records: A practical guide for professionals and organizations* (5th ed.). Chicago: American Health Information Management Association.

Centers for Medicare and Medicaid Services. (2010). Medicare & Medicaid EHR incentive program: Meaningful use stage 1 requirements overview. Retrieved from http://www.cms.gov/Regulations-and-Guidance/Legislation/EHRIncentivePrograms/Downloads/MU_Stage1_ReqOverview.pdf

Centers for Medicare and Medicaid Services. (2013a). Economic Recovery Act. Retrieved from http://www.cms.gov/Regulations-and-Guidance/Legislation/Recovery/index.html?redirect=/recovery/

Centers for Medicare and Medicaid Services. (2013b). Meaningful use. Retrieved from http://www.cms.gov/Regulations-and-Guidance/Legislation/EHRIncentivePrograms/Meaningful_Use.html

Centers for Medicare and Medicaid Services. (2013c). Medicare electronic health record incentive payments for eligible professionals. Retrieved from http://www.cms.gov/Regulations-and-Guidance/Legislation/EHRIncentivePrograms/Downloads/MLN_MedicareEHRProgram_TipSheet_EP.pdf

Centers for Medicare and Medicaid Services. (2013d). Eligible professional's guide to stage 2 for the EHR incentive programs. Retrieved from http://www.cms.gov/Regulations-and-Guidance/Legislation/EHRIncentivePrograms/Downloads/Stage2_Guide_EPs_9_23_13.pdf

Centers for Medicare and Medicaid Services. (2013e). Progress on adoption of electronic health records. Retrieved from http://www.cms.gov/eHealth/ListServ_Stage3Implementation.html

Learning Outcomes

After reading this chapter, the student will:

- Define Pay-for-Performance.
- Identify the impact of Pay-for-Performance on the healthcare organization.
- Define Value-Based Purchasing.
- Identify the impact of Value-Based Purchasing on the organization.
- Define Hospital Consumer Assessment of Healthcare Providers and Systems (HCAHPS).
- Identify the impact of Hospital Consumer Assessment of Healthcare Providers and Systems (HCAHPS).
- Understand Patient-Centered Medical Home (PCMH).
- Understand the Independence at Home project.

■ Introduction

In another chapter, Electronic Health Records and Meaningful Use were discussed and demonstrated the commitment to quality patient care and the incentive program associated with the program that would offer an incentive to healthcare professionals and hospitals alike. The interest in the program is validated by the commitment of 85 percent of eligible hospitals and over 50 percent of eligible professionals that had received an incentive payment from the Meaningful Use program (CMS, 2013). There are other programs offered by the government that look to incentivize healthcare providers through demonstrating the delivery of quality healthcare and a commitment to quality patient outcomes. There are several programs that provide incentives for healthcare providers for quality outcomes and the first one is Pay-for-Performance (P4P) for healthcare providers that can reward efficient providers and penalize inefficient providers; this program can potentially help save Medicare millions or billions of dollars yearly. Second, there is a program called Hospital Value-Based Purchasing (VBP) that is an incentive program that rewards acute care hospitals based on the quality that they provide to beneficiaries with Medicare. Third, there are Medical Homes, which are intended or designed to provide accessible, continuous, and coordinated family-centered care to certain high-need populations. Finally, there is a program called **Hospital Consumer Assessment of Healthcare Providers and Systems (HCAHPS)** that collects data from the patient's perspective that allows objective and meaningful comparisons between hospitals on areas that are important to consumers or patients. In addition, HCAHPS has a public reporting system of the results and levels of accountability that increases the transparency of care given by hospitals.

▪ Pay-for-Performance

Introduction

In the past, Medicare and other payers reimbursed healthcare providers on a fee-for-service basis. Through this system, these healthcare providers were reimbursed for all the services that they provided to the patient. The more services that were provided, the more money the healthcare provider was paid. This higher payment did not necessarily mean that the patient received better care with the increased costs. In the 1990s, the payer system went to a managed-care approach, where the payers used primary care physicians and case managers as gatekeepers to reduce costs by eliminating unnecessary tests and to find the lower-cost approach to care first, before the more expensive tests and/or procedures were used. Then by the 2000s, **pay-for-performance (P4P)** came into being as an option to fight the escalating costs of healthcare. Definitions of P4P can vary, but Leapfrog Group defines P4P as:

> Performance-based provider payment arrangements, including those that target performance on cost or efficiency measures. Typically, pay-for-performance programs offer financial incentives to physicians and other healthcare providers who meet defined performance targets which tend to focus on quality, efficiency, or related areas (Leapfrog, 2006).

Characteristics of Pay-for-Performance (P4P)

The typical pay-for-performance program will provide a bonus to healthcare providers for meeting or exceeding agreed-upon **quality measures** or performance goals. An example of a goal would be a reduction in hemoglobin A1c in a diabetic patient. The program could also reward a provider for improving performance such as year-over-year decreases in the rate of avoidable hospital readmissions (James, 2012).

In addition to incentives for good care or better performance year-over-year, P4P programs can penalize a provider for not providing quality care along with cost savings. In addition, they can penalize a provider for performance that is not improving, such as an increase in the amount of avoidable readmissions year-over-year. A penalty that Medicare has imposed on hospitals is when a patient acquires a pressure sore during the hospital admission, Medicare will no longer pay for the treatment of the pressure sore during the patient's hospital stay as they did in the past (James, 2012).

The purpose for P4P is to have quality incentives that will be where the payment reflects the process and has an impact on the outcome of care. P4P strives for "the right care for every patient every time" (CMS, 2005, p. 2). Basically, the care needs to be safe, effective, patient-centered, timely and efficient in its delivery, and equitable for the patient. This is a different approach to payment for healthcare services because in the past, payment was based on the process or provision of care and did not look at specific outcomes and tie those to the payment for services or procedures (CMS, 2005, p. 2).

Quality Measures

There are four **quality measures**, and they are **Process**, **Outcome**, **Patient Experience**, and **Structure**. Process is where the provider is measured on the activities that contribute to the positive quality outcomes of a patient stay. An example of this is if aspirin was given to heart attack patients or if the patient was educated on how to quit smoking. The second measure is the Outcome. This is where the healthcare provider is measured on the effectiveness of the care provided. For example, outcomes for a patient that has diabetes could be measured by looking at the lab results to see if the patient's diabetes is under control. This type of measurement can be inconsistent in that the patient has a role in the outcomes, as with the diabetic patient, and some factors are outside of the provider's control, such as the patient's eating and exercise habits. Third is Patient Experience, and this measures the patient's perception of care that they received during their stay in the hospital or the care given as an outpatient. This can range from how the patient viewed the communication from the hospital staff to how they liked the food provided. Finally, Structure measures how well the facilities, equipment, and personnel were used in the treatment of the patient (James, 2012).

P4P incentive programs will differentiate payment for services to providers based on services, quality, and efficiency measures so that the desired outcomes are achieved (Leapfrog, 2006). There are many payers that are utilizing evidence-based medicine as their benchmark or measurement tool. Evidence-based medicine is defined as "Healthcare services based on clinical methods that have been thoroughly tested through controlled, peer-reviewed biomedical studies." (LaTour & Eichenwald Maki, 2013, p. 914) There is also evidence-based management, which is a system where practices are based on research showing that the practices will be effective and will produce the outcomes that they are intended to produce.

Stakeholders Using P4P

There are Public Sector initiatives that include Medicare and Medicaid that have been the leaders in the P4P environment. In 2006, President Bush put into effect an executive order that stated healthcare programs that are sponsored by the federal government will promote quality and efficient health care. As a result of this, there has been a focus with the federal programs on the quality and efficiency of healthcare delivery, the use of health information technology, the transparency of healthcare quality and price, and better or more effective incentives for program beneficiaries including enrollees and providers (Leapfrog, 2006).

This type of activity has many public and private purchasers committing to and participating in value-driven health care through Value-Based Purchasing and P4P. CMS started a pilot project in 2003 that lasted 3 years and focused on providing incentives to hospitals that delivered the highest quality of care to the patients that they served. The project focused on hospital quality performance in areas such as pneumonia, heart bypass, heart attack, heart failure, and hip and knee replacement measures. The result of the project was that quality was raised by 11.8 percent in the first 2 years. CMS awarded incentive payments in year 2 of $8.7 million dollars to the top 115 performing hospitals. CMS decided in 2007 to extend the project another 3 years to allow time to develop more ways to measure quality and design and implement new incentive models (Leapfrog, 2006).

In addition to extending the project, CMS also created the Physician Quality Reporting Initiative (PQRI) that was established through the Tax Relief and Health Care Act of 2006. This is a voluntary program that allows physicians to earn incentive or bonus payments of 1.5 percent of the total allowed charges for covered services if the physician meets the standards. The quality measures for the program are diabetes, heart failure, coronary artery disease, depression, stroke, heart attack, and other various age-related conditions (Leapfrog, 2006).

In some of the Medicaid Managed Care Organizations (MCOs) there has been positive activity such as in California offering financial rewards based on quality of preventative services and in Rhode Island where they use a P4P plan to target asthma care. Unfortunately, Medicaid has historically had a lower reimbursement than other plans and this has driven away providers from the plans. With fewer providers, it is hard to get the results that other plans get with higher reimbursements as the providers tend to stay where the better reimbursement is and stay away from the lower reimbursement plans such as Medicaid.

Private Sector Initiatives

P4P initiatives are also sponsored by private employers, health plans, groups of employees, and Health Information Exchanges (HIEs). In order to take control of rising healthcare costs employer groups have aided in helping to organize and implement P4P programs. Coalitions, or employee groups such as unions, have brought stakeholders together to highlight the importance of safe and effective care for consumers in their groups. Health plans have also initiated P4P programs that financially reward physicians for quality care, appropriate care, accountability, and transparency through reporting publically their results. HIEs have also joined in and have become leaders in the transformation of healthcare. The HIEs help to facilitate the effective and safe transfer of information across organizations, systems, and regions. The sharing of information can help providers to be more effective in the delivery of care to the patient that ultimately can reduce costs and increase quality for the patient (Leapfrog, 2006).

Purchasers thinking of using or implementing P4P need to take into consideration the idea of payment incentives and make sure that they fit into current strategies that may be in place such as private and public report cards, disease management, and technical assistance to make sure that they align with all the physician and patient incentives already in place. Moreover, there may already be in place payment systems that may increase utilization such as fee-for-service or a capitation arrangement where utilization may be reduced to fit the payment model. The overall success of the P4P in any model is how does it fit into the current way of doing business and is it an incentive or a deterrent to the current payment system that the provider operates within.

Return on Investment Calculators

Return on Investment (ROI) calculators are used by P4P programs to identify the financial benefits realized, or dollars saved, by participating in these programs. These tools can also predict associated benefits by measuring lives saved or the outcomes of the program. Financial benefits are not the only measure of a successful plan. There are improved outcomes for consumers that can entail more efficient care and better productivity on the side of the provider that leads to overall improvement for the patient and the employee. The goal for the P4P program is to properly align the incentive program and payments to the providers' operations and goals to ultimately produce better quality outcomes for the patient that will ultimately result in lower costs for the payer, provider, and patient.

Quality Indicators

Quality indicators (QI) and process measures have been developed for the healthcare industry and are continually being refined. These measures, such as web-based portals, increase consumer awareness. There are web-based portals for many of the types of providers in our healthcare system and allow the patient to compare providers on different quality measures. Some of the different sites to compare providers are as follows (Thomas & Caldis, 2007, p. 1–2):

1. Dialysis Facility Compare: https://data.medicare.gov/data/dialysis-facility- compare

   This site allows the patient to compare dialysis centers on quality measures such as anemia, hemodialysis, and patient survival.

2. Medicare's Hospital Compare: http://www.medicare.gov/hospitalcompare/search. html

   This site gives the patient the opportunity to compare hospitals on the basis of heart attack, heart failure, pneumonia, or surgery.

3. Nursing Home Compare: http://www.medicare.gov/nursinghomecompare/?Aspx AutoDetectCookieSupport=1

   This site will allow the consumer to compare services available between nursing homes.

■ Hospital Value-Based Purchasing Program

Introduction

The **Hospital Value-Based Purchasing (VPB)** Program is a CMS initiative that rewards acute-care hospitals with incentive payments based on the quality of care that they provide to the beneficiary/patient that is on Medicare while they are in their care (MLN, 2013, p. 1). In order to achieve this goal, CMS is committed to provide care for the Medicare patient that is safe, effective, timely, patient-centered, efficient, and equitable. In a fee-for-service the payment rewards the healthcare provider for the quantity of care and not the quality of care. VBP links payment to the quality of care provided in order to convert the current payment system through rewarding the healthcare provider for delivering quality and efficient clinical care. VBP has been made available for hospitals, physician offices, nursing homes, home health services, and dialysis centers. (CMS, 2007, p. 3).

History

The Deficit Reduction Act specified that the Secretary of Health and Human Services shall develop a VBP program, similar to the P4P program, for hospitals beginning with the Fiscal Year 2009 and specified that the plan will be an on-going process for developing, selecting, and modifying measures of quality for acute-care (inpatient) settings, the reporting of quality data, the structure of payments, and the disclosure of information on hospital performance (CMS, 2007, p. 4).

Through this process, CMS created an internal group that was charged with developing the VBP plan that would be for Medicare hospital services. This group was divided into four subgroups in order to address the required planning items: measures, data infrastructure and validation, incentive structure, and public reporting (CMS, 2007, p. 5).

The development of the plan was to take place between September 2006 and June 2007. CMS initiated listening sessions to facilitate an ongoing consultative process to help with proposing changes and getting them posted in the *Federal Register*, which that will allow the public to comment on the proposed regulations.

Goals of the Program

Overall, with healthcare spending out of control and deficiencies in the quality of care delivered to the patients, along with safety of care in the U.S. healthcare system, a new system needed to be developed that would improve the care delivered to the patient that would in turn improve the value of care delivered to the beneficiary. The current payment structure did not adequately supply incentives for high quality and efficient care and CMS needed to better align the payment for care delivered with the overall quality of care delivered.

CMS has defined the following goals for the VBP program (CMS, 2007, p. 6):

- Improved clinical quality
- Reduction in adverse events and improve patient safety
- Encourage a more patient-centered care
- Avoid unnecessary costs incurred in the delivery of care
- Stimulate investments in structural components or systems such as IT and Care Management Tools
- Make performance results transparent and comprehensible so that consumers can be better equipped or empowered to make value-based decisions about their healthcare. In addition, to encourage hospitals and clinicians to improve the quality of care delivered to the patient.

In the design of the VBP program, CMS will adhere to various overarching principles such as making sure that the program is budget neutral. The program will build on existing Medicare performance measurement tools, expand to create a comprehensive performance measurement program, have VBP performance measures apply to a broad range of care delivered in the acute care setting all the while addressing the domains of clinical quality, patient centered care and efficiency. CMS will continue to work with agencies such as the National Quality Forum (NQF) and Joint Commission on Accreditation of Healthcare Organizations (JCAHO), the VBP will measure and reward performance in the outpatient setting, the design of the VBP will look to begin reducing existing disparities in the healthcare system and avoid creating any new disparities, and CMS will develop an ongoing evaluation process to assess the impact of the program and monitor for any unintended consequences arising as a result of the program (CMS, 2007, p. 7).

How Does VBP Work

The VBP Program was established by the Affordable Care Act of 2010 (ACA) and begins applying payments for the fiscal year 2013 and has an impact on payments for 2,985 hospitals across the country. Incentive payments are based on how well the hospital performs on each measure or how much they have improved in a measure that they were previously measured on in a previous period or baseline period (MLN, 2013, p. 1).

Quality Domains

Overall, there are four applicable domains for hospitals to be measured on: Clinical Process of Care, Patient Experience of Care, Outcome, and Efficiency. Hospitals are measured on applicable domains that are in place based on the fiscal year. For fiscal year 2013, the applicable domains were:

- Clinical Process of Care Domain
- Patient Experience of Care Domain

For fiscal year 2014 the applicable domains are:

- Outcome Domain
- Clinical Process of Care Domain
- Experience of Care Domain

For fiscal year 2015 the hospitals will be measured on all previous domains:

- Clinical Process of Care Domain
- Patient Experience of Care Domain
- Outcome Domain
- Efficiency Domain

The Clinical Process of Care Measures contains the following measures (MLN, 2013, p. 2–3):

- Fibrinolytic therapy received within 30 minutes of hospital arrival
- Primary PCI received within 90 minutes of hospital arrival
- Discharge instructions
- Blood cultures performed in the ED prior to initial antibiotic received in hospital
- Initial antibiotic selection for community-acquired pneumonia (CAP) in immunocompetent patients
- Prophylactic antibiotic received within 1 hour prior to surgical incision
- Prophylactic antibiotic selection for surgical patients
- Prophylactic antibiotics discontinued within 24 hours after surgery end time
- Cardiac surgery patients with controlled 6:00 a.m. postoperative serum glucose

- Urinary catheter removal on postoperative day 1 or postoperative day 2
- Surgery patients on a beta-blocker prior to arrival where the patient received a beta blocker during perioperative period
- Surgery patients with recommended venous thromboembolism prophylaxis ordered
- Surgery patients who received appropriate venous thromboembolism prophylaxis within 24 hours prior to surgery to 24 hours after surgery (MLN, 2013, p. 2–3)

The Patient Experience of Care Domain covers the following items that are "nurse communication, doctor communication, hospital staff responsiveness, pain management, medicine communication, hospital cleanliness and quietness, discharge information, and overall hospital rating" (MLN, 2013, p. 3).

Outcome Domain covers the following measures "acute myocardial infarction (AMI) 30-day mortality rate, heart failure (HF) 30-day mortality rate, pneumonia (PN) 30-day mortality rate, complication or patient safety for selected indicators (composite), central line-associated blood stream infection" (MLN, 2013, p. 4).

Efficiency Domain covers the measure of Medicare Spending per Beneficiary (MSPB). This assesses the Medicare Part A and Medicare Part B payments made for services provided to a Medicare beneficiary that takes place during a spending-per-beneficiary episode that takes place from a period of time from 3 days prior to an inpatient hospital admission through 30 days after the patient is discharged from the hospital. All of the payments included in the Efficiency Measure are price-standardized and risk-adjusted (MLN, 2013, p. 4).

Participating Hospitals

There are more than 3,000 hospitals that are eligible for VBP across the country. This program applies to the hospitals located in the 50 states and the District of Columbia along with acute care hospitals located in the state of Maryland. All of the data is collected through the Hospital Inpatient Quality Reporting (IQR) Program.

There are hospitals that are excluded from the VBP Program; and they are hospitals that are excluded from the Inpatient Prospective Payment System (IPPS), any hospitals that do not participate in the IQR Program during the performance period, any hospitals that are cited for posing an immediate threat to patient health or safety, and any hospital that does not meet the minimum standards (cases, measures, or surveys) required by the VBP Program (CMS, 2012, p. 9).

Scoring of Hospital Performance

Hospitals are assessed on their performance by their Achievement and Improvement for each measure in the VBP Program. The minimum number of cases that a hospital must have during a Performance Period is 10 cases per measure (CMS, 2012, p. 10).

The Achievement points are awarded during the performance period and then compared to the hospital's baseline period. Improvement points are awarded in the same way as the Achievement points. They are awarded during the performance period and then compared to the hospital's baseline period. In addition to the Achievement and Improvement points, there are Consistency points and they are awarded during the performance period and then compared with all hospitals' Patient Experience of Care rates from a baseline period. The Total Performance Score is calculated taking the greater of either the Achievement or Improvement points for each measure and then multiplying each of the greater scores for each domain by a specified weight, or percentage, and then adding all the weighted domain scores together (MLN, 2013, p. 5).

VBP Program Periods

There are two periods that are used in capturing data on how well a hospital is performing. This data that is collected is done in a Performance Period and a Baseline Period. The Performance Period is where the data is captured and is different for each year from Fiscal Year (FY) 2013 to FY 2015. For example, the Baseline Period in FY 2013 was July 1, 2009 to March 31, 2010; for FY 2014, the Baseline Period was April 1, 2010 to December 31; 2010; and for FY 2015, the Baseline Period was January 1, 2011 to December 31, 2011. The Performance Period for FY 2013 was July 1, 2011 to March 31, 2012; for FY 2014, the Performance Period was April 1, 2012 to December 31, 2012; and for FY 2015, the Performance Period was from January 1, 2013 to December 31, 2013 (MLN 2013, p. 7).

The Reward Process for Hospitals

The VBP Program is funded through a process that withholds a percentage of the Diagnosis-Related Group (DRG) payments from participating hospitals. The percentage range from 1 percent in 2013 to 2 percent in 2017 and thereafter. The funding specifics also include that the total amount of VBP incentive payments that are obtained from the percentage withheld be equal to the amount of funds available for the VBP payments. CMS also uses a linear exchange function to translate the Total Performance scores into a VBP incentive payment (MLN, 2013, p. 8).

Public Reporting

A hospital's performance in the VBP will be made available to the public and will include the hospital's performance on each measure that applies, the hospital's performance on each condition or procedure, and the hospital's total performance.

This information will be posted periodically on the Hospital Compare website and will include the number of hospitals receiving VBP incentive payments and the range and amount of the incentive payments, number of hospitals receiving less than the maximum payment available under the VBP for that FY, and the range and amount of all the payments (CMS, 2012, p. 28).

■ Hospital Consumer Assessment of Healthcare Providers and Systems (HCAHPS)

The Hospital Consumer Assessment of Healthcare Providers and Systems (HCAHPS) is a standardized survey and data collection tool that has been used since 2006. The goal of HCAHPS was to measure the patient's perspective of the hospital care that they received. HCAHPS created a national standard for collecting, and reporting to the public, information that produces valid comparison for patients to make a choice between hospitals to support their choice of hospitals (CMS, 2010, p. 1).

There are three goals that define or shape the HCAHPS Survey. First, the survey is designed to produce consistent data that can be compared by the patients to allow objective and meaningful comparisons between hospitals on topics that are important to the patient. Second, public reporting of the survey results are done so that the hospitals are incentivized, by public opinion, to improve the quality of care and therefore improve their results. And third, the idea of public reporting will enhance public accountability of the hospital as the healthcare delivery model is becoming more and more transparent (CMS, 2010, p. 1).

Survey Content

The HCAHPS Survey asks recently discharged patients about their experience while in the hospital. The questions contain 21 items that ask whether and how often the patient experienced a critical aspect of hospital care, as opposed to if they were "satisfied" with the care provided. There are also four items that will direct the patients to relevant questions in the survey and five items that will adjust for the patient mix across hospitals. And finally, there are two items that support reports that are mandated by Congress. If a hospital chooses, they may add questions after the core questions on the survey (HCAHPS, 2013, p. 2).

HCAHPS is a survey that is administered as a random sample that includes adult inpatients who were discharged from an inpatient hospital between 48 hours and 6 weeks and were admitted to a medical, surgical, or maternity floor or wing. This survey is not restricted to just Medicare patients as the hospital may send this survey to patients other than Medicare beneficiaries who were recently discharged. The hospital providing the survey may, at their own choice, collect the data on their own or contract with an approved CMS vendor to provide this part of the survey for them. The survey itself can be either by mail, telephone, mail with telephone follow-up, or active interactive voice recognition (IVR). All of these must be able to provide multiple attempts to reach the patient to complete the survey.

Hospitals are required to continually survey the recently discharged patients every month of the year and complete at least 300 surveys over the past 4 consecutive quarters. The survey is also required to be available in multiple languages, such as official English, Chinese, Spanish, Russian, and Vietnamese versions (HCAHPS, 2013, p. 2).

What HCAHPS Measures

Overall, the HCAHPS Survey measures eight areas/items. There are six summary measures, two individual and two global items that are reported on the website Hospital Compare, www.medicare.gov/hospitalcompare. The summary measures are also considered composites, or combinations, that are constructed from two or three survey questions. According to HCAHPS, "Combining related questions into composites allows consumers to quickly review patient experience data and increases the statistical reliability of these measures" (HCAHPS, 2013, p. 2).

Basically, the six composites will summarize how the nurses and doctors communicate with the patient, how responsive the staff at the hospital are to the patient's needs, how well the staff helps to manage the pain that the patient is experiencing, how well the staff communicates with the patient when a new medicine is being administered to the patient, and if the key information regarding the patient and their leaving the hospital is provided upon discharge. There are two individual items that will address the cleanliness and quietness of the patient's room while they were in the hospital and the two global items capture the two areas of their overall rating and would they recommend the hospital to family or friends (HCAHPS, 2013, p. 3).

There are adjustments made to the data that will make for fair and accurate comparisons from hospital to hospital. Factors that are not directly related to hospital performance are adjusted; the intent is to eliminate any advantage or disadvantage in the scoring process that may be a result of something in the survey that is totally out of the hospital's control. In addition, there are site visits of the survey vendors to make sure that the administration process, trace records, and analyses of submitted data are being done to ensure that the HCAHPS Survey is being administered consistently and in a proper fashion (HCAHPS, 2013, p. 3).

HCAHPS Public Reporting

As stated earlier, the HCAHPS scores are based on four consecutive quarters of patient surveys and are reported on the Hospital Compare website. Every time a new quarter of data is put on the website, the oldest quarter that was being reported is removed. Summaries and analyses of HCAHPS scores can be found on another website called HCAHPS On-line and the web address is www.hcahpsonline.org. This website will report current and historical results for the state and nationally, a "Top-Box" that will include the most positive survey responses and a "Bottom-Box" that will include the least positive responses for each measure, and comparisons of HCAHPS results by hospital characteristics. In addition to the reporting and tallying of data, HCAHPS is the basis for the VBP Patient Experience of Care Domain that represents 30 percent of the total score for a hospital (HCAHPS, 2013, p. 3).

■ Patient Centered Medical Homes

The **Patient Centered Medical Home (PCMH)** started as a Demonstration Project to help in the redesign of the healthcare delivery model. The goal was to "provide targeted, accessible, continuous and coordinated, family-centered care to high-need populations under which care management fees are paid to persons performing services as personal physicians and incentive payments are paid to physicians participating in practices that provide services as a medical home" (CMS, 2006, p. 1).

A high-need population is one where it consists of individuals with multiple chronic illnesses that require ongoing monitoring, advising, or treatment for their condition. The focus of the project is to engage small physician practices that have three or fewer full time equivalents (FTEs) or larger physician practices in rural settings.

Comprehensive Care

A PCMH is responsible for supplying a large portion of a patient's physical and mental healthcare needs. This includes prevention, wellness, acute care, and chronic care of a patient under their care. This will require a team of providers and can include physicians, advanced practice nurses, physician assistants, pharmacists, nutritionists, social workers, physical therapists, and the like. A smaller practice may not have the same size or composition of a clinical team, but will have the ability to bring in or work with the individuals necessary to provide the same type of care as that of a larger practice.

Patient Centered Care

The PCMH will provide primary care to their patients and this will be focused around the relationship with the patient and will treat the whole person. Each patient is unique in their needs and wants when it comes to their relationship with their primary care physician. In addition to the patient, the practitioner will need to manage the relationship with the patient with regards to their culture, values, and preferences along with allowing them the ability to organize and manage their own care as they choose. Moreover, the patient's family will also be a core member of the care team as much of a person's care can come from family members. The ability to make all parties involved fully informed will assist in establishing comprehensive care plans for the patient (PCMH, 2014).

Coordinated Care

Coordinated care is a major part of a PCMH as the practice will need to facilitate care across a larger portion of the patient's care plan. This will include coordinating specialty care, inpatient hospital care, home health care, and community care. In addition, the PCMH will need to make sure that the patient's care is coordinated when a patient is transitioning between different levels of care or different providers and this can be accomplished by keeping clear lines of communication between all providers, the PCMH, and the patient and their family.

Accessible Services

The PCMH is responsible for delivering accessible services to their patient base that come with shorter wait times for urgent needs, enhanced office hours where a patient can see a clinician or the physician, and 24-hour access through telephone or electronic communications such as e-mail or texting. The PCMH is responsible for being responsive to all the patient's needs and their preferences in how they wish to receive care and not limiting the patient's access to the practice based on those needs.

Quality and Safety

The PCMH needs to demonstrate a high level of commitment to quality care and to Continuous Quality Improvement. This ongoing commitment to quality will be in using evidence-based medicine and clinical decision-support tools through the use of tools such as the EHR. This shared decision process that includes multiple practitioners and the patient and family members will require measuring patient satisfaction and responding to patient experiences as they arise. In addition, the PCMH will need to adapt their care model to meet the population's needs that they practice in and serve. As stated in the VBP, the transparency of healthcare data and patient satisfaction will show the level of commitment that the PCMH has towards the community in which they operate and actively serve and look to make their health outcomes better on a consistent basis.

■ Independence at Home Demonstration Project

The **Independence at Home project** was created by the Affordable Care Act and is a delivery and payment incentive model that is using home-based primary care teams. These teams are focused on improving health outcomes and ultimately reduce healthcare costs for Medicare beneficiaries that have chronic conditions. The homecare team is managed, or directed, by primary care physicians and nurse practitioners. Incentive payments will be awarded to the providers that are successful in reducing costs and meeting the quality measures set for the program. The Independence at Home program allows for home-based primary care that gives the practitioner the ability to spend more time with their patients while in their home setting and to be better able to manage all aspects of the patient's care. This will be accomplished by making in-home visits tailored to the individual patient needs and preferences. Another outcome of this program will be the constant monitoring of quality care delivered to the patient and how this quality reduces costs for the Medicare program (CMS IHD, 2013, p. 1).

Requirements for Participation

To be part of the Independence at Home program the practice must demonstrate that they are familiar with and have adequate experience in delivering primary care in a patient home setting. The practice can be a primary care practice or a multidisciplinary practice that are led by a physician or nurse practitioner, the focus of care is on primary care or physician services, have experience in providing primary care in the home setting, and the practice must serve at least an average of 200 patients or eligible beneficiaries.

Due to this the size of the minimum savings requirement (MSR) is inversely related to the size of the IAH practice. With this challenge for small practices CMS provides three options for participation in the program. They are Option 1 where any practice that meets the eligibility criteria may apply as a sole legal entity. Second, Option 2 allows multiple primary care practices in a specific geographic area to join a consortium, or association, to enable them to participate. And Option 3 allows practices with a patient load of 200–500 eligible beneficiaries to select to be part of a national pool of providers. Practitioners that choose to be part of the national pool will have the savings realized calculated on a national pool level as opposed to a single practice level.

Eligible Beneficiaries for the Independence at Home Program

To be an eligible beneficiary to participate in the Independence at Home program the beneficiary must have two or more chronic conditions; have health coverage from Medicare fee-for-service (FFS); the patient needs help with at least two functional dependencies such as walking, bathing, or feeding; have had a "nonelective" inpatient hospital admission within the last 12 months; and have received acute or subacute rehabilitative services within the last 12 months (CMS IHD, 2013, p. 2).

Financial Incentives

To receive the financial incentives for the practice they must succeed in offering a high level of quality care to the patient that results in reducing the costs for the Medicare program. By demonstrating that the practice expenses are lower for the calculated target expenditure this would be present if the Independence at Home program was not in place. Moreover, the practices are required to meet the stringent quality standards that are established by the program.

■ Conclusion

The emphasis on quality of patient care is demonstrated with the introduction of P4P and Value-Based purchasing. Positive quality outcomes in both programs are rewarded. Negative outcomes will impact the financial health of the organization. In addition the HCAHPS program documents the patient perception of quality. Organizations must address the quality issues and manage the delivery of care in such a way that the perception of the patient is positive. Medical Homes and the Independence at Home project are entering the delivery system and impact access to quality care. The healthcare leader needs to provide a service that demonstrates quality outcomes and provides access to care.

References

Casto, A.B., & Forrestal, E. (2013). *Principles of healthcare reimbursement* (4th ed.). Chicago: AHIMA.

Centers for Medicare and Medicaid Services. (2005). Pay-for-performance/Quality incentives. Retrieved from https://www.cms.gov/Regulations-and-Guidance/Guidance/FACA/downloads/tab_H.pdf

Centers for Medicare and Medicaid Services. (2006). Tax Relief and Health Care Act of 2006: Medicare Medical Home Demonstration Project. Retrieved from http://www.cms.gov/Medicare/Demonstration-Projects/DemoProjectsEvalRpts/downloads/MedHome_TaxRelief_HealthCare.pdf

Centers for Medicare and Medicaid Services (CMS). (2007). Medicare hospital value-based purchasing plan development: Issues paper: 1st public listening session. https://www.cms.gov/Medicare/Medicare-Fee-for-Service-Payment/AcuteInpatientPPS/downloads/hospital_VBP_plan_issues_paper.pdf

Centers for Medicare and Medicaid Services (CMS). (2010). The HCAHPS survey: Frequently asked questions. http://www.cms.gov/Medicare/Quality-Initiatives-Patient-Assessment-Instruments/HospitalQualityInits/downloads/HospitalHCAHPSFactSheet201007.pdf

Centers for Medicare and Medicaid Services. (2012). Frequently asked questions: hospital value-based purchasing program. Retrieved from http://www.cms.gov/Medicare/Quality-Initiatives-Patient-Assessment-Instruments/hospital-value-based-purchasing/Downloads/FY-2013-Program-Frequently-Asked-Questions-about-Hospital-VBP-3-9-12.pdf

Centers for Medicare and Medicaid Services. (2013). Independence at home demonstration project. Retrieved from https://www.cms.gov/Medicare/Demonstration-Projects/Demo-ProjectsEvalRpts/downloads/IAH_FactSheet.pdf

Hospital Consumer Assessment of Healthcare Providers and Systems. (2013). HCAHPS fact sheet. Retrieved from http://www.hcahpsonline.org/files/August%202013%20HCAHPS%20Fact%20Sheet2.pdf

James, J. (2012). Health policy brief: Pay-for-performance. *Health Affairs*, October 11. Retrieved from http://www.healthaffairs.org/healthpolicybriefs/brief.php?brief_id=78

LaTour, K.M., & Eichenwald Maki, S. (2013). *Health information management: Concepts, principles, and practice* (4th ed.). Chicago: AHIMA.

Leapfrog Group. (2006). P4P background/summary. Retrieved from http://www.leapfroggroup.org/compendium_dt_home/4692933

Medicare Learning Network. (2013). Hospital value-based purchasing program. http://www.cms.gov/Outreach-and-Education/Medicare-Learning-Network-MLN/MLNProducts/downloads/Hospital_VBPurchasing_Fact_Sheet_ICN907664.pdf

Patient Centered Medical Home. (2014). Patient centered medical home resource center. Retrieved from http://pcmh.ahrq.gov/page/defining-pcmh

Thomas, F.G., & Caldis, T. (2007). Emerging issues of pay-for-performance in health care. *Health care financing review*, 1(29), 1–2.

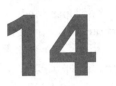

14 | Recovery Audit Contractors

Learning Outcomes

After reading this chapter, the student will be able to:
1. Explain the history and purpose of the Recovery Audit Contractor (RAC) demonstration project.
2. Define the process of the RAC and understand the impact on healthcare organizations.
3. Analyze work flow to identify areas of improvement in a healthcare organization Evaluate, track, respond, and appeal RAC requests for records are handled effectively from initial request to appeal.
4. Identify key members of a healthcare organization to be a part of the RAC focus team to investigate and respond to RAC requests.
5. Understand the five levels of appeals in the RAC process.

■ Introduction

Recovery Audit Contractors (RAC) is the term defined by Centers for Medicare and Medicaid Services (CMS) program that is responsible for detecting and correcting Medicare improper payments. This chapter covers the origins and history of the RAC. In this chapter, further information will be provided regarding the goals of the RAC and outlining the process as it can be very complicated. In addition, helping the healthcare administrator understand the processes involved and implement effective tools for the organization will assist in the appeals process with the RACs and help to avoid a negative impact to the financial health of the organization.

■ Origin and History

Many times a month, or at least on a regular basis in a healthcare facility in the Finance Department and Health Information Management Department, is mention of the "RAC" requesting charts for an audit. The term RAC is short for the Centers for Medicare and Medicaid Services (CMS) program called the Recovery Audit Contractor. This program is responsible for detecting and correcting improper Medicare payments. This is a program that came out of a successful demonstration program that used auditors, or Recovery Auditors, to go into healthcare settings and look for overpayments and underpayments and help with identifying future improper payments and lowering the overall error rate for processing a Medicare claim. CMS conducts a number of demonstration projects to evaluate the program and any changes needed. A demonstration project is one that assesses the effectiveness of a service offered by CMS and is defined by the "methods of service delivery, coverage of new types of service, and new payment approaches on beneficiaries, providers, health plans, states, and the Medicare Trust Funds" (CMS, 2012a).

These evaluation projects confirm the findings of the demonstration project and allows CMS to effectively monitor the efficacy of the program. Currently, there are many types of demonstration projects that are being run by CMS such as Alternative Approaches to Measuring Physician Resource Use, Assessing the Impact of Licensed Clinical Pharmacists to improve quality of care for Medicare beneficiaries, Designing a System to Monitor Medicare Beneficiaries' Access to Care, and one from a few years ago starting in 2005 and running to 2008, the Recovery Audit Demonstration (CMS, 2012b).

The background on the Recovery Audit Demonstration is that it was a part of Section 306 of the Medicare Prescription Drug, Improvement, and Modernization Act of 2003 or otherwise known as the Medicare Modernization Act (MMA). Congress directed the Department of Health and Human Services (DHHS) to conduct a demonstration project that would run for 3 years and they were to use Recovery Audit Contractors or as they are called, RACs. They were empowered to go in the field and detect and correct improper payments in the Medicare Fee-for-Service (FFS) program.

According to the RAC Status Document for FY 2006, the CMS has been calculating improper payment estimates and coming up with strategies to protect the Medicare program from these types of issues. In 2003, the CMS program called the Comprehensive Error Rate Testing Program (CERT) began to produce error reports that were designed to evaluate individual contractor and program performance. Since the inception of this program CMS has reduced improper payments from 9.8 percent in 2003 to 3.9 percent in 2007. According to the Improper Medicare Fee-for-Service (FFS) Payments Report for November 2007, approximately 3.9 percent of the Medicare dollars paid out to providers did not comply with one or more of the Medicare payment rules. This equates to an amount of $10.8 billion that the Medicare Fee-for-Service programs made in overpayments and underpayments (CMS, 2013a).

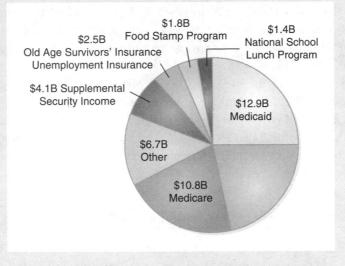

$1.8B Food Stamp Program

$1.4B National School Lunch Program

$2.5B Old Age Survivors' Insurance Unemployment Insurance

$4.1B Supplemental Security Income

$12.9B Medicaid

$6.7B Other

$10.8B Medicare

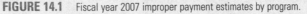

FIGURE 14.1   Fiscal year 2007 improper payment estimates by program.

Reproduced from Office of Management and Budget, Improving the Accuracy and Integrity of Federal Payments (January 31, 2008), Available at: http://www.whitehouse.gov/omb/financial/fia/2007_ipia_final.pdf. Accessed April 4, 2014.

Figure 14.1 (CMS, 2013b) displays the top federal programs with improper payments in fiscal year 2007. Medicare and Medicaid combined topped out the list of federal programs that experienced improper payments.

This RAC program was designed to establish whether or not this type of program would be a cost-effective means of adding resources to determine if correct payments were being made from Medicare to various providers and suppliers. The overall goal was to protect the Medicare Trust Fund as there were many that felt if CMS did not do anything to slow spending in the FFS program the availability of funding in the future could be compromised. The demonstration project was held in five states and they were New York, Massachusetts, Florida, South Carolina and California. The demonstration project lasted for 3 years and ended on March 27, 2008.

The identification of incorrect payments is the first step in the process of reducing unwarranted payments from CMS. The next step is to develop a way to identify where the problems are and to get improvement. According to CMS RAC Status Document in 2007, the cornerstone of these efforts is CMS' Error Rate Reduction Plan (ERRP), which includes agency level strategies to clarify CMS policies and implement new initiatives to reduce improper payments. In addition to these strategies, CMS also directs the claims processing contractors to provide education to local providers to reduce improper payments, request and review the medical record that is associated with the claim for services to determine proper reimbursement, develop medical necessity criteria, or billing instructions to assist providers in what is a clean claim for submission and remind them of the billing errors that have been identified in the past (CMS, 2013a).

According to the Medicare Prescription Drug, Improvement, and Modernization Act of 2003, Congress gave directions to the Department of Health and Human Services (DHHS) to start the demonstration program. Then in the Tax Relief and Healthcare Act of 2006 (TRHCA), Congress required that the RAC program become permanent by no later than January 1, 2010.

■ Goals of the Recovery Audit Contractor

The RAC Status Document for FY 2007 states that the RACs were established to detect and correct improper Medicare payments. They follow the same guidelines and policies that are followed by the Medicare claims processing contractors. Most importantly, RAC contractors are paid via a contingency fee paid, based on the amount of improper payments that they correct both overpayments and underpayments. There is not a consistent fee that the Centers for Medicare and Medicaid Services (CMS) pays each contractor as this is determined by the negotiation process for each vendor. CMS was given the authority to pay the RACs, using a different method than in the past, through a contingency fee (CMS, 2013a).

The goal of the program is that, even with paying a contingency fee to the RAC auditors, that the integrity of the Medicare Trust Funds would be maintained. CMS, during the demonstration phase of this project, committed to address all concerns raised along with identifying successes and opportunities for improvement to the program before expanding to any further states.

According to the RAC Status Document for FY 2007, improvements to the RAC program were identified such as changing the look-back period from 4 years down to 3 years, making a maximum look-back date of October 1, 2007; making it possible for the RAC to review claims in the current fiscal year, making it mandatory that the RACs have Certified Coding Specialists (CCS), setting mandatory limits on the number of medical records requested, making it mandatory to discuss with the Medical Director regarding claim denials, making it mandatory to report problem areas that are identified more frequently, holding the RAC accountable to pay back contingency fees from all level of appeals and not just the Level 1 appeals, utilizing a web-based portal to view the status of the appeals, and making it mandatory to have a validation process to keep everything standardized and uniform (CMS, 2013b).

The RAC Status Document of 2007 states that improper payments from the Medicare Fee-for-Service (FFS) are a result of services that were not medically necessary based on the criteria of medical necessity and the setting in which the service took place, incorrectly coded services, claims that have improper or insufficient documentation, providers using the improper fee schedule, and providers being paid twice for the same service (CMS, 2013a).

The RACs were given a total dollar value to review at the end of the FY 2007 totaling $239.6 billion including Physician Evaluation and Management Coding, Hospice and Home Health Services, claims reviewed by another Medicare Contractor, claims involved in a potential fraud investigation, and payments that were made during a CMS conducted demonstration (CMS, 2013c).

The RAC Process from Review to Response

The RACs were not told which claims they had to review, or even how they went about identifying claims to review. The RACs would often use their knowledge that they have gained through the auditing process to identify claims to review. The RACs would often look at services that were identified by the Office of the Inspector General (OIG) or the General Accounting Office (GAO). There is a good deal of reporting coming from the OIG and the GAO that highlight Medicare payments that are suspect or services that are traditionally associated with improper payments. The goal of the RAC was to identify claims that would most likely contain improper payments. This would be accomplished by using their proprietary techniques to identify improper payments and errors in claims.

Once an improper payment is identified, the RAC would contact the provider and notify them of an overpayment that they received and look to collect that amount from the provider or an underpayment that the provider received from CMS and pay that amount to the provider. This process is called an Automated Review. According to Schramm (2012), "one of the most notable changes was the requirement that RACs use web-based systems that enable providers to send medical documentation to support audited claims electronically and view the status of a claim at any stage of the audit process online."

The next type of review is the Complex Review. The main part of this process, after identifying an improper payment, is to request the medical records for the patient's stay that is in question. The medical record will assist the RAC in determining if there was an overpayment or underpayment. This process is not uncommon in the Medicare environment as the claims processing contractors follow the same steps to identify improper overpayments and underpayments.

RACs are guided by Medicare guidelines and they review claims based on accepted clinical standards, follow Medicare coding and billing processes, can't develop their own coverage guidelines for coding and billing processes. They employ nurses, therapists, and certified coders to review medical claims and have a physician acting as medical director to oversee the review process with the medical records. Moreover, the physician will assist nurses and coders during a complex review, manage the quality assurance procedures, and inform provider associations about the RAC Program. Another area that the RACs work on is education. They will educate the providers and provider community so that they can look at improving their own processes. There are a few items that are required of a RAC such as having a toll-free number for provider inquiries and holding monthly conference calls, which helped the providers to identify area of improvement on behalf of the RACs (CMS, 2013c).

Long-Term Care Facilities

Mary Ann Leonard states that there are some different focuses on Long-Term Care Facilities. The issues that are specific to skilled nursing facilities that have been identified are as follows (Leonard, 2010):

- The use of acute care diagnoses without services provides that are in relationship to the type of care and services the diagnosis may warrant
- A higher resource utilization group score
- The acceptance of the procedural codes from the hospital record
- Therapies not medically supported by the diagnosis

Overpayments

According to the RAC Status Document of 2007 the RACs identified and corrected $371 million dollars of improper payments during the fiscal year 2007 (CMS, 2013c). Over 96 percent of the claims found were overpayments. The other 4 percent were underpayments that were repaid to the provider. The reason for such a low percentage of underpayments was that the RACs did not have experience in working the private industry and CMS only had 9 percent estimated as underpayments based on the Improper Medicare FFS Payments Report.

Underpayments

In fiscal year 2007 the RAC succeeded in correcting over $1.03 billion of Medicare improper payments. Over 96 percent of these claims were overpayments, and the remaining 4 percent were underpayments that were repaid to providers.

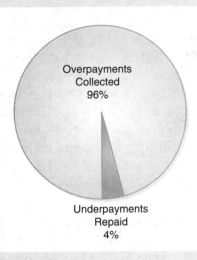

FIGURE 14.2   Overpayments vs. underpayments.
Reproduced from The Medicare Recovery Audit Contractor Program: An Evaluation of the 3-Year Demonstration, June 2008. Source: For
Claim RACs, RAC invoice files and RAC Data Warehouse. For MSP RACs, Treasury deposit slips.

TABLE 14.1   Improper payments corrected by the RAC demonstration: cumulative through 3/27/08, both claim RACs and MSP RACs.

RAC	Overpayments Collected[a]	Underpayments Repaid[b]	Total Improper Payments Corrected
Connolly	$266.1	$4.3	$270.4
HDI	$396.1	$20.8	$416.9
PRG	$317.8	$12.7	$330.5
Claim RAC Subtotal	$980.0	$37.8	$1,017.8
HMS	$1.3	$0.0	$1.3
DCS	$11.4	$0.0	$11.4
MSP RAC Subtotal	$12.7	$0.0	$12.7
Grand Total	$992.7	$37.8	$ 1,030.5

[a] Collected is defined as overpayments that have been recovered from providers and deposited.

[b] Repaid is defined as underpayments that have been paid back to the provider. MSP RACs were not tasked with identifying under-payments.

Note: For this Evaluation Report, CMS lists all dollars actually collected and repaid between March 2005 and March 2008. In contrast, reporting for the FY 2006 RAC Status Document was based on overpayment and underpayment notification letters that were sent to providers and to the Medicare claims processing contractor during the fiscal year.

Appeals of RAC Determinations

The Medicare appeals process consists of five levels of appeal. Once an initial claim determination is made the right to appeal is initiated. The First Level of Appeal is the Redetermination and this can be requested by physicians, suppliers, and beneficiaries. This appeal must be requested within 120 days and submitted to the contractor. The Second Level of Appeal is where a party to the redetermination may request another review if they are dissatisfied with the original ruling. The Third Level of Appeal is established when at least $140 remains in controversy following a Qualified Independent Contractor (QIC) decision. A request for reconsideration through an Administrative Law Judge (ALJ) hearing must be filed within 60 days of receipt of the reconsideration decision. The ALJ will generally issue a decision within 90 days of receipt of the hearing request. The Fourth Level of Appeal is when an organization or party is unhappy with the ALJ decision, the party may request a review by the Appeals Council. This request must be submitted within 60 days of receipt of the ALJ's decision and must specify the issues and findings that are being contested. In general, the Appeals Council will issue a decision within 90 days of receipt of a request for review. The Fifth Level of Appeal is a Judicial Review in the U.S. District Court. If at least $1,400 or more is still in controversy following the Appeals Council, a party involved may request a review in a federal district court. The request must be filed within 60 days of receipt of the ALJ's decision (CMS, 2013b).

Lessons Learned

According to *The Medicare Recovery Audit Contractor (RAC) Program: An Evaluation of the 3-Year Demonstration,* the results were that many of the key questions regarding the feasibility and merits of applying recovery audit principles has shown the following Lessons Learned (CMS, 2013c):

- Claim RACs are able to find a large volume of improper payments.
- Providers do not appeal every overpayment determination.
- Overpayments collected were significantly greater than program costs.
- Claim RACs are willing to spend time on provider outreach activities, developing strong relationships with provider organizations.
- It is administratively possible to have a RAC work closely with a Medicare claims processing contractor.
- RAC efforts did not disrupt Medicare or law enforcement antifraud activities.
- It is possible to find companies willing to work on a contingency fee basis.

Cost of Operating the RAC

The amount to run the RAC program was much less than the amount that it returned to the Medicare Trust Funds through the audit process (CMS, 2013c). The costs fall into three categories:

- RAC contingency fees that include the fees paid to the RACs for detecting and collecting overpayments plus the fees paid for detecting and refunding underpayments.

- Medicare claims processing contractor costs are the funds paid to the carriers, fiscal intermediaries, and Medicare Administrative Contractor (MAC) for processing the overpayment/underpayment adjustments, handling appeals of RAC initiated denials and other costs incurred.

- RAC evaluation, validation, and oversight fees are funds paid to the RAC Evaluation Contactor, the RAC Data Warehouse Contractor, the RAC Validation Contractor, and the federal employees who oversee the RAC demonstration (CMS, 2013c).

The report goes on to say that the RAC project only spent 20 cents for each dollar collected and this total for all the RACs was $201.3 million (CMS, 2013c). See Figure 14.3 below.

Impact on Providers

According to Leonard (2010), inpatient hospitals, inpatient rehabilitation facilities, skilled nursing facilities, and hospices, RACs can request records for 10 percent of the average monthly Medicare claims per 45 days. The maximum amount of records that the RAC can request is a maximum of 200 records. Leonard goes on to show an example of a local community hospital that had 1,200 Medicare Claims in 2007. The average number of claims per month is 100. This is calculated by taking the 1,200 claims per year and dividing by 12 months. Ten percent of that monthly average amount would be 10. Therefore the RAC medical requests would be limited to 10 medical records per 45 days (Leonard, 2010).

According to the American Health Information Management Association (AHIMA, 2009), it is important for every facility to have policies and procedures that will ensure corporate support, clear communication, and systematic procedures based on the hierarchy of authority (AHIMA, 2009). Figure 14.3 shows the Recovery Audit Contractor (RAC) Timelines starting with the initial request to the Fifth Level Appeal in the U.S. District Court.

Along with policy and procedures healthcare organizations need to have adequate tracking systems so as to make sure that all requests are identified, responded to, and, when appropriate, the appeal is filed. AHIMA lists the considerations for a tracking system in their Recovery Audit Contractor Toolkit to include the following (AHIMA, 2009):

- The volume of requests the healthcare entity will likely be handling for each batch of requests. Will there be a way to enter requests into the system automatically or in a very efficient manner?

- Types of data needed to track requests, including items like dates (request, delivery, determination, appeals, final disposition); location of records (especially if records need to be obtained from off-site and stored locally until review is complete); and individuals responsible for retrieving, reviewing, copying, and sending records.

- Who will be responsible for entering or updating and reviewing information into the tracking system? Will it be multiple individuals requiring a system that can be shared or accessed via a network?

- Types of reports needed to monitor the status of each batch of requests, notify the user of pending due dates, and provide trending data for productivity, turnaround times, and disposition of cases. Can the system create custom reports and send e-mails for follow-up to individuals in the healthcare entity?

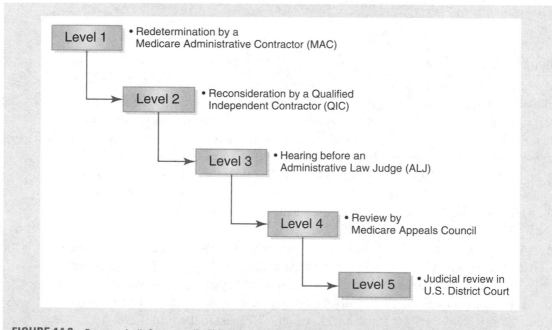

FIGURE 14.3   Recovery Audit Contractor (RAC) Timelines starting with the initial request to the 5th level appeal in the US District Court. (*continued*)

Modified from Center for Medicaid Services, Medicare Learning Network, Medicare Appeals Process. http://www.cms.gov/Outreach-and-Education/Medicare-Learning-Network-MLN/MLNProducts/downloads/MedicareAppealsprocess.pdf

Level of Appeal	What takes place	Review performed by	Time frame to request appeal	Time frame for decision	Amount in Controversy
Level 1 Redetermination	Review of documents from initial claim determination	MAC	Up to 120 days after receipt of initial determination	60 Days	No
Level 2 Reconsideration	Review of documents for redetermination. Submit any documentation that was not sent in previously	QIC	Up to 180 days after receipt of MRN	90 days	No
Level 3 ALJ Hearing	May be a situation where the review is "on-the-record" or an interactive hearing between both parties	ALJ	Up to 60 days after notice received from QIC of their decision. Or after time has expired for QIC to make their decision and notify provider	Time frame may be delayed due to volume of requests in processing at this level.	Yes. (this threshold is updated annually and should be checked on the CMS website)
Level 4 Medicare Appeals Council Review	Document review of ALJ's decision. At this time oral arguments may be requested	Appeals Council	Up to 60 days after receipt of the ALJ's decision or after time has expired for ALJ to make their decision and notify provider of a decision	90 days if appealing the ALJ's decision

Or

180 days if ALJ review time has expired without notifying provider | No |
| Level 5 Judicial Review | Judicial Review | U.S. District Court | Up to 60 days after receipt of the Appeals Council decision or after time has expired for the Appeals Council to notify the provider of a decision | No statutory time frame is established for a decision | Yes. (this threshold is updated annually and should be checked on the CMS website) |

FIGURE 14.3 Recovery Audit Contractor (RAC) Timelines starting with the initial request to the 5th level appeal in the US District Court. Modified from Center for Medicaid Services, Medicare Learning Network, Medicare Appeals Process. http://www.cms.gov/Outreach-and-Education/Medicare-Learning-Network-MLN/MLNProducts/downloads/MedicareAppealsprocess.pdf

- The type of system required to support this type of data tracking and reporting. Simple spreadsheet applications are not enough.

- Additional software purchases for the system. Can it easily be updated to add or modify data elements based on changes in the RAC requirements?

- Be sure the tracking system is capable of handling multiple audit requests as CERT, PERM, etc. Note: The RAC Scope of Work prevents repeat audits.

Overall, the goal of a healthcare organization is to develop a tracking system that is easy to implement, provides access to all the required data, helps to ensuring that the healthcare entity can meet deadlines for the audit, and will help to identify opportunities for improvement in the RAC process at the healthcare facility.

According to Schramm, other impacts on healthcare providers is that it is taking extra time and money to substantiate a RAC claim, and this is having a significant impact on budgets that are already stretched thin. On the flip side, in a recent hospital survey of more than 125 hospitals regarding their perceptions of the RAC program, 60 percent feel the audit process is not fair. But most of those hospitals that have actually been through a RAC audit, 64 percent felt that the appeals process was fair (Schramm, 2012).

■ Review of the RAC

In the past there have been complaints on the RAC. In 2009, Lester J. Perling, Esq., identified characteristics and issues surrounding the RAC in his article, *Recovery Audit Contractors: They're Back!* Perling addressed current issues providers were experiencing in 2009 such as how RACs were paid on a contingent-fee basis and they received a portion of the overpayment that they discovered even if their determination was ultimately overruled. In addition, the RACs were not required to engage the services of a medical director when assessing the medical necessity of claims, they could request an unlimited amount of records from a particular provider, and were only required to do limited reporting on the problem areas they identified. As a result, CMS has attempted to address many of the perceived flaws in the RAC demonstration program by amending the statement of work for the program. Ultimately, they made the changes to the number of medical records requested by the RAC based on the type and size of the provider, required documentation of the credentials of individuals making medical review determinations, specifying the limits of the RAC reviews to a look back period of a maximum of three years, required each RAC to hire a physician medical director that must be available to discuss claims with providers, all claim denials need to be independently audited for accuracy, and finally that the RACs pay back the contingency fee if they lose at any level of appeal (Perling, 2009).

The Centers for Medicare and Medicaid Services are being asked to improve the performance of the RACs going forward. The Department of Health and Human Services Office of the Inspector General (OIG) did a study on the RAC and published *Medicare Recovery Audit Contractors and CMS's Actions to Address Improper Payments, Referrals of Potential Fraud, and Performance.* The reason for the study is that there have been inconsistencies found with CMS's actions to address payment vulnerabilities and prior to this report CMS's actions to address referrals of potential fraud were flawed. In addition, the OIG found issues with CMS's oversight of its contractors. The OIG felt that identifying improper payments and effective oversight of the RAC is very important. The OIG collected data from the RACs to review the activities of the RACS to identify improper payments. The OIG also collected data from CMS regarding activities to address vulnerabilities such as improper payments exceeding $500,000 and any referrals of potential fraud. Finally, they collected RAC performance evaluations and then collected metrics from CMS and determined the extent that RAC performance evaluations addressed these metrics (Levinson, 2013).

What they found was that in fiscal years 2010 and 2011, RACs identified half of all the claims that they reviewed resulted in improper payments to providers totaling $1.3 billion dollars. Although CMS took corrective actions to address the reasons for the improper payments, they did not evaluate the effectiveness of these actions. In addition, there were six referrals of potential fraud that CMS received from the RACs for which there was no action taken. Finally, CMS's performance evaluations did not include metrics to evaluate the performance of the RACs (Levinson, 2013).

What was recommended from the OIG was to take action as appropriate, assess vulnerabilities that are pending corrective action, ensure refer all cases that represent potential fraud, review and ensure timely action on RAC referrals or potential fraud, and develop additional evaluation and management matrix. CMS stated that they agreed with the majority of the recommendation, but they did not render a decision on the third option (Levinson, 2013).

■ Tools for the Healthcare Administrator

One of the first tools to have in the RAC audit process, outside of solid policy and procedures, is the identification of a RAC Coordinator for your facility. The next step is to identify a team of key players to be part of a RAC Team. This person will be the lead person on all RAC audits. In addition, the RAC Coordinator will be in charge of education for each member of the RAC Team. This team will consist of a member of Administration; a Health Information Management professional from Operations,

Coding, and Release of Information; the Business Office; Information Technology (IT); Clinical Department Managers; Quality Management and Performance Improvement; Utilization Review; Research; Compliance; Finance; Contract Management; General Council; and Registration will finish out the team (AHIMA, 2009).

■ Conclusion

The healthcare administrator has a variety of responsibilities related to the financial health of the organization. An important program that the healthcare administrator will be dealing with is the RAC program. This chapter has outlined the goals of the RAC and the process in which they operate. It is the facility's responsibility, ultimately the Health Information Management and healthcare administrator, to ensure accurate documentation and coding of the health record and to respond promptly after the necessary research is complete on each request for refund by the Recovery Audit Contractor.

There have been many changes since the inception of the program, and the healthcare administrator must understand the changes and share these changes with the appropriate staff. Moreover, if the healthcare administrator is not aware of the changes, they need to get to the appropriate staff to make sure that everyone is working off of the most current program guidelines.

Understanding of this process will lead to implementation of effective tools to manage the Recovery Audit Contractor process and minimize the risk through managing this process effectively and timely. The final outcome will be that the healthcare administrators will have a financially healthy organization.

References

American Health Information Management Association. (2009). Recovery Audit Contractor (RAC) toolkit. Retrieved from http://library.ahima.org/xpedio/groups/public/documents/ahima/bok1_044065.pdf

Centers for Medicare and Medicaid Services. (2012a). Medicare demonstration projects & evaluation reports. Retrieved from http://www.cms.gov/Medicare/Demonstration-Projects/DemoProjectsEvalRpts/index.html

Centers for Medicare and Medicaid Services. (2012b). Master Demonstration, Evaluation, and Research Studies for ORDI System of Record 09-70-0591: List of Reports. Retrieved from http://www.cms.gov/Medicare/Demonstration-Projects/DemoProjectsEvalRpts/Downloads/MasterSORList.pdf

Centers for Medicare and Medicaid Services. (2013a). Historical programs. CMS RAC status document FY 2007 (p. 3). Retrieved from http://www.cms.gov/Research-Statistics-Data-and-Systems/Monitoring-Programs/recovery-audit-program/downloads/2007RACStatusDocument.pdf

Centers for Medicare and Medicaid Services. (2013b). Original Medicare fee-for-service appeals. The Medicare appeals process fact sheet. Retrieved from http://www.cms.gov/Outreach-and-Education/Medicare-Learning-Network-MLN/MLNProducts/downloads/MedicareAppealsProcess.pdf

Centers for Medicare and Medicaid Services. (2013c). Historical programs. Recovery audit demonstration: An evaluation of the 3-year demonstration (p. 23). Retrieved from http://www.cms.gov/Research-Statistics-Data-and-Systems/Monitoring-Programs/recovery-audit-program/downloads/RACEvaluationReport.pdf

Levinson, D. R. (2013). Medicare recovery audit contractors and CMS's actions to address improper payments, referrals of potential fraud, and performance. *Department of Health and Human Services Office of the Inspector General*, 2–17. OEI-04-11-00680. Retrieved from http://oig.hhs.gov/oei/reports/oei-04-11-00680.pdf

Leonard, M. (2010). A RAC primer for LTC facilities. *Journal of AHIMA*, *81*(1), 56–68. Retrieved from http://search.ebscohost.com/login.aspx?direct=true&db=ccm&AN=2010520205&site=ehost-live

Perling, L. J. (2009). Recovery audit contractors: They're back!. *South Florida Hospital News and Healthcare Report*, *5*(11). Retrieved from http://southfloridahospitalnews.com/page/Recovery_Audit_Contractors_Theyre_Back/3993/1/

Schramm, M. (2012). Strategies for responding to RAC requests electronically. *Healthcare financial management*. Retrieved from http://search.ebscohost.com/login.aspx?direct=true&db=ccm&AN=2011534229&site=ehost-live

List of Acronyms

ABN: Advance Beneficiary Notice

ACA: Affordable Care Act of 2010 (also called PPACA)

AHI: Apnea–Hypopnea Index

AHIMA: American Health Information Management Association

AI: Assessment Indicator

ALJ: Administrative Law Judge

ALS: Amyotrophic Lateral Sclerosis

APC: Ambulatory Payment Classification

ARRA: American Recovery and Reinvestment Act of 2009

ASC: Ambulatory Surgical Centers

BBA: Balanced Budget Act

CAH: Critical Access Hospital

CBO: Congressional Budget Office

CCI: Correct Coding Initiative

CCIIO: Center for Consumer Information and Insurance Oversight

CCP: Coordinated Care Plan

CCR: Cost-to-Charge Ratio; Charge-to-Cost Ratio

CCS: Certified Coding Specialists

CDI: Clinical Documentation Improvement

CDM: Charge Description Master

CEHRT: Certified Electronic Health Record Technology

CF: Conversion Factor

CHAMPVA: Civilian Health and Medical Program of the Department of Veterans Affairs

CMG: Case Mix Groups

CMI: Case Mix Index

CMS: Centers for Medicare and Medicaid Services

CoP: Conditions of Participation

CPAP: Continuous Positive Airway Pressure

CPI: Center for Program Integrity

CPOE: Computerized Provider Order Entry

CPT: Current Procedure Terminology

CQM: Clinical Quality Measures

CWF: Common Working File

DAB: Departmental Appeals Board

DCN: Documented Control Number

DEERS: Defense Enrollment Eligibility Reporting System

DHS: Designated Health Services

DME: Durable Medical Equipment

DMEMAC: Durable Medical Equipment Medicare Administrative Contractors

DMEPOS: Durable Medical Equipment, Prosthetics, Orthotics and Supplies

DRG: Diagnosis Related Group

DSH: Disproportionate Share Hospital

E/M: Evaluation and Management

EGHP: Employer Group Health Plan (EGHP)

EHR: Electronic Health Record

EMR: Electronic Medical Record

EOC: Episode of Care

EP: Eligible Professionals

EPO: Exclusive Provider Organization

eRX: E-Prescribing (eRx)

ESRD: End-Stage Renal Disease

FASAB: Federal Accounting Standards Advisory Board

FCA: False Claims Act

FECA: Federal Employees' Compensation Act

FI: Fiscal Intermediary

FICA: Federal Hospital Insurance Trust Fund

FPL: Federal Poverty Level

GAAP: Generally Accepted Accounting Principles

GAO: General Accounting Office [of Congress]

GBA: Government Benefits Administrators

GDP: Gross Domestic Product

GPCI: Geographic Practice Cost Indices

HCAHPS: Hospital Consumer Assessment of Healthcare Providers and Systems

HCPCS: Healthcare Common Procedure Coding System

HEAT: Health Care Fraud Prevention and Enforcement Action

HEDIS: Healthcare Effectiveness Data and Information Set

HIPAA: Health Insurance Portability and Accountability Act

HHPPS: Home Health Prospective Payment system

HHA: Home Health Agency

HHRG: Home Health Resource Groups

HHS: Department of Health and Human Services

HI: Hospital Insurance

HIM: Health Information Management

HINN: Hospital-Issued Notices of Noncoverage

HIPAA: Health Insurance Portability and Accountability Act

HIPPS: Health Insurance Prospective Payment System

HMO: Health Maintenance Organization

HOPPS: Home Health Prospective Payment System

IAH: Independence at Home

ICD-10-PCS: International Classification of Diseases, Tenth Revision, Procedural Classification System

ICD-10-CM: International Classification of Diseases, Tenth Revision, Clinical Modification

ICD-9-CM: International Classification of Diseases, Ninth Revision, Clinical Modification

IDE: Investigational Device Exemption

IDS: Integrated Delivery System

IHS: Indian Health Services

IME: Indirect Medical Education

IOM: Institute of Medicine

IPA: Independent Practice Association

IPO: Integrated Provider Organization

IPPS: Inpatient Prospective Payment System

IRF: Inpatient Rehabilitation Facilities

IRF PPS: Inpatient Rehabilitation Facility Prospective Payment System

IRS: Internal Revenue Service

KPI: Key Performance Indicator

LCD: Local Coverage Determinations

LMRP: Local Medical Review Policy

LUPA: Low Utilization Payment Adjustments

M+C: Medicare+Choice

MA: Medicare Advantage

MCO: Managed Care Organization

MDS: Minimum Data Set

MLR: Medical Loss Ratio

MMA: Medicare Prescription Drug, Improvement, and Modernization Act of 2003

MPFS: Medicare Physician Fee Schedule

MSA: Medicare Medical Savings Account

MS-DRG: Medicare Severity DRG

MSN: Medicare Summary Notice

MSO: Management Service Organization

MUE: Medically Unlikely Edit

NBI MEDIC: National Benefit Integrity Medicare Drug Integrity Contractor

NCCI: National Correct Coding Initiative

NCD: National Coverage Determination

NCQA: National Committee for Quality Assurance

NF: Nursing Facility

NPI: National Provider Identifier

OASIS: Outcome and Assessment Information Set

OIG: Office of the Inspector General

OPPS: Outpatient Prospective Payment System

P4P: Pay-for-Performance

PA: Prior Authorization

PACE: Programs of All-inclusive Care for the Elderly

PBM: Prescription Benefit Manager

PCMH: Patient-Centered Medical Home

PCP: Primary Care Physician

PEN: Parental and Enteral Nutrition

PEP: Partial Episode Payment

PFFS: Private Fee-for-Service

PHI: Protected Health Information

PHO: Integrated Provider Organization

POC: Plan of Care

POS: Place of Service, Point of Service

PPACA: Patient Protection and Affordable Care Act

PPO: Preferred Provider Organization

PPS: Prospective Payment System

PSO: Provider Sponsored Organizations

QC: Quarters of Coverage

RAC: Recovery Audit Contractors

RAP: Request for Anticipated Payment

RCM: Revenue Cycle Management

RDI: Respiratory Disturbance Index

RFB: Religious Fraternal Benefit

RPPO: Regional PPO

RRB: Railroad Retirement Board

RUG: Resource Utilization Group

RVU: Relative Value Unit

SBC: Summary of Benefits and Coverage

SCHIP: State Children's Health Insurance Program (also known as CHIP)

SEC: Securities and Exchange Commission

SMI: Supplementary Medical Insurance

SNF: Skilled Nursing facility

SNP: Special Needs Plans

SSA: Social Security Administration

TANF: Temporary Assistance for Needy Families

Title XIX: Medicaid Program (Title XIX of the Social Security Act)

Title XVIII: Medicare Program (Title XVIII of the Social Security Act)

UCR: Usual, Customary, and Reasonable

UHDDS: Uniform Hospital Discharge Data Set

UMWA: United Mine Workers of America

UPIN Number: Unique Physician Identification Number

UMWA: Unique Physician Identification Number

UR: Utilization Review

VBP: Value-Based Purchasing

ZPIC: Zone Program Integrity Contractors

Glossary

Abuse Unintentional or unknowing submission of an inaccurate medical claim to an insurance company for payment.

Accountable Care Organization A primary care physician and hospital organization that has formed a network to provide care for a population which will receive a share of the savings it realizes and at the same time delivering the highest quality of care to the patient.

Accounts Payable An accounts payable is an amount due to outside vendor for the purchase of supplies, equipment, or services.

Accounts Receivable If an organization sells a product or service to a customer and they do not pay at the time of delivery, this sale amount is considered to be an accounts receivable due to the organization.

Accrual Accounting Method There is an important factor in the accrual accounting method for the healthcare administrator to understand and that is in the accrual concept the organization will account for revenue in the period it was realized even though it was not paid for yet. Moreover, for the expense part of the equation, if there are expenses realized during a period but they were not paid for as of yet, they too will be accounted for in the accrual method.

Acid-Test Ratio The acid-test ratio will take into account cash, short-term investments and net current receivables and divide by total current liabilities. The example is as follows:

$$\frac{(\text{Cash} + \text{short-term investments} + \text{net current receivables})}{\text{Total current liabilities}}$$

Activity-Based Budget These budgets are based on projects instead of departments.

Advance Beneficiary Notice (ABN) An Advance Beneficiary Notice (ABN) is a form used to inform a Medicare beneficiary, before he or she receives specified items or services that otherwise might be paid for, that Medicare certainly will not or probably will not pay for the item on that particular occasion.

Allowable This is the net amount of reimbursement that is paid by an insurance company based on a fee schedule or a discount off of the charge amount of a claim.

Ambulatory Surgical Center (ASC) An ASC for Medicare is defined as an entity that operates exclusively for the purpose of furnishing outpatient surgical services.

Anti-Kickback Statute The Anti-Kickback Statute is found in 42 U.S.C. Section 1320a-7b(b) and makes it a criminal offense to knowingly and willfully offer, pay, solicit, or receive any remuneration to induce or reward referrals of items or services reimbursable by a federal healthcare program.

Asset As a result of past transactions a positive economic benefit is realized by the organization such as an increase in accounts receivable, cash, or inventory.

Assignment of Benefits This is a document that is signed by the patient before services are rendered and is a contract between the health care provider and payer that states the provider will bill the payer for the services and the patient for their copayment or deductible amount.

Authorized Representative An authorized representative of the beneficiary in regards to receiving notice should be a person that can be reasonably expected to act in the best interest of the beneficiary.

Average Length of Stay This is the average number of days that patients are hospitalized. The calculation is to take the total number of hospital bed days in a period and dividing that number by the number of admissions or discharges during the same time frame.

Bad Debt This is where a healthcare facility provides services to a patient and fully expects to be paid. When the payer does not pay, the amount for the service is charged off to this account.

Balance Sheet The statements of financial positions, otherwise known as the balance sheet, display information about the organization's assets and owner's equity along with the financing structure of liabilities and equity in accordance with GAAP. The balance sheet shows, at a certain point in time, the impact that all the transactions organizations have had on the assets, liabilities, and owner's equity of the organization (Flood, 2014a, p. 43).

Benefit Period The Benefit Period is the time frame that is part of a hospital stay and is subsequently discharged.

Budget To forecast revenue and expenses for the department or organization to meet the mission and vision of the organization.

Budget Cycle The budget cycle is generally related to a fiscal year of a company. The process takes into account the projected revenues generated from sales by the organization and expenses for the organization to manufacture product or deliver these services.

Budget Variance A budget variance is the mathematical difference between what was budgeted versus what actually happens.

Calendar Year This is the financial time frame for reporting that is based on the calendar year (January 1 to December 31).

Capable Recipient A capable recipient is considered to be a beneficiary that can comprehend the notice.

Capital Budget A capital budget is one that looks mainly at large purchases in the upcoming year.

Capitation This type of payment is not based on a specific procedure or hospital stay, as it is based on a per-member-per-month (PMPM) methodology. In the managed care environment the plan will negotiate with a large group, employer, or a government agency and contracts to cover the agreed upon population and provide all contracted services listed in the agreement for a set fee per-member-per-month.

Case Management Case management is defined by the Case Management Society of America as a collaborative process of assessment, planning, facilitation, care coordination, evaluation and advocacy for option and services to meet an individual's and family's comprehensive health needs through communication and available resources to promote quality, cost-effective outcomes (CMSA, 2014).

Case Mix Index (CMI) The Case Mix Index is measurable and analyzable and allows the organization to compare the cost of providing services to its DRG mix and compare it to other like or similar hospitals. The CMI is calculated by summing up the Medicare DRG's weight for the number of patients in the DRG. Then the sum of the weights is divided by the total number of discharges.

Cash Cash is considered to be cash on-hand or items that can be converted into cash easily and in a short period of time.

Cash Flow Statement The cash flow statement will only track cash in and cash out and this includes cash equivalents such as investments that are considered to be liquid, or easily turned into cash.

Center for Consumer Information and Insurance Oversight (CCIIO) The Center for Consumer Information and Insurance Oversight is responsible for assisting in implementing various parts of the Patient Protection and Affordable Care Act.

Center for Program Integrity (CPI) The Center for Program Integrity (CPI) was created in 2010 and brought together the Medicare and Medicaid program integrity groups under one management structure to strengthen and better coordinate existing activities and to detect fraud, waste, and abuse.

The Civilian Health and Medical Program of the Department (CHAMPVA) The Civilian Health and Medical Program of the Department of Veterans Affairs

(CHAMPVA) is a comprehensive healthcare program where the Veterans Affairs (VA) shares the cost of care for covered services and supplies.

Charge This is the amount that the healthcare facility bills the insurance company for services rendered to a patient.

Charge Capture Charge Capture is defined as "a method of recording services and supplies or items delivered to a patient and the directing them to be billed on a claim form" (LaTour & Eichenwald Maki, 2013d, p. 465).

Charge Description Master (CDM) The Charge Description Master (CDM) is "an electronic file that represents a master list of all services, supplies, devices, and medications that are charged for inpatient or outpatient services" (LaTour & Eichenwald Maki, 2013e, p. 467).

Charity Care This is where a patient receives care and does not have the means in which to pay for the care delivered. The patient, or guarantor, will have to fill out financial paperwork to support the patient to be deemed as charity.

Clinical Documentation Improvement (CDI) The Clinical Documentation Improvement (CDI) is a program to assure that the health record accurately reflects the condition of the patient. According to The American Health Information Management Association (AHIMA) the definition of the CDI program is "to initiate concurrent and, as appropriated, retrospective reviews of inpatient health records for conflicting, incomplete, or nonspecific provider documentation" (AHIMA, 2010a, p. 4).

Comorbidity Comorbidities are a specific patient condition that is secondary to a patient's principle diagnosis.

Compliance Program A compliance program is a guide that is intended to assist individual and small group physician practices in developing a voluntary compliance program that promotes adherence to statutes and regulations applicable to the federal healthcare programs.

Components of Revenue Cycle Management The first part of the revenue cycle is the front-end, and this entails payer negotiation that happens outside the patient encounter, the patient access component that includes the scheduling of the patient for inpatient or outpatient services, registration, insurance verification, obtain a prior authorization or a precertification if necessary, and patient financial counseling. The middle process in the revenue cycle is where case management is involved, charge capture, hard coding and soft coding of diagnoses and procedures that are all based on clinical documentation. The back end of the revenue cycle usually resides in the patient financial services or business office area. This area will handle processing bills, posting payments, correcting any claims that were denied for errors, appeal any denials that are incorrect, supply additional documentation when needed, and make corrections to the charge description master if needed.

Contract Management Contract management is a very important part of the episode-of-care payment method and it requires that the providers of care, along with the plans have to be as precise as possible in projecting expenditures in order to negotiate a contract that will cover the costs involved in treating the members of the plan.

Coordinated Care Plan (CCP) A Coordinated Care Plan (CCP) includes a network of providers that are under a contractual arrangement to deliver the benefit package that is approved by CMS.

Corporation A corporation is a legal entity that is in existence, but separate from the owners. A corporation will pay its own taxes and will experience its own legal rights and responsibilities (LaTour & Eichenwald Maki, 2014b, p. 767).

Cost of Goods Cost of Goods is defined as "made up of all costs allocated to inventory sold during the period, including labor, materials, and overhead" (Bandler, 1994b, 35).

Cost-to-Charge Ratio The Cost-to-Charge Ratio (CCR) is applied to the covered charges for a case to determine whether the costs of a case exceeds the fixed-loss outlier threshold.

Criminal Health Care Fraud Statute The Criminal Health Care Fraud Statute is found in 18 U.S.C. Section 1347 and prohibits knowingly and willfully executing or attempting to execute and scheme or artifice to defraud any healthcare benefit program or to obtain by means of false or fraudulent pretenses, representations, or promises any of the money or property owned by or under the custody or control of any healthcare benefit program that is in the connection with the delivery of or payment for healthcare benefits, items, or services.

Current Procedural Terminology The CPT is a uniform coding system that is made up of descriptive terms and codes that are primarily used to identify medical services and procedures that are furnished by physicians and other health care professionals. Also referred to as Level I.

Current Ratio This ratio determines the ability of the organization to pay their current liabilities with the use of their current assets. The current ratio is calculated as follows:

$$\frac{\text{Total current assets of the organization}}{\text{Total current liabilities of the organization}}$$

Debt Ratio In the debt ratio the lender will take a look at the total assets and the total liabilities that an organization may have on their balance sheet.

Depreciation Depreciation is where the company takes the value of the asset and spreads out the cost over a period of time that is consistent with the accounting practices of the company.

Diagnosis-Related Groups (DRG) Diagnosis-Related Groups (DRG) that are assigned to each patient based on their diagnosis at the time of discharge (LaTour & Eichenwald Maki, 2013a, p. 16).

Direct Cost A direct cost is one that is able to be tracked back to a specific service provided or a product that was manufactured.

Discharge Planning Under the Medicare Conditions of participation for Hospitals: Discharge planning, (42 CFR, §482.43 [b] [3] and [6]), hospitals must have a discharge process in place that applies to all patients and must include the evaluation or likelihood of the patient needing post-hospital services and of the availability of the services.

Disproportionate Share Hospital If a hospital treats a high percentage of low-income patients, it will receive a percentage add-on payment that will be applied to the DRG-adjusted base payment rate that is known as a disproportionate share hospital (DSH) adjustment.

Electronic Health Record (EHR) "An electronic record of health-related information on an individual that conforms to nationally recognized interoperability standards and that can be created, managed, and consulted by authorized clinicians and staff across more than one healthcare organization" (Amatayakul, 2013b, p. 5).

Electronic Medical Record (EMR) "An electronic record of health-related information on an individual that can be created, gathered, managed, and consulted by authorized clinicians and staff within one healthcare organization" (Amatayakul, 2013b, 5).

Employer Group Health Plan (EGHP) An Employer Group Health Plan (EGHP) is a group plan that is sponsored by an employer or labor organization.

Encounter An encounter is where a patient and provider engage in an instance where the provider delivers service to a patient. For example, a primary care physician has an appointment with the patient and his/her primary responsibility is to take care of the patient and their particular condition.

Episode of Care Payment This payment mechanism referred to as Episode-of-Care (EOC) payment, or sometimes called a bundled payment, method involves making a lump sum payment to healthcare providers to cover all services that were delivered to a patient for a specific illness that was treated during a specific period of time.

Equity This amount is what is left in an asset after removing any liability from its value. For example, in a partnership equity is considered to be the owner's interest.

Established Patient An Established Patient is one who has received professional services from the physician or qualified healthcare professional or another physician or qualified healthcare professional of the exact same specialty and subspecialty who belongs to the same group practice within the past 3 years (AMA, 2013f, p. 4).

Event The use of raw materials by a company to be provided to a customer and in exchange is made.

Exclusive Provider Organization (EPO) An Exclusive Provider Organization (EPO) is similar to the PPO, except that the patients enrolled in the plan are to receive healthcare services only from the EPO network providers.

Expenses These are items that are satisfied by the discharge of assets, such as cash, to the organization or entity that supplied it to the company.

False Claims Act The False Claims Act (FCA) of the United States Code Sections 3729–3733 protects the government from being overcharged or sold substandard goods or services.

Federal Accounting Standards Advisory Board (FASAB) The FASAB is an independent organization that works towards setting the accounting standards for all businesses that operate in the private community (LaTour & Eichenwald Maki, 2013a, p. 766).

Fee-for-Service Provider will bill for all services rendered to the third-party payer after the services have been provided and then the third-party payer, retrospectively, will pay the provider.

Financial Accounting Financial Accounting is defined as "the branch of accounting that provides general-purpose financial statements or reports to aid many decision-making groups, internal and external to the organization, in making a variety of decisions" (Cleverley, 2012a, p. 182).

Financial Counselors The healthcare organization is required to educate the patient on their responsibility for his or her encounter with the healthcare provider. This can be accomplished by using Financial Counselors.

Financial Relationship A financial relationship includes both ownership and investment interests along with compensation arrangements that include contractual arrangements between a hospital and a physician for physician services.

Financial Reporting Financial reporting is a tool that is used for providing information to decision makers that will allow them to make choices based on this information that will be useful in the decision-making process.

Financial Statements Financial statements are considered to be the principal means of communicating useful financial information and the statements that are included cover the financial position of the organization at the end of the period, the earnings of the period, overall income for the period, cash flows during the period, and the investments by and distributions to the owners (Flood, 2014d, p. 21).

Fiscal Intermediary (FI) Medicare payment branch that is local and they are the ones that are contracted with the public or private providers and act as agents of the federal government.

Fiscal Year Yearly accounting period that is not based on the calendar year starting on January 1. This is where the accounting period runs from October 1 to September 30 for federal agencies. And some state fiscal years are from July 1 thru June 30.

Fixed Budget This type of budget is designed based on expected activity in the upcoming year based on historical data.

Fixed Cost The classification of a fixed cost is one that will remain constant and will not be influenced by volume.

Flexible Budget A flexible budget is one that is created based on productivity that is projected based on historical data.

Forecasting Forecasting goes hand in hand with planning as this too looks at future trends based on historical data.

Formulary Listing of drugs/medications that are on a preferred listing where the patient will pay less in out-of-pocket than if the drug/medication was not on the formulary.

Gains Gains are increases in equity, or net assets, from the process of completing transactions to external customers.

Gatekeeper A Primary Care Physician (PCP) in a Gatekeeper role is defined as "a primary care physician who controls a patient's access to certain tests, treatments, and specialty physicians in a managed care plan (Patient Advocate Foundation, 2014c).

General Ledger The general ledger is part of the accounting system where all the entries are recorded in chronological order.

Generally Accepted Accounting Principles (GAAP) Accounting principles that are used in the preparation of financial reports and statements for businesses or entities.

Geographic Practice Cost Indices (GPCI) The GPCI stands for Geographic Practice Cost Indices and this is the means in which each payment is adjusted based on the geography or payment locality.

Geometric Mean Length of Stay The Geometric Mean Length of Stay takes an adjustment for the outliers, transfer cases, and negative outlier cases and gives a statistically adjusted value for the length of stay. In addition, it is used to calculate transfer case payments.

Global Payment Method The global payment methodology can be applied to procedures that are associated with technical components. This global payment is a lump-sum payment that can be distributed among all the physicians who either performed the procedure or interpreted the results of the procedure.

Gross Profits The difference between the sales of an organization and the cost of goods sold will be the gross profit.

Group Model HMO Group Model HMOs are considered a closed panel where the physicians are not permitted to treat other managed care patients outside the managed care plan that they are contracted with. The Group Model HMO is where the HMO enters into an agreement with the physician group that is a multispecialty group that can provide medical services to the plan members.

Health Care Fraud Prevention and Enforcement Action (HEAT) Team The HEAT Team is a joint initiative between the Department of Health and Human Services and the Department of Justice. This was to improve interagency collaboration on reducing fraud in federal healthcare programs.

Health Care Reconciliation Act of 2010 The PPACA was enacted on Mach 23, 2010 and shortly after the name of the act was changed to Health Care Reconciliation Act of 2010.

Health Insurance Marketplace The Marketplace is a new way to shop for healthcare coverage if you currently have coverage or are looking for coverage and you need options.

Health Insurance Prospective Payment System (HIPPS) Health Insurance Prospective Payment System (HIPPS) rate codes represent specific sets of patient characteristics or case-mix groups on which payment determinations are made under several prospective payment systems. For the payment systems that use HIPPS codes, clinical data is the basic input used to determine which case-mix group applies to a particular patient (CMS, 2010, p. 1). HIPPS codes are used for Inpatient Rehabilitation Facilities (IRF) and Home Health Agencies (HH) along with Skilled Nursing Facilities (SNF).

Health Maintenance Organization (HMO) An HMO is a voluntary health plan that will provide healthcare services to its members in return for a monthly premium their coverage. A Health Maintenance Organization (HMO) is generally a more restrictive model than the others offered as it controls utilization through the use of referrals from the primary care practitioner (PCP) and restricts the patient's access to a network of providers to receive routine, nonurgent, or emergency services.

Health Record The source of information on all aspects of an individual's health care. The health record is vital to patient care as it includes demographics, reasons for visits, results of tests, treatments ordered, and plans for follow-up. In short, the health record explains the who, what, when, where, why, and how of patient care (Kuehn, 2013a, p. 2).

Healthcare Common Procedure Coding System (HCPCS) The Healthcare Common Procedure Coding System (HCPCS) was established in 1978 to provide a standardized coding system for describing the specific items and services provided in the delivery of health care.

Healthcare Effectiveness Data and Information Set (HEDIS) The Healthcare Effectiveness Data and Information Set (HEDIS) was originally developed by

National Committee for Quality Assurance (NCQA) along with a group of various health plans and employers. One of the main ideas with the development of HEDIS was to allow employers to see what they are getting for their healthcare dollars. The Health Care Financing Administration (HCFA) contracted with the NCQA to develop a database of HEDIS measures that would be used to measure the performance of the Medicare Program (Lied, 2001, p. 150).

Home Health Care The physician needs to attest that the patient in fact needs home care and is confined to his or her home. They do not have to be bedbound, but considered to be confined to their home environment.

Home Health Prospective Payment System (HHPPS) The HHPPS was initially mandated by law in the Balanced Budget Act of 1997. Home health agencies provide skilled nursing care to patients that are considered to be homebound. The services that are provided are skilled nursing care, physical therapy, occupational therapy, speech therapy, social work, and home health aide services.

Hospice Hospice care is a benefit under the hospital insurance program. According to CMS, to be eligible to elect hospice care under Medicare, the individual must be entitled to Medicare Part A and be certified as being terminally ill. To be considered terminally ill the patient's medical prognosis is where the individual's life expectancy is 6 months or less if the illness runs its normal course (CMS, 2012a).

Hospital Consumer Assessment of Healthcare Providers and Systems (HCAHPS) The Hospital Consumer Assessment of Healthcare Providers and Systems (HCAHPS) is a standardized survey and data collection tool that has been used since 2006 and the goal of HCAHPS was to measure the patient's perspective of the hospital care that they received.

Hospital Outpatient Prospective Payment system (OPPS) The Hospital Outpatient Prospective Payment system (OPPS) has a set of rules and regulations separate from the delivery of care in the acute setting. Outpatient, home health, physician and nonphysician practitioners, and ambulatory surgery have rules and regulations related to billing.

Hospital Wage Index The Wage Index is an adjustment based on the geographical location of a hospital and their area wage level as compared to the national average and this is adjusted annually.

Hybrid Medical Record As the progression over the years from a completely paper file to a hybrid file containing paper that was scanned into a file combined with electronic images that created this hybrid format.

Income Statement The income statement is also known as the profit and loss statement. The profit and loss statement is intended to demonstrate how much money a company is making or losing and it accomplishes this "by subtracting all of the costs of production of goods that have been sold during the period and other expenses of running the company from the revenues generated from sales of products or from services provided" (Bandler, 1994a, p. 34).

Independence at Home Project The Independence at Home project was created by the Affordable Care Act and is a delivery and payment incentive model that is using home-based primary care teams.

Independent Practice Association (IPA) The characteristics of an Independent Practice Association (IPA) are that it operates as an HMO, but not like the Group Model where they are limited in who they can treat.

Indian Health Services (IHS) Indian Health Services (IHS) is an agency within the Department of Health and Human Services that is responsible for providing federal healthcare services to American Indians and Alaska natives.

Indirect Cost An indirect cost is a cost that is incurred in the organization as they provide products or services to a customer, but the cost is not directly related to the manufacturing of goods or services provided by the organization.

Indirect Medical Education Section 1886(d)(5)(B) of the Social Security Act provides that PPS hospitals that have residents in an approved Graduate Medical Education (GME) program will receive an additional payment for a Medicare discharge. This higher payment will reflect the additional costs that are incurred by teaching hospital as opposed to a facility that is not a teaching facility.

Inpatient Hospital Coverage An inpatient stay is defined by CMS as a person who has been admitted to a hospital for bed occupancy for purposes of receiving inpatient hospital services. In addition, they will be formally admitted to the facility with the expectation that he or she will remain at least overnight or transferred to another hospital for care (CMS, 2010a).

Inpatient Prospective Payment System (IPPS) Inpatient Prospective Payment System (IPPS) is designed for an acute care inpatient setting and the single payment does not include payment for any professional services that are provided during the patient's hospital stay.

Inpatient Rehabilitation Facility Prospective Payment System (IRF PPS) In section 1886(j) of the Social Security Act it was authorized that a Prospective Payment System would be implemented for Inpatient Rehabilitation Facilities.

Institutional Claim An institutional claim is any claim that is submitted using the Health Insurance Portability and Accountability Act (HIPAA) mandated transaction ASC X12N 837 – Health Care Claim: Institutional or the UB-04 paper claim form.

Integrated Delivery System (IDS) Integrated Delivery System (IDS) is a healthcare provider that furnishes coordinated healthcare services through a number of affiliated medical facilities.

Integrated Health Record The content of the Integrated Health Record is arranged in strict, chronological order. The order of the record is determined by the date the information was entered or the date of the service which gives the sequence of the care that the patient received during their stay (LaTour & Eichenwald Maki, 2013c, p. 257).

Internal Revenue Service (IRS) IRS is a department of the United States Treasury and is considered to be one of the most efficient tax administrators. Overall, the IRS helps the taxpayer understand the laws that Congress passes and makes sure that they are compliant and for those who are not compliant, the IRS will make sure that they comply and are responsible for their fair share.

Inventory Inventory consists of goods that are purchased by the organization and sold to their customers.

Level II Codes Level II of the HCPCS is a standardized coding system that is used primarily to identify products, supplies, and services not included in the Level I CPT codes.

Liability As a result of a past transaction a negative economic benefit is realized by the organization such as accounts payable, loans payable, and variable expenses.

Losses Losses are a negative impact on an owner's equity in the organization. In addition, this is where the liabilities are greater than the increases in assets during a period.

Low Utilization Payment The normal episode of care covers a 60-day period. However, there are times that a shorter length of stay, or episode, is experienced for a patient. If a home health agency provides four visits or less in an episode, they will be paid a standardized per visit payment instead of an episode payment for a 60-day period. Such payments adjustments and episodes themselves are called Low Utilization Payment Adjustments (LUPAs).

Malpractice (MP) Part of the Resource Based Relative Value Scale (RBRVS) calculations is malpractice. This represents the calculation that covers the malpractice insurance portion of the visit.

Managed Care Managed care is a generic term for prepaid health plans and ultimately the goal of the managed care organizations (MCOs) is to control the cost of health care that is delivered to the member and, at the same time, offer the services their members need and to manage the delivery of these services in a cost effective manner.

Market Basket A mix of goods and services that are appropriate to the setting that they service; for example, home health.

Meaningful Use Meaningful Use is where a provider uses a certified EHR system to improve quality, safety, efficiency, and to reduce healthcare disparities. In addition, the EHR system will allow the provider to engage patients and their families and to improve care coordination to improve the overall health of the population, all the while maintaining privacy and security with regards to Protected Health Information (PHI).

Medicaid The federal/state entitlement program that came out of the Title XIX of the Social Security Act that pays for medical assistance for individuals with low income is called Medicaid and this became law in 1965. This is a jointly funded program by the federal and state governments. The purpose of this funding is to assist in supplying medical coverage for persons that are in need and eligible for the program. For the poor people in America, the Medicaid program is the largest source of funding for health care (Klees, 2009i).

Medical Loss Ratio The 80/20 Rule is where insurance companies are to spend at least 80 percent of the money that they take in through premiums and spend this on health care and quality improvement as opposed to overhead and administrative or marketing costs. This 80/20 Rule is also known as the Medical Loss Ratio (MLR).

Medical Necessity The American College of Medical Quality has defined Medical Necessity as "accepted health care services and supplies provided by health care entities, appropriate to the evaluation and treatment of a disease, condition, illness or injury and consistent with applicable standard of care" (ACMQ, 2010, p. 1).

Medicare Medicare came out of Title XVIII of the Social Security Act. This was designated as being "Health Insurance for the Aged and Disabled," which is commonly known as Medicare.

Medicare Abuse Abuse is when a healthcare provider or supplier does not follow good medical practice that results in unnecessary costs, improper payment, or services that are not medically necessary (CMS, 2013a, p. 10).

Medicare Fraud Medicare defines fraud is an occurrence that someone intentionally falsifies information or deceives Medicare.

Medicare Managed Care The Balanced Budget Act of 1997 created the Medicare Part C plan and in 1999 changed its name to Medicare+Choice (M+C). CMS is able to contract with private or public organizations to offer various health plans to their beneficiaries that include traditional insurance and managed care plans.

Medicare Medical Savings Account (MSA) Medicare Medical Savings Account (MSA) Plans combine a high deductible MA plan and a medical savings account that is used to pay for qualified medical expenses for the account holder.

Medicare National Correct Coding Initiative (NCCI) The Medicare National Correct Coding Initiative (NCCI) or the Correct Coding Initiative (CCI) was implemented to promote a national correct coding methodologies and to control improper coding that can lead to inappropriate payments.

Medicare Part A According to CMS, Medicare Part A provided protection against costs of specific medical care for around 45 million people and paid out in benefits over $232 billion in 2008 (Klees, 2009c). There are several types of care that are covered by Medicare Part A and they are inpatient hospital coverage, skilled nursing facility (SNF), home health care, and hospice care for the terminally ill.

Medicare Part B To obtain Medicare Part B, Supplemental Medical Insurance (SMI), an individual must enroll during an enrollment period and pay the required premiums. SMI provides for payment to participating providers for furnishing covered services after a yearly cash deductible is met (CMS, 2013a). Medicare Part B is designed to supplement voluntary medical insurance that the beneficiary may have coverage with while on Part B.

Medicare Part C Medicare Part C is also known as Medicare Advantage. It is an alternative to the traditional Medicare plan for beneficiaries to choose from instead of Medicare Part A or Part B. The Medicare Part C plans are offered by private insurance companies and they have to offer beneficiaries at least what is offered by Part A and Part B, excluding hospice. The plans may, and in certain instances must, provide extra benefits such as dental, vision, or hearing. In addition, they may reduce cost sharing or premiums in lieu of extra benefits (Klees, 2009d).

Medicare Part D Medicare Part D started out by providing access to prescription drug discount cards for no more than $30 annually. Then the program transitioned into a program that provides subsidized access to prescription drug coverage. This plan is completely voluntary and the beneficiary has a choice to enroll in a standalone prescription drug plan (PDP) or an integrated Medicare Advantage that offers Part D coverage. Part D coverage includes most FDA-approved medications and biologicals. Moreover, there are formularies for the prescriptions covered and the plan offers different levels of coverage (Klees, 2009g).

Medicare Severity DRGs (MS-DRGs) The Medicare Severity DRGs (MS-DRGs) are a patient classification system that provides a means of relating types of patients a hospital treats, for example their case mix, to the costs incurred by the hospital.

Medigap The term "Medigap" is used by a beneficiary to cover healthcare services that are not covered by Part A or Part B. These policies must meet federally imposed standards and are offered by Blue Cross and Blue Shield and various other commercial health insurance companies (Klees, 2009h).

National Benefit Integrity Medicare Drug Integrity Contractor The National Benefit Integrity Medicare Drug Integrity Contractor (NBI MEDIC) program supports

CMS Center for Program Integrity, monitors fraud and abuse in Medicare Part C and Part D programs in all 50 states, the District of Columbia and U.S. Territories.

NCQA NCQA is an accrediting entity as identified by the Department of Health and Human Services (HHS) for Qualified Health Plan.

Network Model HMO The Network Model HMO is similar to the Group Model HMO, however the Network Model HMO will contract with multiple multispecialty groups to provide care for their members.

New Patient New Patient is a patient that has not received any professional services from the physician or qualified healthcare professional or another physician or qualified healthcare professional of the exact same specialty and subspecialty who belongs to the same group practice, within the past 3 years.

Notes Payable A notes payable is considered to be a financial obligation that is supported by a contract and has a time frame for repayment.

OPPS Payment Status Indicator An OPPS payment status indicator is assigned to every HCPCS code and this indicator identifies whether the service identified by the HCPCS code is paid under OPPS.

Programs of All-Inclusive Care for the Elderly (PACE) The Programs of All-Inclusive Care for the Elderly (PACE) is a managed care benefit for the elderly and features a comprehensive medical and social service delivery system using an interdisciplinary team approach. The PACE organization is a not-for-profit, private, or public entity that is primarily engaged in providing PACE services and must have certain characteristics such as a governing board, ability to provide a complete service package, physical site for adult day services, defined service area, safeguards to avoid conflict of interest, fiscal soundness, and a Participant Bill of Rights (CMS, 2011a).

Packaged Services Packaged services under OPPS include items and services that are considered to be an important or critical part of another service that is paid under the OPPS program.

Partial Episode Payment When a patient is discharged, readmitted, transferred to the same agency in a 60-day period it results in a shortened episode of care given by the agency. In this instance, the payment to the home health agency will need to be prorated for the shorter episode. These adjustments are called Partial Episode Payments (PEP).

Partnership This is where two or more people get together to form a partnership. The partners will share duties and responsibilities for running the company and all revenues will be distributed to the partners and they will pay taxes on the money through the reporting of their individual tax returns. In some cases, the partnership can be required to file its own tax return that will show in detail the income distributed to the partners of the company.

Patient-Centered Medical Home (PCMH) The Patient-Centered Medical Home (PCMH) started as a Demonstration Project to help in the redesign of the healthcare delivery model. The goal was to "provide targeted, accessible, continuous and coordinated, family-centered care to high-need populations under which care management fees are paid to persons performing services as personal physicians and incentive payments are paid to physicians participating in practices that provide services as a medical home" (CMS, 2006a, p. 1).

Patient Protection and Affordable Care Act The Patient Protection and Affordable Care Act was designed to ensure that all Americans have access to quality healthcare that is affordable and will ultimately reduce the costs that have been on the rise over the years.

Pay-for-Performance (P4P) "Performance-based provider payment arrangements, including those that target performance on cost or efficiency measures. Typically, pay-for-performance programs offer financial incentives to physicians and other healthcare providers who meet defined performance targets which tend to focus on quality, efficiency, or related areas" (Leapfrog 2006a).

Physician Work (WORK) This is the portion of the Relative Value Unit that covers the physician's salary during a procedure or office visit. This covers the mental effort and judgment, technical skill portion, his/her physical effort, and psychological stress involved with the taking care of the patient.

Planning Based on the Mission Statement, healthcare administrators will need to plan multiple scenarios in the future and track them with current results and make the necessary changes to the plan to reflect the changing environment going forward.

Point-of-Service Collections Point-of-Service (POS) collections are defined as "the collection of the portion of the bill that is likely the responsibility of the patient prior to the provision of services" (LaTour & Eichenwald Maki, 2013c, p. 461).

Point-Of-Service Plan The Point-of-Service Plan is similar to the HMO plans in that the subscriber must select a physician to be what is referred to as the Primary Care Physician (PCP) for the patient. This type of plan is the fastest growing plan in the managed care marketplace and the plan that gives the patient the most flexibility in choices for care.

Practice Expense (PE) Portion of the Relative Value Unit that covers the expenses related to the physician's practice for the visit or procedure that includes wages for office staff, rent, supplies, and equipment.

Preferred Provider Organization (PPO) The Preferred Provider Organization (PPO) is considered to be a large group of hospitals and physicians that are under contract to service members of a managed care plan.

Prescription Benefit Managers (PBMs) There are specialty management organizations, or Prescription Benefit Managers (PBMs), and they administer the prescription portion of health benefit plans.

Prescription Management A prescription formulary, as part of prescription management, can be used as a cost control measure to managing a patient's prescriptions.

Principal Diagnosis The principal diagnosis is defined in the Uniform Hospital Discharge Data Set (UHDDS) as "that condition established after study to be chiefly responsible for occasioning the admission of the patient to the hospital for care." UHDDS definitions have been expanded to include, but not limited to, all nonoutpatient settings such as acute care, short-term, long-term care, psychiatric hospitals; home health agencies; rehab facilities; and nursing homes (CMSI-10, 2010e, p. 90).

Prior Authorization (PA) This process is where a healthcare provider will have to follow an administrative process to obtain a PA for a procedure, test, or hospital stay prior to the services being rendered to the patient.

Private Fee-for-Service A Private Fee-for-Service (PFFS) plan is a MA plan that provides on a fee-for-service basis without placing the provider at risk, and the rates are not subject to vary based on utilization, and does not restrict enrollees' choices of providers that are authorized to provide services and accept the plans payment terms and conditions.

Problem-Oriented Health Record The Problem Oriented Health Record is comprised of a problem list, the database or the history and physical exam and initial lab findings, the initial plan of what tests or treatments the patient will receive during their stay, and progress notes that are organized so that every member of the healthcare team can easily follow the course of the patient's treatment (LaTour & Eichenwald Maki, 2013b, p. 256).

Problem List A list of illnesses that have an impact on an individual's health which usually includes date and/or time of first onset, if it is still being treated, and when it was resolved.

Professional Claim A professional claim is any claim submitted using the HIPAA mandated transaction ASC X12N 837 – Health Care Claim: Professional or the CMS-1500 paper claim form.

Prospective Payment System (PPS) The PPS model is designed to reimburse a hospital an amount based on Diagnosis Related Groups (DRG) that would be assigned to each patient based on their diagnosis at the time of discharge. (LaTour & Eichenwald Maki, 2013a, p. 16).

Provider A provider is a hospital, a Critical Access Hospital (CAH), a skilled nursing facility, a comprehensive outpatient rehabilitation facility, home health agency, hospice agency that has agreed to participate in Medicare, clinic, rehabilitation agency or public health agency that has a similar agreement to provide outpatient physical therapy or speech-language pathology services, or community mental health agency that has a similar agreement but will only furnish partial hospitalization services (CMS, 2013a, p. 11).

Quality Measures There are four quality measures and they are Process, Outcome, Patient Experience, and Structure.

Quality Measures–Outcome Outcome is where the healthcare provider is measured on the effectiveness of the care provided.

Quality Measures–Patient Experience Patient Experience measures the patient's perception of care that they received during their stay in the hospital or the care given as an outpatient.

Quality Measures–Process Process is where the provider is measured on the activities that contribute to the positive quality outcomes of a patient stay.

Quality Measures–Structure Structure measures how well the facilities, equipment, and personnel were used in the treatment of the patient (James, 2012).

Rate Review The Rate Review is where it protects individuals from excessive or unreasonable rate increases.

Recovery Audit Contractors (RAC) Recovery Audit Contractors (RAC) is the Centers for Medicare and Medicaid Services (CMS) program that is responsible for detecting and correcting Medicare improper payments.

Reimbursement This is the monetary value that a healthcare facility or provider receives in return for providing services to a patient. This is for the most part after the patient has received the care.

Relative Value Unit (RVU) A relative value scale permits comparisons of the resources needed or appropriate for various units of services. Relative value scale takes into account labor, skill, supplies, equipment, space, and other costs associated with each procedure or service in a physician's office (Casto & Forrestal, 2013g, p. 155).

Religious Fraternal Benefit (RFB) The Religious Fraternal Benefit (RFB) plans are MA plans that are offered to a society that is a religious fraternal society. The enrollment is limited to only the members of the RFB society.

Request for Anticipated Payment The home health agency can submit a Request for Anticipated Payment (RAP) after the OASIS assessment is complete, export ready, or finalized for transmitting to the state. Second, after a physician's verbal orders for home care have been received and documented. Third, a POC is established and sent to the physician for signature. Finally, the first service visit has been completed by the home health agency (CMS, 2013b, p. 16).

Revenue Cycle Management (RCM) Revenue Cycle Management can be defined as "a complex process that involves balancing people, processes, technology, and the environment in which the process takes place" (LaTour & Eichenwald Maki, 2013a, p. 460).

Revenues This is where an organization increases accounts receivable or cash in exchange for products or services provided by the organization.

Securities and Exchange Commission (SEC) Mission to "protect investors, maintain fair, orderly and efficient markets, and facilitate capital formation" (SEC, 2014a). It has become an even greater need to regulate the market to sustain continued economic growth.

Semi-Fixed Cost There are some costs that are impacted by volume, but are not extremely sensitive to volume changes.

Senior Housing Facility Plan The Affordable Care Act established Senior Housing Facility Plans that limit enrollment to residents of Continuing Care Retirement Communities and are receiving health related services under an agreement that is in place for a specified period or the life of the enrollee.

Skilled Nursing Care Care covered by Medicare Part A and the skilled nursing facility (SNF) provides care similar to that of an inpatient hospital at a lower level and can include rehabilitation services.

Skilled Nursing Facility (SNF) A facility that meets specific regulatory requirements and the primary focus is to provide inpatient skilled nursing care and rehabilitation services such as physical therapy and occupational therapy.

Sole Proprietorship This type of organization consists of one person who owns the company.

Source-Oriented Health Record Source-oriented health record consists of a conventional or traditional method of maintaining paper-based health records. In this method, heath records are organized according to the source or originating department that provided the service to the patient (LaTour & Eichenwald Maki, 2013a, p. 255).

Special Needs Plan Special Needs Plans (SNPs) are Medicare Advantage coordinated care plans that meet all the requirements for CMS and offers a Part D plan for prescriptions and has an approval as an SNPs.

Staff Model HMO In a Staff Model the HMO will directly employ the physicians and various other healthcare professionals to provide healthcare services to their members. The Staff Model HMO is a closed panel which means that the practice does not see any patients outside those of the HMO.

Stark Law The Physician Self-Referral Law, known as the Stark Law, is found in 42 U.S.C. Section 1395nn, and this law prohibits a physician from making a referral for certain designated healthcare services to an entity in which the physician, or an immediate member of his or her family, has an ownership or investment interest, or with which he or she has a compensation arrangement, unless an exception applies.

Supplier A supplier is a physician or other practitioner, or an entity other than a provider that furnishes healthcare services under Medicare. A supplier must meet certain requirements as outlined in the Medicare Program Integrity Manual. A provider may also enroll as a supplier if they meet applicable conditions and bill separately for that service where Medicare payment policy allows for these separate payments (CMS, 2013a, p. 11).

Temporary Assistance for Needy Families (TANF) TANF provides states with grant money that is to help low-income families with case assistance. Due to the many changes in Medicaid eligibility, some individuals may not know that they are eligible for this benefit (CMS, 2011).

Transaction A transaction is an external event that involves transferring something of value such as services or products to another company for in exchange the company will receive payment.

TRICARE TRICARE offers a comprehensive and affordable healthcare coverage to active duty service members and retirees of the seven uniformed services, their family members, survivors and others who are registered in the Defense Enrollment Eligibility Reporting System (DEERS).

TRICARE for Life TRICARE for Life offers secondary coverage to all Medicare beneficiaries that have both Medicare Part A and Medicare Part B.

TRICARE Prime TRICARE Prime is the managed care option offered by the Department of Defense and offers the most affordable and comprehensive coverage for its beneficiaries.

TRICARE Standard and Extra TRICARE Standard and Extra is a fee-for-service plan available to all nonactive duty beneficiaries in the United States and enrollment is not required as coverage is automatic as long as the beneficiary is registered in DEERS. TRICARE Standard and Extra provide coverage for emergency care, outpatient and inpatient care, preventive care, maternity care, mental and behavioral health, and prescription coverage. The beneficiary and their family have both in-network and out-of-network benefits and will experience out-of-pocket costs for care after they meet their annual deductible. The TRICARE Extra option will reduce the out-of-pocket costs for the beneficiary and their family (TRICARE, 2013b).

Utilization Management Utilization Management is defined as "the evaluation of the medical necessity, appropriateness, and efficiency of the use of healthcare services, procedures, and facilitates these under the provisions of the applicable health benefits plan" (URAC, 2014).

Utilization Review Utilization Management is sometimes called Utilization Review (UR) and this is responsible "for the day-to-day provisions of the hospital's utilization plan as required by the Medicare Conditions of Participation (LaTour & Eichenwald Maki, 2013c, p. 464).

Value-Based Purchasing (VBP) The Value Based Purchasing (VPB) Program is a CMS initiative that rewards acute-care hospitals with incentive payments based on the quality of care that they provide to the beneficiary/patient that is on Medicare while they are in their care (MLN, 2013a, p. 1).

Variable Cost Variable costs are influenced by volume and can change each month based on those changes in volume.

Workers' Compensation The workers' compensation benefit is made available to most employees to help cover healthcare costs that are due to a work related injury.

Zero-Based Budget This type of budget is where an organization will decide to continue or discontinue a service based on each department justifying and prioritizing activities each year.

Zone Program Integrity Contractors (ZPICs) The Zone Program Integrity Contractors (ZPICs) were created to perform program integrity functions in zones for Medicare Part A and Part B, Durable Medical Equipment (DME), Prosthetics, Orthotics, Supplies, Home Health and Hospice, and Medicare-Medicaid data matching.

Index

Note: Page numbers followed by *f* or *t* indicate materials in figures or tables, respectively.